Child Behavior
Therapy Casebook

Child Behavior Therapy Casebook

Edited by
Michel Hersen and
Cynthia G. Last

Western Psychiatric Institute and Clinic
Pittsburgh, Pennsylvania

Plenum Press • New York and London

Library of Congress Cataloging in Publication Data

Child behavior therapy casebook.

Includes bibliographies and index.
1. Behavior therapy for children — Case studies. I. Hersen, Michel. II. Last, Cynthia
G. [DNLM: 1. Behavior Therapy — in infancy & childhood — case studies. WS 350.6
C5362]
RJ505.B4C46   1988   618.92′89142   88-15125
ISBN 0-306-42868-7

© 1988 Plenum Press, New York
A Division of Plenum Publishing Corporation
233 Spring Street, New York, N.Y. 10013

Printed in the United States of America

To Vicki and Barry

Contributors

GEARY S. ALFORD   Department of Psychiatry and Human Behavior, University of Mississippi Medical Center, Jackson, Mississippi

ROBERT T. AMMERMAN   Western Psychiatric Institute and Clinic, University of Pittsburgh School of Medicine, Pittsburgh, Pennsylvania

IVAN L. BEALE   Department of Psychology, University of Auckland, Auckland, New Zealand

GORDON W. BLOOD   Division of Special Education and Communication Disorders, The Pennsylvania State University, University Park, Pennsylvania

JEFFREY BOLLARD   The Adelaide Children's Hospital, North Adelaide, South Australia

GLENN R. CADDY   Department of Psychology, Nova University, Fort Lauderdale, Florida

BETTY E. CHESLER   Western Psychiatric Institute and Clinic, University of Pittsburgh School of Medicine, Pittsburgh, Pennsylvania

PAUL M. CINCIRIPINI   Department of Psychiatry, The University of Texas Medical Branch, Galveston, Texas

DANIEL M. DOLEYS   Behavioral Medicine Services, Birmingham, Alabama

BRENDA S. EGAN   Western Pennsylvania School for Blind Children, Pittsburgh, Pennsylvania

EDNA B. FOA   Department of Psychiatry, Temple University, Philadelphia, Pennsylvania

CYNTHIA L. FRAME   Department of Psychology, University of Georgia, Athens, Georgia

GRETA FRANCIS   Western Psychiatric Institute and Clinic, University of Pittsburgh School of Medicine, Pittsburgh, Pennsylvania

LARRY R. FRIEDT   Department of Psychology, Louisiana State University, Baton Rouge, Louisiana

SUE ANN FULTZ   Western Psychiatric Institute and Clinic, University of Pittsburgh School of Medicine, Pittsburgh, Pennsylvania

DAVID M. GARNER   Department of Psychiatry, Toronto General Hospital, Toronto, Ontario, Canada

MARKHAM S. GIBLIN   Department of Psychology, University of Georgia, Athens, Georgia

ALAN M. GROSS   Department of Psychology, University of Mississippi, University, Mississippi

JAN S. HANDLEMAN   Douglass College, Rutgers, The State University of New Jersey, Piscataway, New Jersey

SANDRA L. HARRIS   Rutgers, The State University of New Jersey, Piscataway, New Jersey

MICHEL HERSEN   Western Psychiatric Institute and Clinic, University of Pittsburgh School of Medicine, Pittsburgh, Pennsylvania

STEVEN A. HOBBS   Department of Pediatrics, University of Oklahoma, Tulsa Medical College, Tulsa, Oklahoma

L. K. GEORGE HSU   Western Psychiatric Institute and Clinic, University of Pittsburgh School of Medicine, Pittsburgh, Pennsylvania

ALLEN C. ISRAEL   Department of Psychology, The University at Albany, State University of New York, Albany, New York

JAMES H. JOHNSON   Department of Basic Dental Sciences, University of Florida, Gainesville, Florida

BRICK JOHNSTONE   Department of Psychology, University of Georgia, Athens, Georgia

ALAN E. KAZDIN   Western Psychiatric Institute and Clinic, University of Pittsburgh School of Medicine, Pittsburgh, Pennsylvania

DAVID J. KOLKO   Western Psychiatric Institute and Clinic, University of Pittsburgh School of Medicine, Pittsburgh, Pennsylvania

CYNTHIA G. LAST   Western Psychiatric Institute and Clinic, University of Pittsburgh School of Medicine, Pittsburgh, Pennsylvania

RONALD A. MADLE Early Intervention Program, The Pennsylvania State University, University Park, Pennsylvania

JOHNNY L. MATSON Department of Psychology, Louisiana State University, Baton Rouge, Louisiana

PAUL R. McCARTHY Department of Psychiatry, Temple University, Philadelphia, Pennsylvania

F. DUDLEY McGLYNN Department of Basic Dental Sciences, University of Florida, Gainesville, Florida

JOHN T. NEISWORTH Early Intervention Program, The Pennsylvania State University, University Park, Pennsylvania

N. JENNIFER OKE Department of Psychology, University of California-San Diego, La Jolla, California

THOMAS H. OLLENDICK Department of Psychology, Virginia Polytechnic Institute and State University, Blacksburg, Virginia

BERTRAM O. PLOOG Department of Psychology, University of California-San Diego, La Jolla, California

ANDRES J. PUMARIEGA Department of Psychiatry, The University of Texas Medical Branch, Galveston, Texas

MARK D. RAPPORT Department of Psychiatry and Behavioral Science, State University of New York, Stony Brook, New York

WILLIAM M. REYNOLDS Department of Educational Psychology, University of Wisconsin, Madison, Wisconsin

JOHANNES ROJAHN The Nisonger Center, The Ohio State University, Columbus, Ohio

LAURA E. SCHREIBMAN Department of Psychology, University of California-San Diego, La Jolla, California

NIRBHAY N. SINGH Educational Research and Services Center, Inc., De Kalb, Illinois

LORI A. SISSON Western Psychiatric Institute and Clinic, University of Pittsburgh School of Medicine, Pittsburgh, Pennsylvania

DEBORAH L. SNELL Department of Psychology, University of Canterbury, Christchurch, New Zealand

LAUREN C. SOLOTAR Department of Psychology, The University at Albany, State University of New York, Albany, New York

CYD C. STRAUSS   Western Psychiatric Institute and Clinic, University of Pittsburgh School of Medicine, Pittsburgh, Pennsylvania

VINCENT B. VAN HASSELT   Department of Psychiatry and Human Behavior, University of California, Orange, California

DON P. WILSON   University of Oklahoma Tulsa Medical College, Tulsa, Oklahoma

Preface

Some years ago we edited a general casebook on behavior therapy that was well received. However, those professors who used the book as an adjunct text in child behavior therapy courses were concerned that only 9 of the 26 chapters dealt with the clinical application of behavioral principles to children. Their contention was that a specific casebook on the topic was very much warranted. In considering their comments we took a closer look at the child behavior therapy area and were struck with how diverse it was, how it had expanded, and how it had matured over the last three decades. Given this apparent gap in the literature, we decided to devote an entire casebook to both the standard and the more innovative clinical applications to the behavioral problems presented by children.

The resulting book, containing 28 chapters, is divided into two parts. In the first part, in a chapter entitled "How the Field Has Moved On," we briefly trace the historical roots of child behavior therapy, detail the relationship of psychiatric diagnosis and behavioral assessment, and consider the importance of developmental norms, psychological testing, efforts at prevention, and behavioral medicine. The bulk of this book, of course, appears in the 27 cases presented by our respective experts.

Each of the treatment cases is presented in identical format for purposes of clarity, consistency, and comparability. The sequence of sections is as follows: (1) Description of the Disorder, (2) Case Identification, (3) Presenting Complaints, (4) History, (5) Assessment, (6) Selection of Treatment, (7) Course of Treatment, (8) Termination, (9) Follow-up, and (10) Overall Evaluation.

Presentation of the details of behavioral treatment for so many cases allows the student and the practitioner alike to have a better understanding of how child behavior therapists operate when confronted with difficult clinical problems. Although a firm theoretical understanding is requisite to carrying out effective child behavior therapy programs, we argue that good models of clinical care are equally important for new therapists to become fully effective. And it is to that end that our casebook is directed.

Many people have contributed to this book, and we would like to acknowledge their efforts. First, we thank our contributors for sharing their expertise with us. Second, we appreciate the secretarial and technical help by Jenifer McKelvey, Mary Newell, and Kim Sterner. Finally, once again, we thank our editor at Plenum, Eliot Werner, who makes all of this possible.

Michel Hersen
Cynthia G. Last

Pittsburgh

Contents

CHAPTER 1

How the Field Has Moved On

MICHEL HERSEN and CYNTHIA G. LAST

HISTORICAL ROOTS

Within the context of behavior therapy in general, there is a relatively long tradition of assessing and treating a wide variety of disorders and problems presented by children and adolescents. The usual historical antecedents cited include the work of John B. Watson, Rosalie Rayner, and Mary Cover Jones on the acquisition and removal of fears in very young children (Jones, 1924a, 1924b; Watson, 1924; Watson & Rayner, 1920) and that of Mowrer and Mowrer (1938) in deconditioning nighttime enuresis in children. However, the more careful reviews of the field (Hersen & Van Hasselt, 1987; Kazdin, 1978) acknowledge the importance of Lightner Witmer's pioneering efforts in the Psychological Clinic at the University of Pennsylvania, established in 1896, where children were treated using principles derived from theories of learning and perception.

The greatest upsurge in the application of behavioral principles to the treatment of children occurred in the 1960s and early 1970s, fueled by the Skinnerian conception as to how behavior is developed, maintained, and removed (Skinner, 1953). Following the operant paradigm of behavior that argued for a functional analysis of the controlling variables, specified motoric targets for modification were selected, with the goal of their being increased or decreased in accordance with clinical needs. In the earlier days, such demonstrations, often evaluated in single-case experimental designs (see Barlow & Hersen, 1984; Hersen & Barlow, 1976),

MICHEL HERSEN and CYNTHIA G. LAST • Western Psychiatric Institute and Clinic, University of Pittsburgh School of Medicine, 3811 O'Hara Street, Pittsburgh, Pennsylvania 15213.

were much more concerned with the viability of the short-term therapeutic effects than with the ultimate importance of response maintenance, generalization into the natural environment, and the possibility of negative concurrent effects of some of the strategies being carried out. However, these earlier behavioral applications, many of which were published in the *Journal of Applied Behavior Analysis* effective 1968, served as basic models for later child behavior therapists. Indeed, many of the earlier papers still prove to be exemplars of (1) the careful measurement of motoric behavior, (2) the precise delineation of therapeutic application, and (3) the clear documentation of how change in the targeted behavior is directly related to implementation of the treatment (i.e., the functional relationship between the dependent measure and the independent variable).

By current standards in the late 1980s, some of the work of our colleagues of the 1960s seems to be a bit simplistic. Moreover, some of the writing suggests a certain insularity and immunity to other empirical currents that were extant in the field. But when considering the historical climate into which child behavior therapy emerged, "the somewhat strident 'breast-beating' that then took place is understandable today" (Hersen, 1981, p. 18).

In this introduction to our *Casebook* we will not, once again, document the outstanding accomplishments of the child behavior therapists of the 1960s and 1970s, since this task has been done with considerable care and detail in several specific books (e.g., Kazdin, 1978; Ollendick & Cerny, 1981) and in many chapters of the 21 volumes of *Progress in Behavior Modification*. Rather, we will briefly show how the field has moved on, how it is more complex, how it is willing to incorporate the empirical findings from psychiatry (i.e., diagnosis), developmental psychology, psychometrics, and neuropsychology, how it is concerned with the critical area of prevention, and how it is interested in developing nonmedical strategies for dealing with some of the medical problems of children.

Unfortunately, some misconceptions as to how child behavior therapists currently operate still abound. For example, during the course of interviewing candidates for our Clinical Psychology Internship Training Program, one of the graduate students recently visiting us expressed much surprise that we had a rotation involving long-term outpatient behavior therapy. She erroneously thought that "all behavior therapy was of the short-term variety." Obviously, she was not aware of the complexity of the contemporary behavioral enterprise (cf. Hersen, 1981), nor was she probably cognizant of the thousands of hours that Lovaas (1987), for example, had spent on treating autistic children with behavior therapy procedures.

PSYCHIATRIC DIAGNOSIS AND BEHAVIORAL ASSESSMENT

The behavior therapists of the 1960s were most critical of psychiatric diagnosis (cf. Hersen, 1976), especially given the many deficiencies of the first two official nosological schemes put forth by the American Psychiatric Association (DSM-I and DSM-II; APA, 1952, 1968). However, with the advent of DSM-III (APA, 1980) and its attendant modifications in DSM-III-R (APA, 1987), many of the original concerns about reliability, validity, and the utility of the categories no longer hold. As articulated by Hersen and Turner (1984), "The emergence of DSM-III . . . has influenced all clinical practitioners, irrespective of theoretical allegiance, including behavior therapists" (p. 485). Similar positions have been taken by Hersen and Last (in press) and Kazdin (1983) for a number of reasons. First, the behavioral assessment schemes, offered as alternatives to psychiatric diagnosis (e.g., Adams, Doster, & Calhoun, 1977; Cautela & Upper, 1973), have never been adopted for use, even by behavior therapists, and they have had no impact on the field of diagnosis in general. Second, it is important that child behavior therapy become a part of child psychiatry, and if behavioral findings are to be integrated into the mainstream of practice, a common language system is needed (i.e., the DSM). And third, there is the growing recognition that the clients and patients seen by child behavior therapists present with complicated problems that require a greater breadth of approach than a "narrow-band" behavioral assessment. "That is, a narrow-band behavioral evaluation frequently does not consider: (1) the etiology of the disorder, (2) precipitating stresses, (3) specific onset, (4) chronicity and past episodes, (5) severity, and (6) the complicated interrelationship of targets and symptoms that may be subsumed under a particular diagnostic label (e.g., childhood depression)" (Hersen & Van Hasselt, 1987, p. 8).

With regard to the six aforementioned points, use of the multiaxial system in DSM-III ensures that the assessor will maintain a broader perspective on how particular behaviors in clients and patients came about in the first place. The reader will note that, for the most part in our *Casebook*, we adhere to the nomenclature used in DSM-III and DSM-III-R. However, this is not meant to imply that the DSM (including its revisions), as applied to the problems of children, is considered to be flawless. Indeed, as has been repeatedly pointed out elsewhere (Hersen, in press; Hersen & Bellack, 1988; Hersen & Last, in press; Hersen

& Van Hasselt, 1987), behavioral assessors have much to offer the field of child psychiatric diagnosis, particularly when improvements in the precision of the categories could be achieved.

First of all, once a psychiatric diagnosis has been established, there is absolutely no reason why a behavioral analysis of the problems cannot follow (see Hersen & Last, in press). Indeed, in a two-tiered assessment, consisting of psychiatric diagnosis and behavioral assessment, the broad summary statements emanating from the diagnostic procedure are complemented by the subsequent fine-grained analysis of specific targets that then are slated for modification with particular technical strategies.

Second, behavioral assessment strategies can be used to advantage to improve the precision of the criteria for categories subsumed under DMS-III. In particular, in a seminal contribution to the literature, Tryon (1986) contends that activity measures, subsumed under vague psychiatric diagnostic referents (e.g., "increase," "decrease," "more," "slowed down"), need to be quantified. To illustrate, in the diagnostic category of Attention Disorder with Hyperactivity (314.01), several of the five hyperactivity criteria relate to increased motor activity (e.g., runs or climbs on things excessively). With the technology of behavioral assessment, activity norms for a large variety of such diagnostic categories can be determined for both nonpathological and pathological populations. In each instance the lower and upper limits would be ascertained empirically. Unfortunately, however, this work has not yet been carried out.

DEVELOPMENTAL NORMS

When dealing with children and adolescents, the importance of knowing which behaviors are appropriate from an age-norm perspective cannot be sufficiently underscored. This is especially the case when the behavior therapist is intent on modifying the child's responses so that they fall within the normal limits of his or her peer group. Kazdin (1977) refers to the setting of such specified criteria (based on a normed-reference group) as the "process of social validation." However, in children and adolescents an important *caveat* is in order. Given the incredibly complex biological and maturational changes that occur during this time period, many of these norms alter rapidly as the child is developing, indeed sometimes within a matter of months. Thus, it behooves each child behavior therapist to have a firm grounding in developmental psychology.

Developmental psychology is a well-established discipline with a time-honored methodology steeped in rigor. Moreover, within the archival literature of developmental psychology there is a vast reservoir of information that is of much value to the practicing child behavior therapist. However, to date there has been very little discourse between child behavior therapists and developmental psychologists, with the exception of a few calls for integration by a few child behavior therapists (see Harris & Ferrari, 1983; Hersen & Van Hasselt, 1987). We fully agree with Harris and Ferrari (1983) that child behavior therapists could avoid mistakes if they incorporated the findings of developmental psychology in their work. Indeed, "Developmental capacities in children . . . have a large impact on what we can expect our child clients to do in the therapeutic setting. Given that the behavioral approach to treatment is an active one that involves full participation of the client, it is critical for child behavior therapists to know their client's intellectual and developmental capabilities at varying age levels" (Hersen & Van Hasselt, 1987, p. 9). For example: (1) When can mental imagery be used effectively in children? (2) How old does the child have to be for him/her to understand the notion of self-control and be willing to carry out such strategies? (3) How old does a child have to be for a therapist to encourage assertive responding to adults in an adult-controlled environment? (4) At what developmental stage is the child able to carry out extratherapeutic assignments in the natural environment (i.e., homework) without parental assistance and/or guidance?

PSYCHOLOGICAL TESTING

At first, child behavior therapists eschewed the use of standard psychological tests, literally "throwing out the baby with the bath water," in their reaction to the then prevalent use of projective devices. Indeed, throughout the 1960s and most of the 1970s there appeared to be very little interest in integrating intelligence tests and neuropsychological batteries with the strategies of behavioral assessment. However, more recently such calls for interaction have appeared from a number of quarters (e.g., Goldstein, 1979; Horton & Miller, 1985; Kaufman & Reynolds, 1984; Nelson, 1980). At this time the importance of intellectual evaluations (including IQ and achievement testing) and neuropsychological evaluations to a more comprehensive understanding of a given child or adolescent has been acknowledged.

Kaufman and Reynolds (1984) outline a model for the judicious use of intellectual and academic achievement tests in child clinical cases where there are cognitive or affective disorders. They argue, "Intelligent testing is a challenging, difficult enterprise but one that we believe offers the best model for using test scores for children and not merely as vehicles to classification'' (p. 217). Indeed, in their model, Kaufman and Reynolds use tests to help generate "remedial and therapeutic hypotheses" (p. 217). This, of course, is vastly different from the sterile use of tests in which there is little, if any, relationship between what is uncovered by the test and future treatment.

In an earlier paper, Nelson (1980) outlined a number of applications of intellectual evaluations under the broader umbrella of behavioral assessment. She pointed out that (1) an IQ score can serve as a dependent measure in a behavioral treatment program, (2) the intellectual evaluation can identify children in need of academic remediation (with test patterns determining specific targets for modification), and (3) the use of IQ scores will enhance communication between and among researchers and clinicians who have different theoretical positions.

Turning to neuropsychological evaluations, Goldstein (1979) astutely observed that the complex patterns of neural disorganization in brain-damaged individuals are not fully reflected in the mere observations of their overt behavior. That being the case, he envisages a partnership between the neuropsychologist and the behavior therapist in which the neuropsychologist assists in selecting targets for modification by carefully evaluating data resulting from standardized batteries.

EFFORTS AT PREVENTION

It is only in recent years that child behavior therapists have concerned themselves with the area of prevention, albeit in the field of therapeutics this approach has an extensive history. Child behavior therapists apparently are cognizant of Caplan's (1964) tripartite model, and they have carried out efforts at the primary, secondary, and tertiary levels (see Table 1 for definitions). For example, Schinke's (1984) work in teaching adolescent girls assertive refusal skills to prevent unplanned pregnancy is a good example of a behavioral effect in primary prevention. Similarly, Rivera-Tovar and Jones's (in press) recent investigation dedicated to teaching children how to use the telephone in an emergency is also exemplary of the primary prevention approach.

An example of secondary prevention carried out by child behavior therapists is seen in Epstein, Koeske, Zidansek, and Wing's (1983) study, in which obese preadolescents were taught appropriate nutritional practices and exercise to decrease weight and ameliorate improved physical fitness. Nutritional practices and exercise were directed to prevent future cardiovascular problems in basically healthy, albeit obese, children. Another excellent example of secondary prevention involves teaching pa-

Table 1
Levels of Prevention

Primary prevention—The major goal here is to diminish the number of new cases of a given disorder (i.e., decrease the incidence). Indeed, issues for an entire population are addressed before the problem can arise. Preventative intervention is accomplished by teaching individuals strategies for dealing and coping with stress and ways to anticipate problems.

Secondary prevention—The major goal here is the early identification of at-risk individuals before problems attain major proportions. Early intervention is accomplished through specific behavioral treatment strategies in addition to teaching individuals how to anticipate problems for which they are vulnerable.

Tertiary prevention—The major goal here is for the individual to recover from the problem or disorder and be reintegrated in smooth fashion into the community. This is accomplished through specific behavioral treatment strategies, with particular attention paid to ensuring generalization into the natural environment (i.e., usual treatment procedures).

---

tients who have abused their children (but not caused serious physical harm) appropriate child management strategies to ensure that abuse will no longer occur (see Gambrill, 1983). Efforts here are to prevent the possibility of serious physical harm in an at-risk population.

We will not identify individual examples of tertiary prevention, since the field of child behavior therapy, in principle, has been devoted almost entirely to remediating childhood psychopathology and reintegrating children and adolescents to the fullest extent possible in family and school environments. However, in the future we anticipate that a much more concerted effort will be directed to primary and secondary prevention. Preventing teenage pregnancy, child abuse, and the dire consequences of accidents and fires is just a first step for child behavior therapists.

BEHAVIORAL MEDICINE

In the realm of pediatric behavioral medicine, child behavior therapists have conducted some of the most socially relevant work in the entire field of behavior therapy. It is only in the last decade or so that the talents of child behavior therapists have been applied to the medical problems of children. But already an impressive array of achievements have been documented, including the interruption of a seizure chain not controlled by medication (Zlutnick, Mayville, & Moffat, 1975), decreasing of pain prior to and following surgical procedures (Hickman, Thompson, Feldman, & Varni, 1985), teaching a leukemia patient to swallow pills

(Walco, 1986), strategies for reducing and eliminating enuresis and encopresis (Doleys, 1978), relaxation techniques for reducing fear of the dental setting (Melamed, 1979), and improved adherence to medical prescriptions (Epstein, *et al.*, 1981).

The above-mentioned list reflects only a very small portion of this burgeoning field. There can be no doubt that the emergence of pediatric behavioral medicine is one of the most exciting developments in child behavior therapy. We certainly anticipate the continued collaboration between child behavior therapists and their pediatric colleagues to be extremely fruitful. Indeed, the work in pediatric behavioral medicine once again underscores the dictum that physiologically and/or medically based disorders can benefit from nonmedical interventions such as behavior therapy.

OVERVIEW OF THE CASES

The bulk of this book is concerned with the description of a wide variety of behavioral applications to children, some being typical and others, of course, representing the more atypical. The breadth of case material herein is equally matched by the diversity of technical applications and theoretical positions of our contributors. However, irrespective of the unique aspects of each case, an underlying feature of all of the therapists represented is a concern for the efficaiousness of their strategies and a willingness to subject them to public scrutiny. In so doing our contributors explicate how they conceptualize their cases and why particular strategies were selected at given times. Some of the treatments are of a short-term nature (consistent with the stereotypical views that are held about behavior therapists), but other treatments are more protracted (consistent with the complexity of the case material). In either instance, the technical operations implemented are presented in such a manner that colleagues in the field should be able to replicate when they encounter similar clinical problems.

On the basis of our prior experience in developing a more general casebook (i.e., *Behavior Therapy Casebook*: Hersen & Last, 1985), we have found that an identical format across chapters enhances readability and cross-case comparison. Therefore, in our *Child Behavior Therapy Casebook* each contribution follows a set format: (1) Description of the Disorder, (2) Case Identification, (3) Presenting Complaints, (4) History, (5) Assessment, (6) Selection of Treatment, (7) Course of Treatment, (8) Termination, (9) Follow-up, and (10) Overall Evaluation.

REFERENCES

Adams, H. E., Doster, J. A., & Calhoun, K. S. (1977). A psychologically based system of response classification. In A. R. Ciminero, K. S. Cahoun, & H. E. Adams (Eds.), *Handbook of behavioral assessment* (pp. 47–48). New York: Wiley.

American Psychiatric Association. (1952). *Diagnostic and statistical manual of mental disorders*. Washington, DC: Author.

American Psychiatric Association. (1968). *Diagnostic and statistical manual of mental disorders* (2nd ed.). Washington, DC: Author.

American Psychiatric Association. (1980). *Diagnostic and statistical manual of mental disorders* (3rd. ed.). Washington, DC: Author.

American Psychiatric Association. (1987). *Diagnostic and statistical manual of mental disorders* (3rd. ed.-revised). Washington, DC: Author.

Barlow, D. H., & Hersen, M. (1984). *Single case experimental designs: Strategies for studying behavior change* (2nd ed.). New York: Pergamon Press.

Caplan, G. (1964). *Principles of preventive psychiatry*. New York: Basic Books.

Cautela, J. R., & Upper, D. (1973, December). *A behavioral coding scheme.* Paper presented at the Association for Advancement of Behavior Therapy, Miami.

Doleys, D. M. (1978). Assessment and treatment of enuresis and encopresis in children. In M. Hersen, R. M. Eisler, & P. M. Miller (Eds.), *Progress in behavior modification* (Vol. 6, pp. 85–121). New York: Academic Press.

Epstein, L. H., Beck, S., Figueroa, J., Farkas, G., Kazdin, A. E., Daneman, D., & Becker, D. (1981). The effects of targeting improvements in urine glucose on metabolic control in children with insulin dependent diabetes. *Journal of Applied Behavior Analysis, 14,* 365–375.

Epstein, L. H., Koeske, R., Zidansek, J., & Wing, R. R. (1983). Effects of weight loss on fitness in obese children. *American Journal of Diseases of Children, 137,* 654–657.

Gambrill, E. D. (1983). Behavioral intervention with child abuse and neglect. In M. Hersen, R. M. Eisler, & P. M. Miller (Eds.), *Progress in behavior modification* (Vol. 15, pp. 1–56). New York: Academic Press.

Goldstein, G. (1979). Methodological and theoretical issues in neuropsychological assessment. *Journal of Behavioral Assessment, 1,* 34–41.

Harris, S. L., & Ferrari, M. (1983). Developmental factors in child behavior therapy. *Behavior Therapy, 14,* 54–72.

Hersen, M. (1976). Historical perspectives in behavioral assessment. In M. Hersen & A. S. Bellack (Eds.), *Behavioral assessment: A practical handbook.* New York: Pergamon Press.

Hersen, M. (1981). Complex problems require complex solutions. *Behavior Therapy, 12,* 15–29.

Hersen, M. (in press). Behavioral assessment and psychiatric diagnosis. *Behavioral Assessment.*

Hersen, M., & Barlow, D. H. (1976). *Single-case experimental designs: Strategies for studying behavior change.* New York: Pergamon Press.

Hersen, M., & Last, C. G. (Eds.). (1985). *Behavior therapy casebook.* New York: Springer.

Hersen, M., & Bellack, A. S. (1988). DSM-III and behavioral assessment. In A. S. Bellack & M. Hersen (Eds.), *Behavioral assessment: A practical handbook* (3rd ed.). New York: Pergamon Press.

Hersen, M., & Last, C. G. (in press). Psychiatric diagnosis and behavioral assessment in children. In C. G. Last & M. Hersen (Eds.), *Handbook of child psychiatric diagnosis.* New York: Wiley.

Hersen, M., & Turner, S. M. (1984). DSM-III and behavior therapy. In S. M. Turner & M. Hersen (Eds.), *Adult psychopathology and diagnosis.* New York: Wiley.

Hersen, M., & Van Hasselt, V. B. (Eds.). (1987). *Behavior therapy with children and adolescents: A clinical approach.* New York: Wiley.

Hickman, C. S., Thompson, K. L., Feldman, W. S., & Varni, J. W. (1985). Pediatric medical problems. In M. Hersen (Ed.), *Practice of inpatient behavior therapy* (pp. 267–282). New York: Grune and Stratton.

Horton, A. M., & Miller, W. G. (1985). Neuropsychology and behavior therapy. In M. Hersen, R. M. Eisler, & P. M. Miller (Eds.), *Progress in behavior modification* (Vol. 19, pp. 1–55). New York: Academic Press.

Jones, M. C. (1924a). The elimination of children's fears. *Journal of Experimental Psychology, 7,* 382–390.

Jones, M. C. (1924b). A laboratory study of fear: The case of Peter. *Journal of Genetic Psychology, 31,* 308–315.

Kaufman, A. S., & Reynolds, C. R. (1984). Intellectual and academic achievement tests. In T. H. Ollendick & M. Hersen (Eds.), *Child behavioral assessment* (pp. 195–220). New York: Pergamon Press.

Kazdin, A. E. (1977). Assessing the clinical and applied importance of behavior change through social validation. *Behavior Modification, 1,* 427–452.

Kazdin, A. E. (1978). *History of behavior modification.* Baltimore: University Park Press.

Kazdin, A. E. (1983). Psychiatric diagnosis, dimensions of dysfunction, and child behavior therapy. *Behavior Therapy, 14,* 73–99.

Lovaas, O. I. (1987). Behavioral treatment and normal educational and intellectual functioning in young autistic children. *Journal of Consulting and Clinical Psychology, 55,* 3–9.

Melamed, B. G. (1979). Behavioral approaches to fear in dental setting. In M. Hersen, R. M. Eisler, & P. M. Miller (Eds.), *Progress in behavior modification* (Vol. 7, pp. 171–203). New York: Academic Press.

Mowrer, O. H., & Mowrer, W. M. (1938). Enuresis—A method for its study and treatment. *American Journal of Orthopsychiatry, 8,* 436–459.

Nelson, R. O. (1980). The use of intelligence tests within behavioral assessment. *Behavioral Assessment, 2,* 417–423.

Ollendick, T. H., & Cerny, J. A. (1981). *Clinical behavior therapy with children.* New York: Plenum Press.

Rivera-Tovar, L. A., & Jones, R. T. (in press). An extension and refinement of telephone emergency skills training: A comparison of training methods. *Behavior Modification.*

Schinke, S. P. (1984). Preventing teenage pregnancy. In M. Hersen, R. M. Eisler, & P. M. Miller (Eds.), *Progress in behavior modification* (Vol. 16, pp. 31–64). New York: Academic Press.

Skinner, B. F. (1953). *Science and human behavior.* New York: Free Press.

Tryon, W. W. (1986). Motor activity measurements and DSM-III. In M. Hersen, R. M. Eisler, & P. M. Miller (Eds.), *Progress in behavior modification* (Vol. 20, pp. 35–66). Orlando, FL: Academic Press.

Walco, G. A. (1986). A behavioral treatment for difficulty in swallowing pills. *Journal of Behavior Therapy and Experimental Psychiatry, 17,* 127–128.

Watson, J. B. (1924). *Behaviorism.* Chicago: University of Chicago Press.

Watson, J. B., & Rayner, R. (1920). Conditioned emotional reactions. *Journal of Experimental Psychology, 3,* 1–14.

Zlutnick, S., Mayville, W. J., & Moffat, S. (1975). Modification of seizure disorders: The interruption of behavioral chains. *Journal of Applied Behavior Analysis, 8,* 1–12.

CHAPTER 2

Separation Anxiety

CYNTHIA G. LAST

DESCRIPTION OF THE DISORDER

Separation anxiety is a childhood anxiety disorder that is characterized by excessive anxiety (fear, worry) concerning separation from a major attachment figure and/or home. Although clinical reports of this syndrome have appeared in the literature for decades, it was not until the publication of DSM-III in 1980 that the disorder was included in the DSM classification system. Nine criteria are included for the diagnostic category, three of which must be met for at least a 2-week period to receive the diagnosis: (1) unrealistic worry about possible harm befalling major attachment figures or fear that they will leave and not return, (2) unrealistic worry that an untoward calamitous event will separate the child from a major attachment figure (e.g., the child will be lost, kidnapped, killed), (3) persistent reluctance or refusal to go to school in order to stay with major attachment figures or at home, (4) persistent reluctance or refusal to go to sleep without being next to a major attachment figure or to go to sleep away from home, (5) persistent avoidance of being alone in the home and emotional upset if unable to follow the major attachment figure around the home, (6) repeated nightmares involving the theme of separation, (7) complaints of physical symptoms on school days (e.g., stomachaches, headaches, nausea), (8) signs of excessive distress upon separation, or when anticipating separation, from major attachment figures (e.g., crying, temper tantrums), and (9) social withdrawal, apathy, sadness, or difficulty

CYNTHIA G. LAST • Western Psychiatric Institute and Clinic, Department of Psychiatry, University of Pittsburth School of Medicine, 3811 O'Hara Street, Pittsburgh, Pennsylvania 15213.

concentrating on work or play when not with a major attachment figure (APA, 1980, p. 53).

Recent data suggest that the disorder is most common in prepubertal children (Last, Francis, Hersen, Kazdin, & Strauss, 1987; Last, Hersen, Kazdin, Finkelstein, & Strauss, 1987). While reluctance or refusal to go to school is present in approximately three-quarters of children meeting criteria for separation anxiety disorder (Last, Francis *et al.*, 1987), it should be noted that this behavior is not necessary for meeting DSM-III criteria for the diagnosis. In addition, the symptom expression of this disorder appears to vary according to the developmental level of the child (Francis, Last, & Strauss, 1987). For example, adolescents with this disorder very rarely have repeated nightmares and excessive distress upon separation (criteria (6) and (8) above), unlike younger children with separation anxiety disorder.

The patient reported on below represents a "typical" case of separation anxiety disorder that we see at our child and adolescent anxiety disorder clinic

CASE IDENTIFICATION

Kenny is a 10-year-old boy who was evaluated at the Child and Adolescent Anxiety Disorder Clinic at Western Psychiatric Institute and Clinic. He was referred to the clinic by his parents, who both accompanied him during his initial visit. The patient lives with his parents in a trailer park located in a rural area outside of Pittsburgh. Kenny has two half-siblings, by his mother's previous marriage, who live close by. He attends public elementary school and is in the fifth grade.

PRESENTING COMPLAINTS

Kenny's parents reported that he is extremely fearful of going to school and has refused to go for the past several months. In addition to school refusal, Kenny is unable to enter all other situations that involve his being separated from his parents (e.g., playing in the backyard or at other children's homes, going to little league practice, staying at home with a baby-sitter). When "pushed" to go to school, or to be separated from his parents when at home, Kenny responds with crying and tantrums. He also has threatened to hurt himself (e.g., jump out of the classroom window) if forced to go to school. At the time of the initial interview, both parents felt that they were unable to control Kenny's behavior regarding his separation problems.

HISTORY

Upon interview, it was evident that Kenny's separation problems began about one year prior to his evaluation at the clinic. At that time, Kenny's father was having problems with alcohol and was frequently absent from the home for prolonged periods of time. Kenny's separation anxiety worsened gradually over the course of the year, resulting in complete school refusal. Help had been sought at a local mental health clinic where psychotherapy was provided, but Kenny continued to deteriorate. He developed significant depressive symptomatology, including dysphoric mood, guilty feelings about his problems, occasional wishes to be dead, and periodic early morning awakening.

ASSESSMENT

Kenny and his parents individually were administered a semistructured diagnostic interview schedule. Results from the interviews confirmed a diagnosis of separation anxiety disorder, according to DSM-III criteria. More specifically, Kenny met the following DSM-III criteria for separation anxiety disorder: (1) worry about harm befalling his mother and father (i.e., "they'll be in an accident"), (2) worries about being kidnapped and separated from his parents, (3) somatic complaints when anticipating a separation situation, (4) excessive distress upon separation, and (5) refusal to be alone at home or to stay at home with a baby-sitter. Although Kenny also had significant depressive symptomatology, these symptoms were seen as secondary to his primary anxiety condition and were not numerous enough to meet criteria for a DSM-III diagnosis of major depression. It was anticipated that his depressive symptoms would remit as his separation anxiety improved.

In addition to the diagnostic interview, Kenny completed several self-report questionnaires, including the State-Trait Anxiety Inventory for Children (STAIC; Spielberger, 1973), the Revised Fear Survey Schedule for Children (FSSC-R; Ollendick, 1983), and the Child Depression Inventory (CDI; Kovacs, 1978). Results from the STAIC revealed very high levels of both state (60) and trait (49) anxiety. For specific fears, Kenny reported "intense" fears (ratings of "a lot") for seven items: (1) being alone, (2) being hit by a car or truck, (3) being in a fight, (4) not being able to breathe, (5) strange-looking people, (6) cats, and (7) getting a cut or injury. Finally, Kenny's score on the CDI (25) revealed significant depressive symptomatology.

SELECTION OF TREATMENT

Graduated *in vivo* exposure was selected as the treatment for this patient. This treatment approach previously has yielded positive results with a variety of childhood and adult anxiety disorders, particularly where avoidance behavior is a central feature of the disorder. While imipramine was considered as an adjunct, Kenny's parents were opposed to his taking medication. It was decided that the possibility of adding medication to the treatment program would be reconsidered in one month if Kenny did not show at least some improvement by that time.

It was explained to the patient and his parents that the only way in which Kenny would overcome his fear was by repeatedly confronting the very situations that he feared and avoided. It was further emphasized that these situations would be tackled in a *very* gradual manner, beginning with tasks that cause little or no anxiety and then, in a stepwise manner, moving to increasingly difficult tasks. Kenny was told that he would be in control of the rate at which he would proceed, and that he never would be asked to do anything for which he did not think he was "ready."

COURSE OF TREATMENT

During the first treatment session, a *fear and avoidance hierarchy* was constructed that was to be used in planning the steps in the treatment program. For Kenny, two hierarchies were built—one for school, and one covering all other separation-related situations. Each hierarchy listed 10 situations that caused Kenny increasing levels of anxiety. Each situation was rated by him for degrees of fear and avoidance using a 0–8 scale (0 = no anxiety, never avoid, 8 = panic, always avoid). Kenny's pretreatment ratings for his school hierarchy are presented in Table 1.

Treatment sessions were held once a week. At each session, Kenny was given a "homework assignment," where he was required to practice an item selected from his fear and avoidance hierarchy every day until the next session. Homework assignments were "negotiated," in that the child, his parents, and the therapist mutually agreed on each specific weekly task assigned. It should be noted that in our treatment approach the *child* essentially is in control of his/her treatment and the rate at which

Table 1
Pretreatment Ratings

Description	Rating
1. Entering the school building (no classes)	0
2. Attending class for 10 minutes	1
3. Attending class for 30 minutes	2
4. Attending class for 1 hour	3
5. Attending class for 2 hours	4
6. Attending class for 3 hours	5
7. Attending class for 4 hours	6
8. Attending class for 5 hours	7
9. Going all day	8
10. Taking the school bus to and from school	8

he/she progresses, since in our clinical experience we have found this to be positively related to successful outcome. Kenny was instructed to keep track of his homework sessions on a form designed for this purpose that required him to rate each practice using the 0–8 anxiety scale. At each treatment session progress/problems from the previous week's homework were reviewed, and a new assignment then was given. Assignments increased in level of difficulty, on the basis of Kenny's fear and avoidance ratings, across treatment sessions.

Using the above approach, Kenny's school avoidance was tackled first. During the first 2 weeks of treatment, the therapist maintained frequent telephone contact with Kenny in order to provide opportunities to verbally reinforce him for his progress. In addition, a telephone contact person was established at Kenny's school (his school guidance counselor). The establishment of a school contact person is essential for three reasons. First, it lets the school know what to expect, since the child initially will be going to classes only for a brief period of time and then leaving. Second, it makes it less likely that the child will "cheat" on his/her assignments, since relevant school personnel know what the child is supposed to be doing. Third, school personnel can serve as on-location therapists, if they have an understanding of what the therapist is trying to accomplish and what they can do to be of assistance (e.g., verbal reinforcement).

After 6 weeks of treatment, Kenny was attending half days of school on a regular basis. At this time, it appeared that his progress with school generalized to other non-school-related separation situations. During the next six sessions, Kenny continued to work toward attending full days of school, and also worked on home-related separation items using the same graduated exposure approach. He continued to make consistent progress and showed no signs of separation anxiety problems by the end of the 3-month treatment program.

TERMINATION

Following the end of treatment, Kenny completed the same self-report questionnaires that he had initially completed at the pretreatment assessment (i.e., the STAIC, the FSSC-R, and the CDI). Self-reported anxiety on the STAIC showed marked reductions for both state (21) and trait (22) anxiety. Similarly, Kenny no longer reported "intense" fear on the FSSC-R for any of the items on the questionnaire. Finally, his posttreatment CDI score (0) showed an absence of depressive symptomatology.

In addition to the above, Kenny's posttreatment ratings on his fear and avoidance hierarchies showed an absence of anxiety/avoidance (each item rated as 0).

At the time of termination, Kenny's parents were asked to contact the therapist should any problems arise. Otherwise, the therapist would contact the family following summer vacation to make sure that Kenny did not experience any difficulty with returning to school in the fall.

FOLLOW-UP

When Kenny and his parents were recontacted following summer vacation, his parents reported that he had no difficulty reentering school, and that he seemed to enjoy his classes and interacting with the other children. The family again was contacted following Christmas vacation, and, once more, Kenny appeared to be maintaining his progress. At this time, the family had made plans for Kenny to go away to "basketball camp," to which he was looking forward. No problems with separation or school refusal were reported.

OVERALL EVALUATION

Kenny is a 10-year-old boy whose presenting complaints were fairly typical of a child with separation anxiety disorder. He had difficulty in virtually all activities that involved his being separated from his parents, both at school and at home. His school refusal was targeted first for intervention and was treated with a program of graduated *in vivo* exposure. He showed gradual and consistent progress in returning to school, and some of these gains appeared to generalize to other non-school-related separation situations. The remaining feared situations at home also were treated successfully with graduated exposure. By the end of the 3-month treatment program, Kenny was going to school full time and showing no signs of separation anxiety at home. Follow-up contact up to 1 year indicated that Kenny had maintained his treatment progress and that he was functioning well in academic, social, and home environments.

REFERENCES

American Psychiatric Association. (1980). *Diagnostic and statistical manual of mental disorders* (3rd Ed.). Washington, DC: Author.

Francis, G., Last, C. G., & Strauss, C. C. (1987). Expression of separation anxiety disorder: The roles of age and gender. *Child Psychiatry and Human Development, 18*, 82–89.

Kovacs, M. (1978). *Children's Depression Inventory (CDI)*. Unpublished manuscript, University of Pittsburgh School of Medicine.

Last, C. G., Francis, G., Hersen, M., Kazdin, A. E., & Strauss, C. C. (1987). Separation anxiety and school phobia: A comparison using DSM-III criteria. *American Journal of Psychiatry, 144*, 653–657.

Last, C. G., Hersen, M., Kazdin, A. E., Finkelstein, R., & Strauss, C. C. (1987). Comparison of DSM-III separation anxiety and overanxious disorders: Demographic characteristics and patterns of comorbidity. *Journal of the American Academy of Child Psychiatry, 26*, 527–531.

Ollendick, T. H. (1983). Reliability and validity of the Revised Fear Survey Schedule for Children (FSSC-R). *Behaviour Research and Therapy, 21*, 685–692.

Spielberger, C. D. (1973). *Manual for the State-Trait Anxiety Inventory for Children*. Palo Alto: Consulting Psychologists Press.

CHAPTER 3

Overanxious Disorder

CYD C. STRAUSS

DESCRIPTION OF THE DISORDER

Overanxious disorder is a childhood anxiety disorder subtype characterized by anxiety that is not focused on a specific situation or object. The
hallmark of this disorder is excessive or unrealistic worry about future
events, a symptom that is present in almost all children and adolescents
diagnosed with overanxious disorder (Strauss, Lease, Last, & Francis,
in press). Overanxious children also demonstrate excessive or unrealistic
worry about past events, an overconcern about their performance or evaluation by others, an extreme need for reassurance by others, and marked
self-consciousness. Finally, children with overanxious disorder are almost continuously tense and often have multiple somatic complaints, such
as headaches, stomachaches, fatigue, dizziness, palpitations, and breath-
lessness. This childhood subcategory appears to have many features in
common with the adult-onset diagnosis of generalized anxiety disorder,
but currently there is no information as to whether one is the developmental precursor of the other.

Children and adolescents with overanxious disorder are commonly
referred for clinical outpatient services. In fact, Last, Hersen, Kazdin,
Finkelstein, and Strauss (1987) recently found that 52% of children referred to a child and adolescent anxiety disorder clinic over an 18-month
period met DSM-III criteria for overanxious disorder. The clinical importance of this disorder is underscored by its association with other forms

CYD C. STRAUSS • Western Psychiatric Institute and Clinic, Department of Psychiatry,
University of Pittsburgh School of Medicine, 3811 O'Hara Street, Pittsburgh, Pennsylvania
15213.

of impairment, including major depression, suicidal ideation and attempts, poor social adjustment, and low self-esteem.

Overanxious disorder appears to be equally common in young children and adolescents (Strauss *et al.*, in press). However, interesting age differences in the expression of overanxious disorder have been found to occur (Strauss *et al.*, in press). For instance, older overanxious children are significantly more likely to meet most or all (6 or 7) diagnostic criteria for the disorder than are younger children. Furthermore, patterns of co-morbidity differ for younger versus older overanxious children. Older overanxious children more frequently exhibit a concurrent major depression or simple phobia, whereas younger overanxious children more commonly have coexisting separation anxiety or attention deficit disorders. Finally, older overanxious children report significantly higher levels of general anxiety than young children.

Empirical investigations of overanxious disorder in childhood have been few in number, so that much remains to be learned concerning the etiology, course, prognosis, and treatment for this childhood disorder. The following case report will provide a description of a child whose clinical presentation is typical of children referred for overanxious disorder.

CASE IDENTIFICATION

Ashley is an 11-year-old girl who was referred for an evaluation in the Child and Adolescent Anxiety Disorder Clinic at Western Psychiatric Institute and Clinic by her father. The reasons for referral included excessive worrying, anxiety, and depressed mood. Ashley attends the sixth grade at a small parochial school. She resides with both natural parents and her 6-year-old sister in an urban setting. The mother is 31 years old and currently is a homemaker, although previously she was employed as an accountant. The father is a 33-year-old electrical engineer. Ashley's sister suffers from cerebral palsy, which reportedly had required that the parents devote considerably more time and energy in the past attending to the needs of this child than to Ashley's needs. Both parents expressed a willingness to participate actively in treatment for Ashley to help reduce problems with anxiety and sadness.

PRESENTING COMPLAINTS

Ashley began to demonstrate significant difficulties when she was enrolled in the fifth grade in a new school after a family move. At this time, she worried excessively about upcoming events at school, as well as at home. She frequently ruminated for extended periods of time about incidents that already had occurred, such as what she had said in class, her performance on tests, and her social behavior with other children. Ashley often was overly concerned and perfectionistic about her performance during academic tasks, athletic activities, and social situations. Consequently, she sought reassurance from her parents, on a daily basis, about the correctness of her schoolwork, her decisions about what to say or how to act with peers, and what she should wear. In addition, she reportedly was extremely self-conscious, such that she became easily embarrassed when she spoke during class, refused to participate in activities that required that she assume a leadership role, blushed easily, and was very anxious and uncomfortable whenever she was the center of attention in groups of children. Finally, Ashley was described as frequently tense.

Following the onset of overanxious features, Ashley became increasingly isolative at school and showed sadness. She reported occasional suicidal ideation, although she denied serious suicidal intent. Ashley cried frequently about having to go to school, but her parents insisted that she attend school daily. Both the child and her parents denied any separation anxiety that may have interfered with her ability to attend school; instead, Ashley's fears appeared to be focused on the scrutiny of other children and teachers at school.

Ashley was also described as very anxious and uncomfortable in social situations with unfamiliar peers. She tended to avoid such situations owing to her extreme discomfort. In contrast, Ashley enjoyed close relationships with family members and other very familiar persons. Thus, although it was not a reason for referral, Ashley showed evidence of avoidant disorder.

These problems continued through the beginning of Ashley's sixth-grade year, at which time the parents referred the child for therapy. The child had not received previous psychiatric treatment for these presenting complaints.

HISTORY

Ashley and her parents indicated that Ashley always had been a somewhat shy and sensitive girl. Beginning at age 6, they noted that she began to be generally anxious, overly concerned with her competence, and perfectionistic about her performance at school. She frequently compared her school performance with that displayed by her classmates. As a result, Ashley became reluctant to attend school, often crying in the evenings and mornings prior to school. In efforts to reduce school reluctance, the father accompanied the child to school several hours each week. School reluctance decreased after 2 months. No further interventions were used to alleviate anxiety symptoms.

Subsequently, Ashley attended school regularly and generally enjoyed school. In terms of actual school performance, Ashley has always been an excellent student. She consistently performed at the top of her class academically. With regard to social adjustment, Ashley tended to have one or two close friends and otherwise generally was neither well liked nor actively disliked among her classmates. Ashley presented significant past difficulties with initiating peer interactions and being assertive with other children, although no other social skills deficits were noted.

ASSESSMENT

A multimethod assessment approach was used to evaluate anxiety, depression, peer adjustment, and other behavior problems. In particular, semistructured child and parent interviews, self-report inventories, and teacher questionnaires were administered at the initial assessment and immediately following treatment.

Prior to treatment, Ashley and her parents individually were administered a modified version of the Schedule for Affective Disorders and Schizophrenia for School-Age Children (K-SADS; Puig-Antich, Orvaschel, Tabrizi, & Chambers, 1978). The K-SADS was modified to include questions about all symptoms used in the DSM-III-R (American Psychiatric Association, 1987) for the syndromes of separation anxiety disorder, overanxious disorder, avoidant disorder, phobic disorders, obsessive–compulsive disorder, attention deficit hyperactivity disorder, conduct disorder, and oppositional disorder. According to both parent and child responses to interview questions, Ashley met diagnostic criteria for overanxious disorder and avoidant disorder. She also showed evidence of past diagnoses of a social phobia of school in the first and fifth grades. Information obtained during the semistructured interviews suggested that the onset of overanxious symptoms occurred when Ashley was 6 years old and that avoidant disorder features first were apparent when she was 8 years old.

In addition to data derived from interviews, Ashley completed numerous self-report measures. These included the State-Trait Anxiety Inventory for Children (STAIC; Spielberger, 1973), the Revised Fear Survey Schedule for Children (FSSC-R; Ollendick, 1983), the Children's

Depression Inventory (CDI; Kovacs, 1978), the Loneliness Scale (LS; Asher, Hymel, & Renshaw, 1984), and the Children's Negative Cognitive Error Questionnaire (CNCEQ; Leitenberg, Yost, & Carroll-Wilson, 1986). Ashley's responses on self-report measures of anxiety were consistent with descriptions obtained from interviews. Specifically, she reported high levels of state (score of 30) and trait (score of 45) anxiety on the STAIC. She also indicated that she had an extremely high number of intense fears (i.e., 30) on the FSSC-R. Her total FSSC-R score (169) was substantially higher than the mean (143) obtained for a normative sample. Examination of factor scores on this measure revealed that Ashley showed excessive fearfulness on two dimensions: (1) failure and criticism, and (2) minor injury and small animals.

In addition, Ashley described herself as having concurrent difficulties, including depression and social impairment. In particular, her score of 23 on the CDI was suggestive of significant depressive symptomatology. Furthermore, she reported feelings of loneliness and social dissatisfaction on the LS (score of 48). Finally, Ashley endorsed several types of negative cognitive errors (derived from Beck's cognitive theory of adult depression) on the CNCEQ, including catastrophizing, overgeneralizing, personalizing, and selective abstraction. She primarily reported use of negative cognitive errors in social situations, rather than in academic or athletic contexts.

Teacher perceptions of Ashley's behavior in the classroom were obtained using the Revised Behavior Problem Checklist (Quay & Peterson, 1983). Using this measure, the teacher indicated that Ashley demonstrated high levels of anxious–withdrawn behavior in the classroom setting, but that otherwise she did not display problematic classroom behavior. The teacher's evaluation of Ashley's social adjustment was also obtained using a rating scale assessing peer popularity and social status. Results from this teacher sociometric questionnaire revealed that the teacher perceived Ashley as socially neglected among her classmates. That is, she was described as neither well liked nor actively disliked among her peers.

SELECTION OF TREATMENT

Virtually no published reports have been presented in the literature concerning effective treatments for children or adolescents with overanxious disorder. Instead, interventions have been developed for *specific* fears and phobias in children and adolescents. On the other hand, treatment procedures have been implemented successfully to reduce adult forms of generalized anxiety. Owing to the absence of empirical evidence supporting the use of a specific intervention for overanxious disorder, a treatment package consisting of multiple components was modeled after adult treatment approaches for generalized anxiety. Similar therapeutic approaches have previously been used effectively to treat specific childhood fears and phobias.

The behavior therapy package incorporates the following treatment components: (1) relaxation techniques, (2) cognitive rehearsal and restructuring, and (3) social skills training. First, Ashley was trained in deep muscle relaxation, using a modified technique devised for children and adolescents. She also was asked to imagine a pleasant scene to facilitate relaxation. In terms of cognitive procedures, rehearsal of positive self-statements and substitution of adaptive cognitions for maladaptive thoughts were employed. Social skills training consisted of instructing Ashley in the use of assertive and initiation social skills.

COURSE OF TREATMENT

Ashley was seen individually on a weekly basis for a total of 25 sessions over the course of a 6-month period. Initially, she was trained in deep muscle relaxation. She learned a maximum of three muscle groups each session and practiced these skills twice daily at home. She also chose and imagined a pleasant scene (e.g., walking along the beach), which was used at the end of each relaxation session to enhance relaxation. Instruction in relaxation was completed after six treatment sessions. Owing to Ashley's initial reluctance to practice relaxation skills regularly, a reward (e.g., special outing with her father) was offered to her weekly for successful completion of daily exercises. According to the child's report, regular practice of relaxation exercises did not lead to reductions in feelings of tension, worrying, or other overanxious features.

While learning relaxation techniques, Ashley was asked to keep a daily diary at home of situations that induced anxiety and worrying. In her diary, she reported subjective anxiety and cognitions that preceded or accompanied each situation. Anxiety ratings were made on a scale ranging from 0 to 8 (0 = not at all, 8 = panicky). Records of cognitions were used to identify Ashley's beliefs that were contributing to her anxious states. Subsequently, Ashley was taught to rehearse positive self-statements that could substitute for maladaptive cognitions, such as "I can relax," "I know I am as good as the other kids," or "I studied hard and will just do the best I can."

In addition to the use of cognitive rehearsal, a cognitive restructuring procedure was implemented. First, a cognitive model of anxiety was described to the child; i.e., it was explained that her anxiety resulted from automatic, exaggerated thinking. Because of the child's age, it was necessary to draw diagrams and to repeat the rationale during several sessions to enable her to understand the concepts. Weekly sessions subsequently were focused on substituting more rational, logical thoughts for faulty thinking. The Socratic method of asking questions to lead Ashley to identify irrational thoughts and to replace them with more appropriate thoughts was used whenever possible. Homework assignments were also used to allow Ashley to practice the concepts and skills learned each week.

Several types of faulty thinking repeatedly were demonstrated by Ashley. These included the following:

Catastrophizing. Ashley consistently focused on the worst possible outcome of any situation in which a negative consequence was possible. She dwelled mainly on negative outcomes and exaggerated the probabilities of their occurring. An example of catastrophizing was that when Ashley had minor social difficulties with peers, she anticipated that these children would no longer want to be her friends. She then imagined that she would be left friendless and would be alone and miserable.

Selective Abstraction. Ashley commonly ruminated about unpleasant or negative events that took place each day and overlooked more positive, contradictory pieces of information. She primarily recalled a single negative occurrence and excluded other relevant positive events from her thinking. For instance, if a friend had not included her in a play activity during recess, Ashley would worry for hours about this oversight. She would not think about the many other times during the school day when her friend talked to her and made friendly overtures toward her.

Personalizing. Ashley tended to take personal responsibility for others' negative behavior toward her. For example, if she invited a friend to come over on the weekend and the friend said, "No. I have other plans this weekend," then Ashley would think, "She doesn't want to come over to my house." She would fail to consider that the friend might indeed have made previous plans. If a friend was less talkative than usual, Ashley would conclude that she had done something to make her friend angry at her, instead of considering that the friend might be tired or have her own personal reasons for being quiet.

Cognitive behavior therapy aimed at remediating these faulty ways of perceiving events helped Ashley (1) to consider all possible outcomes and realistically to estimate the probability of each outcome, (2) to focus on positive experiences, and (3) to consider numerous alternative explanations for others' behavior that did not contain a personal element. It was necessary to review these concepts multiple times (a minimum of three sessions each) before Ashley was able to adopt these strategies in an independent manner outside of therapy sessions. Ashley was asked to record three positive events each day to facilitate changes in her thinking.

A final cognitive strategy was utilized, in which Ashley was instructed in the use of distraction (e.g., reading a book) and thought stopping to force herself to discontinue ruminating at bedtime. These techniques were recommended for use at bedtime because worries occurred at a high rate at this time and Ashley was too tired to challenge her automatic negative cognitions.

Although progress in this cognitive phase of treatment initially was slow, Ashley eventually was successful in learning and implementing more effective cognitive strategies. Once she grasped the notion that her thinking was in fact interfering with her adjustment (not until the sixth cognitive therapy session), Ashley easily was able to identify maladaptive thoughts and to replace them with more rational cognitions. This component of therapy appeared to be the most meaningful in terms of reducing overanxious features, including excessive future and past worries, overconcern about competence, self-consciousness, and feelings of tension.

The following is an excerpt from the 15th therapy session, at which time Ashley was showing recognition of maladaptive cognitions:

ASHLEY: Today, Lisa walked with her sister to recess instead of with me.

THERAPIST: How did you feel when she did that?

ASHLEY: Well, I felt okay because I thought maybe she needed to talk to her sister about something. She is her sister and it's okay for Lisa to talk to her, too.

THERAPIST: That's right. And did Lisa talk to you at any other times during the day?

ASHLEY: Yes. We played together at recess. And I stayed after school to talk to her when she waited for her mother to pick her up.

THERAPIST: So you see, even though Lisa talked with her sister instead of you just before recess, she also spent time with you today. There were many times when she wanted to be with you.

In the final phase of therapy, social skills training was used to increase assertiveness and initiations of peer interactions. Role-play practice sessions involved providing a rationale for each skill, modeling of skills, practice of skills by Ashley, and feedback and praise for successive approximations. Ashley was taught to stand up for her rights, to express opinions that might differ from those of others, and to refuse unreasonable demands placed on her. Practice of these social behaviors during therapy sessions resulted in Ashley's becoming significantly more assertive with peers and family members. Daily records of assertiveness and opinions that Ashley revealed to others reflected these gains. During therapy sessions, Ashley also practiced inviting others to join her in recess, inviting friends to her home, and calling friends on the telephone, all of which were absent prior to the onset of therapy. Ashley successfully generalized these initiation skills to her home and school environments.

Ashley showed evidence of having acquired assertive skills and reduced concern about others' perceptions of her during the 21st treatment session. At that time, she provided the following description of her behavior toward a classroom bully that week:

ASHLEY: Well, I did it! I stood up to Robin this week in school. I told her what I thought of her.

THERAPIST: What did you do?

ASHLEY: Well, in front of the whole class, I told her to stop whispering to her friends about me. I told her that I didn't like it that she always said mean things about other people.

THERAPIST: Wow! You really did it, Ashley. You told her how you really felt after all this time. And how did she react?

ASHLEY: The whole class clapped when I said that and she just walked away. But, later she tried to be my friend. But I didn't act friendly back. She hasn't been nice all year, so I don't want to be her friend now.

THERAPIST: The important thing is that you were able to stand up for yourself. How do you feel about having done this?

ASHLEY: (smiling) I feel good.

TERMINATION

Following treatment, assessment measures again were administered to evaluate treatment gains. In particular, the parents and child were interviewed using the K-SADS to assess directly the presence of overanxious symptomatology. In addition, Ashley completed all self-report measures filled out prior to treatment, i.e., the STAIC, FSSC-R, CDI, LS, and CNCEQ. Finally, Ashley and her parents rated the child's overall progress in therapy on a 7-point Likert scale ranging from "very much worse" to "completely well."

Information obtained from the K-SADS interviews revealed that Ashley no longer met DSM-III-R criteria for a diagnosis of overanxious disorder. All symptoms had reduced in frequency and severity to subclinical levels, with the exception of mildly significant self-consciousness. Ashley also reported lower state (score of 10) and trait (33) anxiety on the STAIC.

Substantial reductions in the number and intensity of fears were found on the FSSC-R, such that her number of intense fears decreased from 30 at pretreatment to 18 at posttreatment, and her total FSSC-R score changed from 169 to 152 over the course of treatment. Of particular interest, Ashley's responses on the CNCEQ revealed that her frequency of negative cognitive errors (i.e., catastrophizing, overgeneralizing, personalizing, and selective abstraction) had declined significantly, so that her scores on each subscale had reduced to levels comparable to a normative sample of children with low evaluation anxiety. Dramatic improvement in depressive symptomatology also was evident, with Ashley's CDI score decreasing from 23 at pretreatment to a score of 5 following treatment. Ashley reported that she was less lonely as well following therapy. Finally, both Ashley and her parents provided global progress ratings indicating that she was "much better" at termination of therapy.

FOLLOW-UP

Ashley and her parents were contacted by the therapist 3 months following termination of therapy to assess maintenance of treatment gains. The family reported that Ashley continued to exhibit low rates of worrying, anxiety, and depression. Friendships also were reported to be satisfactory. Thus, no problems with overanxious disorder were evident, and progress in treatment had been sustained during the follow-up period.

OVERALL EVALUATION

Ashley is an 11-year-old girl who showed significant difficulties with overanxious disorder that had impaired her social adjustment and had been associated with depressive symptomatology. Her presentation of overanxious features and concurrent pathology is fairly representative of children diagnosed with overanxious disorder. A multicomponent treatment approach consisting of relaxation training, cognitive behavior therapy, and instruction in social skills resulted in gradual improvement in cognitive strategies, anxiety, depression, and peer relationships. Clinically significant gains were apparent immediately following treatment and were maintained at follow-up.

Thus, this multicomponent treatment approach was successful in reducing overanxious symptoms to subclinical levels. Unfortunately, it is not possible from this case description to determine which specific method(s) were effective in producing these positive changes. However, it is useful to have identified a treatment package that may indeed help to modify overanxious disorder features.

REFERENCES

American Psychiatric Association. (1987). *Diagnostic and statistical manual of mental disorders* (3rd ed., rev.). Washington, DC: Author.

Asher, S. R., Hymel, S., & Renshaw, P. D. (1984). Loneliness in children. *Child Development, 55*, 1456–1464.

Kovacs, M. (1978). *Children's Depression Inventory (CDI)*. Unpublished manuscript, University of Pittsburgh School of Medicine.

Last, C. G., Hersen, M., Kazdin, A. E., Finkelstein, R., & Strauss, C. C. (1987). Comparison of DSM-III separation anxiety and overanxious disorders: Demographic characteristics and patterns of comorbidity. *Journal of the American Academy of Child Psychiatry, 26*, 527–531.

Leitenberg, H., Yost, L. W., & Carroll-Wilson, M. (1986). Negative cognitive errors in children: Questionnaire development, normative data, and comparisons between children with and without self-reported symptoms of depression, low self-esteem, and evaluation anxiety. *Journal of Consulting and Clinical Psychology, 54*, 528–536.

Ollendick, T. H. (1983). Reliability and validity of the Revised Fear Survey Schedule for Children (FSSC-R). *Behaviour Research and Therapy, 21*, 685–692.

Puig-Antich, J., Orvaschel, H., Tabrizi, R. N., & Chambers, W. J. (1978). *Schedule for affective disorders and schizophrenia for school-age children.* New York: New York State Psychiatric Institute.

Quay, H. C., & Peterson, D. R. (1983). *Interim manual for the Revised Behavior Problem Checklist.* Coral Gables, FL: University of Miami.

Spielberger, C. D. (1973). *Manual for the Stait-Trait Inventory for Children.* Palo Alto: Consulting Psychologists Press.

Strauss, C. C., Lease, C. A., Last, C. G., & Francis, G. (in press). Overanxious disorder: An examination of developmental differences. *Journal of Abnormal Child Psychology.*

CHAPTER 4

Social Withdrawal

GRETA FRANCIS and THOMAS H. OLLENDICK

DESCRIPTION OF THE DISORDER

Given the long-term relationship between childhood social functioning and adult adjustment, attainment of social competency has been viewed as critical to normal child development. Excessive social withdrawal during childhood can be viewed as one type of social incompetence; social aggression can be viewed as another. Estimates of the prevalence of social withdrawal in children vary but seem to range from a low of 3% to a high of 38% (e.g., Shepherd, Oppenheim, & Mitchell, 1971). A recent large-scale prospective study of socially withdrawn behavior in children found social withdrawal, when identified at the fourth- or seventh-grade level, to be relatively stable (i.e., .61 to .65 for boys, .42 to .55 for girls) across a 5-year period (Moskowitz, Schwartzman, & Ledigham, 1985). Moreover, the stability of social withdrawal was reported to be comparable to that of social aggression in this sample.

Frequently, children with socially withdrawn behavior are not brought to the attention of mental health professionals. These children seldom are disruptive at school or at home and, as such, their withdrawn behavior may not be apparent immediately to parents and teachers. Therefore, identification of social withdrawal often is secondary to the assessment of other internalizing behavior problems in clinic-referred children.

Empirical evidence suggests that socially withdrawn children often

GRETA FRANCIS • Western Psychiatric Institute and Clinic, University of Pittsburgh School of Medicine, 3811 O'Hara Street, Pittsburgh, Pennsylvania 15213.   THOMAS H. OLLENDICK • Department of Psychology, Virginia Polytechnic Institute and State University, Blacksburg, Virginia 24061.

experience high levels of internalizing behavior problems. Strauss, Forehand, Smith, and Frame (1986) reported that socially withdrawn children frequently have concurrent problems with anxiety and depression.

Typically, there are a number of defining features of social withdrawal in children. The cardinal feature of social withdrawal is a low rate of peer interaction. The socially withdrawn child typically spends much of his/her time engaged in solitary play rather than interactive play with peers. Often, both the quantity and quality of peer interaction are impaired. The socially withdrawn child may not make appropriate and/or effective attempts to initiate interaction with peers. Further, he/she may engage in fewer prosocial behaviors, such as smiling, sharing, and conversing with peers. Other socially withdrawn children may emit these behaviors, but do so at such a low rate that they are equally problematic.

Often, behaviorally withdrawn children also are sociometrically withdrawn or "neglected." Sociometrically neglected children are characterized by low rates of peer acceptance and peer rejection as measured by peer sociometric instruments. In other words, these children are ignored by their peers. Connolly (1983), in her review of the sociometric literature, described sociometrically neglected children as shy children who engage in high rates of solitary play and make few social approaches toward peers.

CASE IDENTIFICATION

Two socially withdrawn children who were identified as part of a clinical research study of group social skills training for social incompetence will be described (Ollendick, 1982). Each child was enrolled in fourth grade in a small, rural, public elementary school. Both children were from the same classroom and were identified on the basis of a teacher nomination procedure. Their teacher identified them using the following definition of social withdrawal: "This child is shy and prefers to be alone most of the time. This child seldom speaks up for him/herself. If this child becomes the center of attention, he/she appears uncomfortable. This child avoids assuming any type of leadership and may appear sad, fearful, and easy to offend."

PRESENTING COMPLAINT

The fourth-grade teacher identified Terri and Susan as being more withdrawn and isolated than their peers. Each child's parents were contacted and agreed that their child was "shy" and in need of help to improve their peer relationships.

Terri was a tall, dark-haired, white female who lived with her parents and two siblings. Susan was a small, blond, white female who was an only child and lived with her parents. The socioeconomic status of both children was lower middle class. Both sets of parents reported that their child was shy, seemed to be nervous about interacting with peers, and had few friends.

Terri appeared to be disliked by her peers, while Susan appeared to be ignored by them. For example, peers often taunted and teased Terri; in contrast, they described Susan as "the shy one" and did not approach her. Both children spent little time engaged in peer interaction and appeared to spend most of their free time either engaged in solitary activity or *observing* the play of other children. Terri did participate in classroom discussions and initiate interactions with peers; however, peers typically responded negatively to these attempts. In contrast, Susan did not participate in classroom discussions or initiate interactions with peers. Typically, Susan's behavior was so quiet and shy that she was overlooked by her peers both in and out of the classroom.

HISTORY

Both Terri and Susan had been enrolled at the same school since kindergarten. As noted earlier, the school was small and there was only one classroom per grade level. Both children's problems with social withdrawal were described as long-standing.

ASSESSMENT

An extensive assessment was conducted for both children. Self-report measures of anxiety, fear, and depression were administered. Peer sociometric measures (rating and nomination) also were obtained in order to assess popularity. In addition, the teacher and parents provided ratings of social isolation and withdrawal. Finally, behavioral observations of peer interaction and a behavioral role-play test were obtained.

Terri's self-reported fear, anxiety, and depression were minimal. In contrast, her peer sociometric rating was very low, suggesting that she was not at all liked by peers; further, no peers nominated Terri as a desired friend. Her teacher rated her behavior as moody and withdrawn; however, parent ratings of social withdrawal were not elevated. Behavioral observations of peer interaction revealed that Terri interacted with peers at a rate much lower than that of her popular classmates. Ratings of Terri's performance on a social skills role-play test indicated that her eye contact was poor, latency to respond was long, and her speech was quite dysfluent. In addition, Terri's responses suggested that she was passive and unassertive.

Susan reported higher than normal levels of anxiety and fear. She did not report significant depressive symptoms, however. Susan's peer sociometric ratings were average, and she was nominated by a few peers as being one of their desired friends. Despite these sociometric endorsements, behavioral observations of peer interaction revealed that Susan spent virtually no time interacting with peers. There clearly was a discrepancy between peers' ratings of Susan's likability and Susan's actual behavior in peer social situations. Both Susan's teacher and her parents reported that she was withdrawn and isolative. Her performance on a social skills role-play test indicated that her eye contact was poor, latency to respond was long, and verbal responses were very short. Susan's responses suggested that she was passive and unassertive. For example, if unreasonable requests were made of her, she typically complied.

SELECTION OF TREATMENT

Since Susan and Terri exhibited deficits in both the quantity and the quality of their peer interactions, involvement in a behavioral social skills training program appeared to be warranted.

COURSE OF TREATMENT

Both children participated in a 12-week group social skills program. The group consisted of four girls from the same classroom. Terri and Susan were in a group with two other girls: one girl identified as socially disruptive/aggressive and another girl identified as socially competent/popular. This group met once per week for 1 hour during the school day. The first author served as the group therapist.

The social skills procedures used in the group were based on principles of social learning theory. As such, instruction, modeling, feedback, practice, and reinforcement were integral parts of each group session. During each session the therapist provided instruction regarding specific social skills so as to include both *information* about the nature of the skill and how to *perform* the appropriate behavior. Moreover, the therapist modeled both appropriate and inappropriate execution of the behaviors and sought feedback from the group. Remediation always followed modeling of inappropriate behaviors so as to point out clearly the differences between appropriate and inappropriate execution. Since the group included a child who was identified as socially competent, this child often served as a model of the appropriate execution of the skill behavior. The majority of each session was spent with children practicing the skills. Each child was given the opportunity to role-play the appropriate behaviors; feedback was provided by the therapist and by group members throughout the session.

The format of the sessions was the same throughout. Each session began with a review of homework that had been assigned the preceding week. A sticker chart was used to monitor homework completion. Following this, social skills training of a particular set of behaviors was conducted. At the end of each session two tasks were accomplished. Homework was assigned and relaxation exercises were conducted. Each week relaxation exercises for one muscle group were presented. By completion of the 12 weeks, the children had learned progressive muscle relaxation.

Social skills training covered a number of different content areas, which have been identified as components of socially competent behavior in children of this age. Content areas included nonverbal behaviors, conversation skills, affect recognition, role-taking, group entry behavior, and assertion skills. Throughout the 12 sessions, prosocial skills, such as sharing and cooperation, were emphasized.

Initial sessions focused on nonverbal components of conversations, including eye contact, voice tone and volume, response latency and duration, posture, and facial expression. These skills provided the basis upon which other skills were built and were used throughout the 12 sessions. In addition, verbal components of conversation-making were covered by delineating four stages of a conversation: greeting, small talk, main topic, and closing. The skills required to begin, perpetuate, and end conversations were practiced using role-play with puppets and then with peers.

Affect recognition and affect expression also were included as a content area. Children were taught how to identify affect using both verbal and nonverbal cues. Children learned to identify various emotions using cues from facial expression, vocal expression, verbal content, and posture. In addition, they practiced expressing a variety of emotions, such as happiness, sadness, embarrassment, shyness, anger, boredom, disgust, and excitement. The relationship between one's emotional reaction and the situation in which one finds oneself was highlighted.

Group entry behavior served as another content area. Children were instructed to use their affect recognition skills to determine whom to approach when asking to join a group of peers. For example, the advantages of asking a peer who looked happy and friendly as opposed to asking a peer who appeared very angry were discussed. Emphasis was placed on maximizing the success of group entry by using appropriate behaviors. Children practiced approaching groups, determining the "frame of reference" (i.e., what the children were doing), choosing a friendly peer to ask, and finally asking if they could join.

Role-taking skills also were covered. Children discussed and practiced "walking in someone else's shoes." Children identified the likely emotions associated with different characters and situations using stories and role-play. For example, one session was devoted to having the group members act out a short play. Periodically during the play they would be required to switch roles and describe what their new character knew, how their new character felt, and how their new character would behave.

A significant amount of time was spent on assertion training. Both positive and negative assertion skills were included. Negative assertion skills include those required to stand up for one's rights and deny unreasonable requests. Both verbal and nonverbal skills were emphasized. For example, children practiced remaining calm, speaking in a firm tone of voice, maintaining eye contact, and saying "no" when faced with unreasonable requests. In contrast, positive assertion skills are those related to giving or receiving compliments, asking for help, and initiating interactions.

The ninth group treatment session, which was devoted to positive assertion, will be described in detail. The purpose of this session was to *introduce* positive assertion skills. Following review and posting of successful homework completion, the therapist introduced positive assertion as the topic for the session. Only those segments of the session pertaining to Terri and Susan are presented.

THERAPIST: Today we are going to talk about something a little bit different. There are times when we want to give someone a compliment or when someone gives us a compliment. Sometimes we want to ask a friend to play with us or ask a classmate for help with our schoolwork. Can anyone think of a time when these things have happened to you? Were these situations easy or hard?

TERRI: Um, I wanted to ask Cheryl to play—on the, um, swings with me yesterday—I asked her, but, ah, she didn't answer me.

THERAPIST: Was it hard or easy to ask?

TERRI: Well—it was, um, hard because I kept—st—stuttering.

THERAPIST: A lot of people feel pretty nervous and find it hard to ask. Susan, have you ever asked someone in the class to help you?

SUSAN: No, but once Jason asked me to help him with a math problem.

THERAPIST: What did you do?

SUSAN: I helped him. . . . Sometimes I tell Mrs. Smith that I like her dress.

THERAPIST: I bet she feels really happy when you give her a compliment. Sometimes it is pretty hard to ask other kids for help or ask other kids to play with you or give other kids a compliment. Today we are going to practice doing those things so they will be easier for you. If you were going to ask a kid for help with a math problem, what would be the best way to look?

SUSAN: Happy—with a smile on your face.

THERAPIST: Terri, how would you want your voice to sound?

TERRI: Loud enough—and happy.

SUSAN: You'd also want to look at the person.

THERAPIST: That's right. You have come up with lots of important things to remember. Now let's pretend that I'm going to ask for help from one of you. Everyone watch and listen carefully, and when I'm done, tell me what you think. Terri, please read the first situation, and Susan can be the other child.

TERRI: Your teacher says that you can work with one other child during math class. You would like to work with your neighbor. You neighbor says—

SUSAN: Do you have a partner?

THERAPIST: (whining voice, good eye contact, scowling face) Nobody wants to work with me. It is not fair!—(pause)—Well, how was that?

TERRI: You looked at Susan—um—but you didn't really ask her. It would have been better to smile—and—um—just ask her if she would be your math partner.

THERAPIST: Anything else that I could have done better?

SUSAN: Yes, your voice didn't sound happy.

THERAPIST: You are right. Susan probably wouldn't want to be my math partner when I act that way. Let me try a different way. Ready? This time, Terri can be the neighbor.

TERRI: Do you have a partner?

THERAPIST: (smiles but says nothing, looks at the ground)—(pause)—What did you think of that one?

SUSAN: You looked pretty shy. There was a nice look on your face.

TERRI: You ignored me when I asked if you had a partner.

THERAPIST: What did you think when I did that?

TERRI: I thought that you didn't want me to talk to you.

THERAPIST: What else did you notice?

SUSAN: You didn't look at Terri.

THERAPIST: Well, these are all good points. Let me try again and see if I can do a better job. I'll try and remember all the things you've said. Terri, go ahead and be my neighbor again.

TERRI: Do you have a partner?

THERAPIST: (smiling, pleasant tone of voice, good eye contact) Not yet. Would you like to work together?

TERRI: (smiles) OK.

THERAPIST: What about that?

SUSAN: That was better.

THERAPIST: What exactly did I do better?

SUSAN: Well, you looked at Terri and you sounded nice and happy.

TERRI: You, ah, asked me to—work with you. Um, that made me think that you li— liked me.

THERAPIST: Yes, I think I did a much better job that time. Looking and sounding happy sure made a big difference—and, like Terri said, it made her feel good because I asked her.

Following the instruction and therapist modeling, the other two group members practiced another scene. The socially competent child served as a child model, while the aggressive child was her role-play partner. Again, Terri and Susan were encouraged to give specific feedback to the other group members. Next, Terri and Susan were chosen as role-play partners.

THERAPIST: OK, this time I'd like Susan to act out a scene and Terri to be her partner. Ready? Susan, pretend that you are painting a picture in art class and Terri says—

TERRI: That really looks nice. It must have taken a lot of work.

SUSAN: (smiles, looks down, voice very soft) Thanks.

TERRI: You're welcome.

THERAPIST: Terri, how did Susan do?

TERRI: She had a nice smile on her face and she thanked me, but it was kind of hard to hear her.

SUSAN: It was hard for me to look at her.

THERAPIST: Yes, I noticed that, too. You did do a nice job thanking Terri. Can you think of anything else you might say?

SUSAN: Well, I could say that her picture is nice—or tell her how long I've been working.

THERAPIST: Those are great ideas. Go ahead and try this scene again. This time, try real hard to look at Terri, speak more loudly, and talk a little bit more. Ready?

TERRI: That really looks nice. It must have taken a lot of work.

SUSAN: (good eye contact, smiling, voice slightly louder) Thanks. Your picture looks nice, too.

TERRI: Thanks.

THERAPIST: Wow, Susan, that was very good! You did a very nice job taking our suggestions. You were easy to hear and looked and sounded friendly and happy. This time we'll have Terri be the actor and Susan can be her partner. Terri, pretend you were absent from school yesterday and need to find out if there was any spelling homework so you can do it tonight. After school you see Susan waiting for the bus. Ready? Go ahead.

TERRI: (good eye contact, no smile, voice loud enough) Susan?—Um—do you—do you know, um, what the sp—spelling homework is?

SUSAN: Yes, we have to finish page twelve.

TERRI: Oh.

THERAPIST: Susan, what did you think of this one?

SUSAN: Terri looked me right in the eye and I could hear her.

THERAPIST: That's right, and she asked you about the homework. Terri did use a lot of
"ums" so it took kind of a long time to ask the question. Terri, try that scene again.
This time take a deep breath before you start and remember to smile when you look
at Susan. Ready?

TERRI: (good eye contact, brief smile, voice loud enough) Susan, um, do you know what
our spelling—homework was?

SUSAN: Yes, we need to finish page twelve.

TERRI: Thanks.

THERAPIST: Very nice job, Terri. What did you think, Susan?

SUSAN: It was good how she said "thanks" at the end.

THERAPIST: It sure was. Terri, you hardly used any "ums" at all that time and that smile
looked friendly.

The session continued in this manner. Each child had the opportunity
to role-play with the other group members and with the therapist. As can
be seen, the majority of the session was devoted to having the children
practice positive assertion skills.

At the end of the session, the children completed the relaxation exercise. The following homework was assigned: "Ask a classmate to play
with you *or* to help you with your schoolwork. Who did you ask? What
did you say? What did the other person say and do?"

TERMINATION

The 12th session was spent discussing termination of the group. The
therapist reinforced attendance, and the children were given the stickers
that they had earned over the 12 weeks. The group discussed briefly all
the content areas, and the therapist praised their efforts and improvement.
Children were encouraged to practice their new skills in order to maintain
their gains. Emphasis was placed on examples of situations in which their
skills could be used. For example, children were instructed to use conversation skills when meeting new kids or to use positive assertion skills
to make friends. Children were told that they would be participating in
booster groups during the next school year. These booster groups would
meet six times over the course of the next school year.

Finally, the group members participated in a social skills game aimed
at assessing their skills. The object was to move around a game board by
correctly answering questions and appropriately responding during role-
play situations.

Both Terri and Susan performed well during the social skills game.
Terri was able to respond to questions more quickly and clearly. She was
able to behave assertively when faced with challenging situations. Sim-

ilarly, Susan was able to speak less quietly and use good eye contact. She, too, was able to behave in a more socially competent manner. Both children easily answered questions regarding the content of the treatment sessions.

FOLLOW-UP

A posttreatment assessment was conducted immediately following completion of the 12 treatment sessions. Both children evidenced improvement on a number of assessment measures. Terri showed increased assertion, decreased teacher-rated moodiness, increased positive peer interaction, decreased solitary play, a slight increase in sociometric rating, and a significant increase in sociometric nominations. Similarly, Susan showed increased assertion, increased positive peer interaction, decreased solitary play, and a slight increase in both sociometric rating and nominations.

Both children participated in booster treatment sessions during the following academic year. As such, they were involved in six booster sessions over the course of fifth grade. The purpose of these sessions was to provide an opportunity for the children to practice their skills and to encourage generalization and maintenance of treatment gains. Both Terri and Susan recalled and were able to use their social skills with ease during the booster sessions. In addition, a considerable amount of time was spent identifying "real-life" situations in which to practice their skills (e.g., how to make new friends when entering the middle school, how to deal with problem situations in their fifth-grade classroom).

OVERALL EVALUATION

This chapter presented a behavioral, group, social skills training procedure for treating childhood social withdrawal. The treatment of two socially withdrawn fourth-grade children was described. In general, the social skills training procedure was successful in helping the children become more assertive, less behaviorally withdrawn, and better accepted by their peers.

REFERENCES

Connolly, J. A. (1983). A review of sociometric procedures in the assessment of social competency in children. *Applied Research in Mental Retardation, 4*, 315–327.

Moskowitz, D. S., Schwartzman, A. E., & Ledingham, J. E. (1985). Stability and change in aggression and withdrawal in middle childhood and early adolescence. *Journal of Abnormal Psychology, 94*, 30–41.

Ollendick, T. H. (1982). *The social competency project.* Unpublished manuscript, Virginia Polytechnic Institute and State University.

Shepherd, M., Oppenheim, B., & Mitchell, S. (1971). *Childhood behavior and mental health.* New York: Grune and Stratton.

Strauss, C. C., Forehand, R., Smith, K., & Frame, C. L. (1986). The association between social withdrawal and internalizing problems of children. *Journal of Abnormal Child Psychology, 14*, 525–535.

CHAPTER 5

Simple Phobia

JAMES H. JOHNSON and F. DUDLEY McGLYNN

DESCRIPTION OF THE DISORDER

Nearly half of children 6 to 12 years of age display multiple fears of sufficient severity to prompt comment by their mothers. Fears of the dark, of strangers, and of animals are found frequently among young children, as are fears of separation, bodily injury, and supernatural beings (e.g., ghosts, monsters). Many of these fears are age- or stage-specific, relatively mild in severity, and transient in nature. As such they can be viewed as benign developmental phenomena. Some childhood fears, on the other hand, are neither age-related nor mild in severity, and among these some pose continuing adaptive hazards. These fears can be viewed as simple phobias provided that they fit DSM-III criteria and that they do not fall under some other diagnostic category (e.g., overanxious reaction of childhood, separation anxiety disorder).

Simple phobia appears only in the adult section of DSM-III. It subsumes that group of anxiety disorders characterized by "a persistent irrational fear of, and compelling desire to avoid an object or situation." Various qualifications also are provided. As it is stated, the DSM-III narrative will not suffice to guide the psychological treatment of phobic children (or, for that matter, phobic adults).

The behavior therapy literature does provide conceptual guidance for the treatment of phobic children. Delprato and McGlynn (1984) described a "multifaceted framework for anxiety disorders" that distills contem-

JAMES H. JOHNSON and F. DUDLEY McGLYNN • Department of Clinical and Health Psychology, J. Hillis Miller Health Center, University of Florida, Box J-165, Gainesville, Florida 32610.

porary behavioral thinking. The framework incorporates the well-known three-systems view of fear in which physiological behavior, overt motor behavior, and private (e.g., cognitive) behavior are substantially independent response classes. It proposes that fear behaviors within any of these response classes can be acquired by at least four ontogenetic processes—that is by aversive respondent conditioning, by operant contingencies, by vicarious experiences, and by other means of information transmission. It suggests also that maintenance of fear behavior is similarly organized. The principal implication of the "multifaceted framework" is that simple phobias involve idiosyncratically patterned physiological, and/or behavioral, and/or private fear behaviors with partially independent ontogenies. This implication does not mean that adequate clinical work must always involve multifaceted assessment and treatment. It does mean that clinicians need to be mindful of various potential complexities and prepared to try successive interventions as the need arises.

In the sections to follow we describe how "simple phobia" was displayed by one child and how behavioral approaches to assessment and treatment were employed in overcoming the problem.

CASE IDENTIFICATION

Jenny was an attractive 6-year-old white female from a middle-class family. At the time of the initial evaluation she had just entered the first grade. An only child, she lived with her natural parents, who were both high school graduates and were employed full time. While Jenny had never received an intellectual evaluation, a recent school readiness testing suggested that her abilities were average for her age.

PRESENTING COMPLAINTS

Jenny was referred to the clinic by her mother, who voiced concern about Jenny's fear of balloons. The mother noted that, when possible, Jenny avoided situations in which balloons were present. She noted also that Jenny became tearful and obviously distressed when she was unavoidably in the presence of balloons. The mother was embarrassed about bringing her daughter to the clinic for a seemingly trivial problem. However, she indicated that it posed enduring problems for her daughter and the family.

Jenny's mother cited several incidents to illustrate the seriousness of the phobia. On one occasion Jenny was unwilling to enter a toy store in the local mall because there was a large balloon display located near the entrance. On another occasion Jenny had to leave an otherwise entertaining parade because of the large numbers of balloons that were present. On still another occasion Jenny refused to enter her school classroom because her classmates were involved in artistic play using papier-maché and inflated balloons. The mother related one incident that occurred just prior to seeking help where, after a wedding ceremony, Jenny had panicked at the sight of a number of festive balloons that had been placed inside the bride and groom's car. Finally, the mother stated that Jenny had recently been having nightmares about balloons. Given the apparent magnitude of fear responses, the adaptive impositions they represented, and the specific nature of the fear-controlling stimulus, the balloon fear was viewed as a simple phobia during childhood. This view, in turn, prompted a classical behavior therapy approach to dealing with the problem (McGlynn & Cornell, 1985).

HISTORY

Jenny's developmental history was unremarkable. She was the product of a normal pregnancy and was said to have developed quite normally and to have met specific milestones within the normal age ranges. There was no evidence of early illness or injury, and the mother reported nothing to suggest anomalous conduct of noteworthy proportions apart from her fear of balloons. The mother did, however, describe Jenny as having been a rather sensitive girl who sometimes tended to overreact to a range of situations.

The mother reported that since the age of 2 Jenny had responded fearfully to diverse inflatable toys. Seemingly these fears had gradually been narrowed to balloons. The mother was unable to recall any aversive encounters with balloons or with other inflatable toys. She did note that the early balloon phobia was paralleled roughly by fearfulness in response to television commercials characterized by loud music and bright lights. She did note also that once, recently, Jenny had appeared afraid of a noisy dragon that appeared on a television game show. Finally, the mother reported that Jenny was somewhat fearful of any type of violence on television, including cartoon violence. None of these fears, however, posed adaptive hazards comparable to those imposed by her fear of balloons.

The mother reported that neither she nor her husband had gone to great lengths to avoid situations where balloons were present, although sometimes in those settings they and other relatives and friends tended to shield Jenny from the balloons. She reported also a history of crude and traumatic parental attempts to treat the fear by direct exposure.

ASSESSMENT

Assessment consisted of a detailed interview with the mother, completion by the mother of the Quay-Peterson Behavior Problem Checklist (see Quay, 1977), an interview with Jenny, and observational assessment of Jenny's fear behaviors. Assessment was directed toward pinpointing the nature and severity of the phobic behavior, the stimulus and/or context variables regulating fear intensity, and any other problem behaviors that might exist.

As noted above, the parental interview suggested that Jenny's fear took the form of motoric agitation and crying in the presence of balloons, along with attempted escape behaviors. Parent reports suggested also that Jenny's fear intensity was regulated importantly by the amount of air the balloons contained and by the extent to which she controlled the inflation parameter. Jenny was described as not fearful of deflated balloons and as very fearful of fully inflated balloons. She was described as most fearful when someone else was blowing up a balloon. Jenny's fear was reportedly unrelated to the colors, sizes, or numbers of balloons, or to the presence of others in settings where inflated balloons were confronted. The mother's responses to the Behavior Problem Checklist were in accord with the interview report that fear of balloons was the only problem of significance.

During the initial appointment, a preliminary attempt was made to substantiate parental report by presenting Jenny with a fairly large transparent plastic bag. She displayed no evidence of fear in response to the empty bag. When asked to blow up the bag, she was able to inflate it approximately three-fourths full and to watch as the top of the bag was tied. Only a moderate amount of fear was shown at this point. The interviewer then squeezed the bag causing it to appear filled to capacity. Jenny in response said she was afraid it would pop and fearfully sought to remove herself from the room. It is of interest to note that Jenny was able to squeeze the bag herself to almost the same extent without appearing so fearful.

In order to assess Jenny's fearfulness more adequately, she was administered a Behavioral Avoidance Test (BAT) during the next visit. The BAT took place in a large room that had 11 steps marked on the floor at 1-foot intervals. At the far end of the room was a "bouquet" made up of

4 large round balloons and 6 long thin balloons. The 10 balloons were attached and all were fully inflated.

Although hesitant, Jenny entered the room and moved slowly to the final step, standing directly in front of the balloons. When she was prompted to touch the balloons, she displayed motoric agitation and said she did not want to, adding that her mother did not allow her to touch balloons. When the therapist picked up the balloons and prompted Jenny to touch them, she touched one reluctantly, said she had to return to her waiting mother, and started to leave the room. These behaviors were ignored and Jenny was prompted to handle one of the balloons. She was able to do this, but when asked if she could pop a balloon she became extremely fearful, turned to leave the room, and again asked to go to her mother. She said that she did not want any of the balloons to pop, adding, "I might cry if they pop." When given the opportunity, Jenny requested that the therapist remove the bouquet of balloons from the room.

The BAT just described was followed by an evaluation of Jenny's behavior vis-à-vis noninflated balloons. Here the therapist took several balloons out of his pocket and gave one to Jenny. When she was prompted to blow up her balloon, she put only one exhalation into it. When the therapist said he was going to blow up his balloon, Jenny became visibly agitated and said, "My brains don't want anyone to blow up balloons. My mommy won't like it if I see anyone blow balloons up." She went on to say, "My mom said that if I see someone blow it up I'll be afraid." Her behavior bordered on panic when the therapist began to put more than one breath of air into his balloon. When further pressed to try and blow up her own balloon, Jenny said she did not want to blow it up. She refused to put more than one breath of air into it and said she was afraid it would pop. She then asked to leave and go back to her mother. Finally, she asked the therapist to put the uninflated balloons back into his pocket and to not take them out again. At this point the assessment session was terminated.

Despite the rather informal nature of the behavioral evaluation, the results were viewed as corroborating the mother's report that Jenny's fear of balloons was indeed sufficient to warrant intervention.

SELECTION OF TREATMENT

Several approaches to the treatment of childhood phobias are described in the clinical child literature. As with adults, numerous case reports describe the effectiveness of systematic desensitization, although well-controlled experimental studies documenting the value of this technique with younger age groups are rare. Brief consideration was given to the use of orthodox systematic desensitization here. That approach was rejected, however, because we did not acquire the type of physiological assessment data that are ideal to recommend desensitization and because imaginal paradigms are largely superfluous when it is convenient to use actual phobic stimuli.

Variations on the reciprocal inhibition concept such as emotive imagery have also been employed with phobic children, particularly in those situations where training in relaxation has been difficult. While case studies support the value of emotive imagery, there have been no controlled studies of the approach. Similarly, there are retrospective case reports on the use of implosive therapy and flooding in treating childhood phobias. Despite the purported usefulness of these and other specific approaches, the treatments receiving the greatest experiment support, in general, are those that provide opportunities for long durations of nonanxious exposure to actual feared stimuli.

During the past two decades a great deal of evidence has accumulated showing that if phobic children observe models interact with phobic stimuli in a consistently or progressively fearless manner, then their anxiety-related behaviors weaken. Some authorities say the fear reduction mirrors vicarious fear extinction. Others argue that fear reduction is mediated by changed performance-outcome and self-efficacy expectations. Additional explanatory models are available. An even more impressive body of evidence shows that when phobic children themselves are induced to interact fearlessly with phobic objects, their anxiety-related behaviors are weakened. Again, this effect can be conceptualized in competing ways (e.g., S-R vs. cognitive theories). Evidence shows also that a set of procedures known as "graduated participant modeling" (Bandura, 1976) is the preferred way to bring about fearless interactions. In this approach, the phobic individual is first provided the opportunity to observe a live model displaying progressively fearless interactions with the phobic object. Then, at each step in the modeling script, the phobic subject is encouraged to imitate the approach behaviors that have just been modeled and is praised for achieving rough topographical equivalence. Some data suggest that using a model similar to the phobic individual enhances the effectiveness of treatment. Other data suggest that modeling the *acquisition* of fearless behavior is more influential than is modeling fearless behavior *per se*. When indicated, "joint simultaneous performance" of the feared activity can be substituted initially for unilateral patient replication of modeled enactments. Here the patient and model jointly and simultaneously perform the aversive behavior after it has been demonstrated and before the patient attempts to perform the behavior alone. In general, a great deal of assistance and support is given in order to help the patient display the targeted performance. Given the data supporting the usefulness of participant modeling in dealing with problems such as Jenny's (Bandura, 1976; Johnson, Rasbury, & Siegel, 1986), a participant modeling approach was selected for use in the present case.

COURSE OF TREATMENT

Jenny's balloon phobia was dealt with in six 1-hour sessions that occurred weekly. The approach involved filmed modeling followed by guided participant modeling. Throughout treatment there was generous use of praise for approaching and for interacting more closely with balloons. A concerted attempt was made also to pair the presence of, and interaction with, balloons with a playful context.

During the first session, Jenny was afforded an opportunity to observe a videotaped model interacting with various sorts of balloons. Because model similarity to an observer enhances modeling outcomes, the model used was a female, and she was roughly Jenny's age. Because an initially fearful and subsequently coping model is seemingly more effective than is an initially fearless model, the modeling film depicted gradual approach behaviors that followed initially fearful responses.

The modeling film was introduced by indicating to Jenny that she was going to be shown a short TV show about a young girl who was afraid of balloons but was able to overcome her fear. In the brief (10–12 minutes) film the model hesitantly entered the room in which the Behavioral Avoidance Test had been administered previously and gradually approached a number of inflated balloons placed on the distant side. Her gradual approach behaviors were accompanied by statements showing mild fearfulness, followed by reassurance from the therapist. After reaching the balloons, she stood in front of them and, when prompted, held the balloons and engaged in increasingly rough play with them (e.g., tossing them up in the air and catching them, throwing them to the therapist, rubbing her hand over them to make noises). In the final behavior depicted, the model initially hesitated then complied with the therapist's request to blow up a balloon and use a pin to pop it. The modeling tape ended with the model receiving a reward (candy) for her performance and with a brief discussion between the model and the therapist that was designed to highlight the idea that one can play with balloons and not suffer adverse consequences.

To provide some index of the impact of videotaped modeling, the therapist subsequently escorted Jenny to the room where the pretreatment BAT had been administered (and where the modeling tape had been filmed). Jenny then was asked to approach the balloons, as in the initial BAT, and was instructed to act just like the girl on TV. As in the initial BAT, Jenny was able to approach, stand in front of, and touch, but not play with, the balloons, stating emphatically that she did not want to use a pin to pop them. As in the earlier assessment, she displayed visible agitation when prompted to put more than one puff of air into the balloon. She jumped up and down, flapped her hands, said "No, no," and begged to return to her mother. She behaved similarly when the therapist attempted to blow up a balloon. On the whole, Jenny's performance on this postmodeling BAT suggested the same degree of fearfulness as was evidenced in the pretreatment assessment.

The next phase of treatment involved graduated participant modeling, utilizing the videotaped model now as a live model. In the second treatment session, Jenny was told that the therapist had asked the girl in the film to help her get over being afraid. In this phase the model entered the room where the BAT had been administered, gradually approached the balloons step by step, and asked Jenny to accompany her and imitate each of her activities (e.g., "Try to do just like I do"). The model then touched the balloons, picked them up, and handled them roughly, and Jenny imitated each behavior in turn. Next, the model encouraged Jenny to join her in various play activities utilizing the balloons. These included jointly picking up the balloons and shaking them, tossing the balloons back and forth, and rubbing them to make them squeak. This resulted in a rather jovial atmosphere, with both girls laughing and apparently enjoying their interaction with each other. Next, the therapist gave the girls several uninflated balloons to play with. The therapist and the model both showed Jenny how these could be blown up to varying degrees and propelled around the room by releasing the stem. Jenny was able to tolerate this and was herself able to put several breaths of air into one of the balloons and act playfully with it. Again, these behaviors were generously rewarded with praise and with candy. Although not able to fully inflate a balloon during this session, Jenny was able calmly to allow the therapist to fully inflate one of the balloons and tie it. The session ended with the therapist, the model, and Jenny again playing with several inflated balloons while singing, to the tune of a well-known children's song, an on-the-spot composition with the lyrics "Who's afraid of the big balloon, the big balloon, the big balloon? Who's afraid of the big balloon? Oh no, oh no, not us." In sum, the first live participant modeling session allowed Jenny to display nonanxious approach behavior for an extended period of time. It appeared to reduce Jenny's fear responses significantly.

In the remaining four sessions, Jenny worked with the therapist individually. There were participant modeling sessions (with the therapist serving as model) that provided additional mastery experiences with balloons such as those just described. By the end of the fourth session, Jenny was able to inflate balloons of various sizes and shapes and to watch calmly as they were tied. At her own request Jenny was allowed to take several balloons home. At this point she demonstrated little in the way of observable fear responses while playing with balloons, although treatment had not progressed to the point where she was required to burst any of the balloons.

TERMINATION

The plan was that treatment include prolonged trials of self-directed mastery to the point where Jenny could burst balloons intentionally. Naturalistic interactions with balloons also were planned, but treatment was terminated before these final stages of the intervention could be completed.

After the sixth treatment session, Jenny's mother called to indicate that bringing Jenny to the clinic was becoming increasingly difficult for a number of practical reasons. She noted also that Jenny had come into contact with balloons outside of the clinic on several occasions during the previous weeks without appearing excessively fearful, and that both she and her husband believed that Jenny's fear no longer needed treatment. Despite suggestions that completing the final stages of treatment would render the fear reduction more durable, the parents chose to discontinue. They were invited to contact the clinic should further problems related to Jenny's balloon fear arise.

FOLLOW-UP

Two years after termination Jenny was again brought to the clinic by her mother. This referral was prompted by school-related difficulties, such as incomplete seatwork and homework and by noncompliance at home. A behavior management program was recommended to aid the parents and the teacher in dealing with these problems. At the time of this referral, Jenny's mother once again completed the Quay-Peterson Behavior Problem Checklist as well as the Personality Inventory for Children (a measure designed to assess a range of childhood problems, such as anxiety, depression, withdrawal, somatic concerns, hyperactivity, inadequate social skills, psychosis, and the like). This was supplemented by interviews. Apart from the presence of mild conduct problems, no major difficulties were suggested by the mother. Responses to the Behavior Problem Checklist confirmed the generally mild nature of Jenny's behavior problems, and all scores on the Personality Inventory for Children were within the normal range. Thus, despite parental concern over Jenny's behavior, there was no evidence of any sort of major conduct problem. Especially noteworthy is that no mention was made of continuing difficulties associated with Jenny's balloon phobia. Hence, no follow-up behavioral test was performed.

OVERALL EVALUATION

The case report just presented exemplifies routine behaviorally oriented clinical work with children. The narrative is based on information (including videotapes) taken from our files for the sole purpose of preparing this chapter retrospectively. Because Jenny's treatment was not part of any research protocol, there are "methodological problems" that constrain the force of empirical claims about treatment efficacy. Nonetheless, an evaluation of our approach and of its success is offered tentatively. Behavior therapy frequently is more protracted and multifaceted than it was here, even for so-called simple phobias. Hence, a brief narrative is also provided about therapy tactics that might have been used had our initial approach been unsuccessful.

Graduated participant modeling apparently succeeded in eliminating Jenny's phobia, even though premature termination precluded important therapeutic experiences such as prolonged self-directed mastery and naturalistic rehearsal. In the absence of follow-up behavioral assessment, success can be argued by the mother's failure to report the phobia as a problem 2 years later and by the fact that she did seek our help for a second (unrelated) behavioral problem.

Obviously the specific therapeutic tactic(s) responsible for clinical success cannot be spelled out confidently. This is so because the approach taken included several behaviorally regnant facets, including observation of a filmed coping model, observation of an *in vivo* mastery model, direct contact with the feared stimulus, praise and appetitive reward for coping and mastery performances, and the temporal pairing of these elements with anxiety-inhibiting play behavior. (No doubt other potentially influential "ingredients" could be listed.) Obviously the clinical use of modeling and guided participation can proceed without any knowledge of the specific ingredients that are most pivotal to clinical success.

Graduated participant modeling was chosen as the intervention here because of the overwhelming literature that supports its technical efficacy.

In the event that the intervention had failed, we would have proceeded in one or both of two alternative directions. In one of these, psychophysiological assessment would have been performed during actual and imagined encounters with inflated balloons. Given evidence of physiological responsivity, especially while imaging, we would have proceeded with systematic desensitization or with some variation on the theme of reciprocal inhibition as overviewed earlier. Quite possibly these interventions would have been used to prepare Jenny for a participant modeling treatment such as the one actually used. In the other alternative approach, we would have adopted a family systems view of the problem. As noted earlier, Jenny was overhead to say, "My mom said that if I see someone blow it [a balloon] up I'll be afraid." Utterances of that sort point to the mother's verbal behavior as maintaining Jenny's fear behavior. Accordingly, intervention with the mother and with other family members might have been undertaken. Probably such interventions would have been used to supplement classical behavior therapy methods.

ACKNOWLEDGMENTS

The authors would like to acknowledge the contribution of Gary Tyson, who, as a clnical psychology intern, served as therapist in the present case. The order of authorship was determined by the toss of a coin and should be considered equal.

REFERENCES

Bandura, A. (1976). Effecting change through participant modeling. In J. D. Krumboltz & C. E. Thoreson (Eds.), *Counseling methods*. New York: Holt, Rinehart & Winston.

Delprato, D. J., & McGlynn, F. D. (1984). Behavioral theories of anxiety disorders. In S. M. Turner (Ed.), *Behavioral theories and treatment of anxiety* (pp. 1–49). New York: Plenum.

Johnson, J. H., Rasbury, W. C., & Siegel, L. J. (1986). *Approaches to child treatment: Introduction to theory, research, and practice*. New York: Pergamon Press.

McGlynn, F. D., & Cornell, C. E. (1985). Simple phobia. In M. Hersen & A. S. Bellack (Eds.), *Handbook of clinical behavior therapy with adults* (pp. 23–48). New York: Plenum.

Quay, H. C. (1977). Measuring dimensions of deviant behavior: The Behavior Problem Checklist. *Journal of Abnormal Child Psychology, 5*, 277–287.

CHAPTER 6

Obsessive–Compulsive Disorder

PAUL R. McCARTHY and EDNA B. FOA

DESCRIPTION OF THE DISORDER

In the DSM-III-R, the official diagnostic manual of the American Psychiatric Association, obsessive–compulsive disorder (OCD) is listed among anxiety disorders. Required for the diagnosis of this disorder are the presence of obsessions and compulsions. Obsessions are recurrent and persistent thoughts, images, or impulses that are experienced as intrusive, unwanted, and senseless, and the individual attempts to ignore or suppress them. They are recognized by the person as a product of his/her mind, not imposed on him/her externally.

Compulsions are defined as repetitive and purposeful behavior performed according to certain rules in a stereotyped fashion. The compulsion is not an end in itself; rather, it is an attempt to neutralize or prevent discomfort that arises from confrontation with a feared situation or a feared cognition. The compulsion must be excessive and irrational and must be recognized as such by the disordered individual. However, such recognition may be absent in obsessive–compulsive (OC) children. In general, the presence of obsessions and compulsions produces marked distress, is quite time-consuming, and interferes markedly with the daily functioning of the individual.

Obsessive–compulsive disorder in childhood has been estimated to

PAUL R. McCARTHY and EDNA B. FOA • Department of Psychiatry, Medical College of Pennsylvania at EPPI, 3200 Henry Avenue, Philadelphia, Pennsylvania 19129.

occur in approximately 1% of child psychiatric inpatients. In a retrospective examination of more than 8,000 inpatient and outpatient records of children, Hollingsworth, Tanguay, Grossman, and Pabst (1980) found an incidence of .2% (17 cases). Because of the extremely low prevalence of this disorder in children, even studies of large populations do not yield a sufficiently large sample to study relevant variables. Despite this low prevalence, the study of OCD children is important. As noted by Rapoport *et al.* (1981), "From a practical clinical view, childhood obsessive–compulsive disorder is rare but malignant. Review of follow-up studies . . . , suggests that up to 50 percent of the children may not make substantial recovery. Therefore, children and adolescents are an appropriate and important group in which to evaluate treatment because their illness is likely to continue and impairment of function justifies experimental intervention" (p. 1545).

CASE IDENTIFICATION

Steve is a 13-year-old boy who worried about causing injuries to family members, failing in school, and being ridiculed by peers. In order to reduce these fears, Steve performed a variety of behavioral and cognitive rituals. Thoughts about failing tests were frequent and intrusive, giving rise to extreme anxiety. To offset his anxiety, Steve either rehearsed test material excessively or performed repeated movements of his head and hands in a prescribed ritualistic manner. In addition, intrusive thoughts of possible accidents or injuries to loved ones triggered repetition of whatever behavior he had been engaged in at the time of the thought. This behavior was repeated until Steve "felt" that the danger was neutralized. In addition to the concerns described above, Steve feared that he would perform poorly in athletics and be ridiculed by his coach and teammates. To neutralize this fear, he again repeated whatever actions were co-occurrent with the thought (e.g., brushing teeth, combing hair, both approximately 20 times). While recognizing the senselessness of the OC patterns, Steve was unable to control his obsessions and compulsions.

PRESENTING COMPLAINTS AND HISTORY

The onset of the OC symptoms occurred 4 years prior to treatment. Steve's parents reported that around age 9, Steve's study patterns became increasingly more demanding; at age 10, they noticed the repetitive occurrence of head and hand gestures. Initially, these movements were infrequent, but they increased rapidly along with Steve's compulsive re-hearsal of schoolwork. Symptoms largely remitted over each summer recess but resumed their intensity when school started again in the fall. Throughout the following year, Steve's parents sought advice from nu-merous mental health professionals. They were advised to help Steve relax and avoid stressful situations. Despite their efforts to follow these instructions, Steve's symptoms became more severe. In addition to OC symptoms, Steve evidenced depression and general anxiety during the school year. The pattern of symptoms' remission during the summer and their return during the school year persisted thereafter, until behavioral treatment was implemented. Pharmacological interventions, tryptophan and clomipramine, were tried prior to behavior therapy, but these were unsuccessful.

ASSESSMENT

The Rating of Fear and Avoidance

To evaluate the specific symptomatology of OCD patients, several forms of assessment are used in our center, including a clinical interview, clinical rating scales, and standardized questionnaires that are described below. Assessment, beginning with careful behavioral analysis of fear and avoidance (i.e., obsessions and compulsions), was conducted along the following guidelines.

The assessment of *obsessions* (anxiety/discomfort-evoking material) is composed of three components: *External cues* refer to objects or sit-uations that arouse high anxiety or discomfort (e.g., urine, pesticides, doorknob, driving over bumps); *internal cues* refer to thoughts, images, or impulses that provoke anxiety, shame, or disgust (e.g., the number 3, thoughts of being contaminated, or bodily sensations); *anticipated harm* comprises feared catastrophes that may ensue from external sources (e.g., disease from touching a contaminated object, burglary if a door is not properly locked) or from internal sources (e.g., "God will punish me," "I may be responsible for harm happening to my parents").

Not every obsession contains all three elements. Contamination ob-sessions typically focus on external cues (e.g., urine or feces and bath-rooms). Many patients who fear contamination fail to identify specific harm, which they try to prevent via the ritualistic cleaning. For checkers, however, the core of the obsession is the anticipated catastrophies.

The assessment of *avoidance* is composed of two components. *Pas-

sive avoidance refers to situations or objects that are shunned (e.g., public bathrooms, stepping on brown spots on the sidewalk, touching doorknobs on the least-used surface). The second component, *ritualistic behavior*, is an active escape from anxiety-evoking cues. For example, the individual who fears contamination by bathroom germs will avoid using public toilets. When such passive avoidance fails to ensure comfort, he/she will resort to washing and cleaning ritualistically; likewise, the person who fears the death of loved ones when thinking a certain number, will try to avoid thinking about this number. When such attempts prove unsuccessful, the person will develop rituals such as praying to protect the people so loved.

Fear, avoidance, and rituals are rated on 8-point Likert scales, where 0 represents no symptoms and 8 denotes extreme severity of symptoms. The ratings of Steve's symptoms on these scales are presented in Appendix A. When evaluating the three main fears, we attempt to rate both the feared situation (e.g., touching public toilet seats) and the anticipated harm (e g , contracting venereal disease). Delineating concrete stimulus situations associated with an obsession provides the basis for a behavioral test, which provides an opportunity to observe the patient's behavior and emotions when confronted with these situations. In selecting avoidance items, we attempt to identify situations that are avoided during everyday life, rather than delineating merely a feared object (e.g., "grass where dogs are likely ot defecate" versus "dog feces"). The severity of compulsions is determined on the basis of frequency and/or duration. (For a further detailed discussion of these scales, see Kozak, Foa, & McCarthy, in press).

Symptom patterns may vary from one individual to another. Some evidence little avoidance and much ritualizing, whereas others may successfully reduce anxiety by passive avoidance, resorting to ritualistic behavior only infrequently. The frequent discordance among these measures may reflect their function: Both avoidance and rituals reduce anxiety; thus, only one or the other may be "needed." Such is reflected in Steve's symptom profile. To reduce anxiety he ritualized quite heavily but did not resort to passive avoidance.

Standardized Instruments

Several standardized instruments have been developed to assess OC symptoms. The most commonly used are discussed below.

The Compulsive Activity Checklist (CAC) is an instrument that focuses on obsessive–compulsive symptoms, rather than on compulsive traits. The name of the instrument has been changed several times from its original one, the Obsessive–Compulsive Interview Checklist. Originally, it contained 62 items describing specific activities, each of which was rated by an assessor on a 4-point scale of severity. Each point on the scale was anchored with quantitative written descriptors. A 37-item version of the CAC also exists and has been found to be sensitive to changes following behavioral treatment. (For a review of the psychometric properties of this instrument, see Freund, 1986.)

The Maudsley Obsessional–Compulsive Inventory (MOCI) is a 30-item self-report questionnaire with a true–false response format that assesses cognitive and behavioral aspects of obsessive–compulsive disorder. It yields four subscales: washing, checking, slowness, and doubting, as well as a total score.

The sensitivity of the MOCI to treatment effects has been documented. In addition, the MOCI has been found to differentiate obsessive–compulsives from normals and neurotics (including phobics) (Rachman & Hodgson, 1980). In a comparison of obsessive–compulsive adolescents with anxious nonobsessional adolescents, Clark and Bolton (1985) found the MOCI to be a valid instrument for differentiating the former from the latter. (For an extended review of OCD measures, see Freund, 1986.)

The Child Behavior Checklist (CBCL) consists of 20 competence items and 118 behavior problem items for children ages 4 to 16 (Achenbach & Edelbrock, 1983). The scale was developed by factor-analyzing parent ratings of disturbed children separately for each sex, at ages 4 to 5, 6 to 11, and 12 to 16. For each group, eight to nine syndromes were identified. Six syndromes were identified in girls ages 4 to 5 and 6 to 11 (somatic complaints, depressed, social withdrawal, hyperactive, sex problems, aggression). Additional distinct syndromes were identified for girls ages 4 to 5 (schizoid or anxious, obese), and for girls ages 6 to 11 (schizoid–obsessive, cruel, delinquent). These syndromes form the scales found in the Child Behavior Profile, which provides normative data for age and sex for each syndrome. The median r across age, sex, and profile was .89 for 1-week test-retest reliability, and .66 for interparent agreement. High correlations were found between total scores on the CBCL and the Conners Parent Rating Scale ($r = .91$) and between total scores on the CBCL and the Peterson-Quay Revised Behavior Problem Checklist ($r = .92$).

While several standardized scales are available for the assessment of OCD symptomatology in adults, there are no data about the reliability of these measures for OCD children.

SELECTION OF TREATMENT

Previous Treatment Studies

To date, no controlled psychosocial treatment studies of OC children have been conducted, although several cases have been described which employ a variety of techniques. A case report of a 9-year-old boy evidencing ritualistic hand washing and frequent checking was presented by Dalton (1983). Treatment emphasized both reinforcement of "normal" (nonritualistic) behaviors and family therapy with a problem-solving orientation. Fifteen sessions were given over a 7-month period. However, evaluation of the child's symptom severity is not possible since no information as to the extent of his symptoms was provided by the author. At 1-year follow-up, it was reported that the child was symptom-free (hand washing and checking) both at home and at school. Queiroz, Motto, Madi, Sossai, & Boren (1981) presented treatment results for two cases, a 9-year-old male with hoarding rituals and a 12-year-old female with repeating rituals. Following a careful behavioral analysis of the ritualistic behaviors, the authors employed extinction procedures coupled with the substitution of reinforced alternative noncompulsive behaviors. The reward structures in the home and school environments were redesigned such that all reinforcement (e.g., attention) for ritualistic behavior was eliminated. While no information about number and frequency of sessions was provided, the authors indicated that treatment for these children spanned approximately 18 months. At 1-year follow-up, one child was much improved, demonstrating "negligible problem behavior" and the other was symptom free. Unfortunately, as with other case reports, no adequate measures of pre- versus posttreatment symptom severity were provided, rendering an evaluation of the actual degree of improvement impossible. However, while both case reports indicate significant improvement, there is no consensus at present as to what form of psychosocial treatment is the most effective for childhood OCD.

Given the scarce information about treatment efficacy with OCD children, the use of knowledge about the treatment of adult OC patients is a reasonable strategy. In Steve's treatment, we employed a variant of exposure and response prevention, a behavioral treatment commonly used with OC adults. A description of this treatment follows.

Exposure and Response Prevention

Our treatment program consists of three components: exposure in imagination, exposure *in vivo*, and response prevention. Treatment typically includes 15 90-minute sessions conducted over a 3-week period. In order to better generalize gains from the clinic to home and school environments, during the fourth week therapy is conducted over 2 consecutive days in the patient's environment for a total of 8 hours. Patients are given written follow-up instructions at the end of the treatment program.

Exposure in imagination takes place during the first 45 minutes of each session and includes six scenes of gradually increasing anxiety-evoking potential. The least disturbing is presented on the first day, the second on the second day, and so forth, until the most disturbing scene is presented on the sixth day. The remaining 10 sessions are devoted to presentation of the most disturbing scene with incorporation of anxiety-evoking material that arises during treatment. All scenes are tape-recorded and replayed by the patient as part of the daily homework assignment. Imaginal scenes include exposure to disturbing stimuli (objects, thoughts, images, situations) and to the catastrophic consequences the patient fears may follow if rituals are not performed. Emission of rituals is prevented in the scenes. Both stimulus and response descriptions are incorporated throughout the scene. An example of a scene used with Steve follows:

It is the morning of your math exam. As you get out of bed you find yourself thinking, "I'm going to flunk my test." You continue to worry about "What if I forget everything I studied? What if I fail my math test? What will Mrs. Green (my teacher) think of me? What will my parents think of me?" After trying to eat breakfast, you dress. As you finish brushing your teeth and are putting your toothbrush back in the rack the thought "I'm going to flunk" occurs to you. You feel you must pick up the toothbrush again and put it back with a "good thought" ("I'm going to pass"). Although you try to fight this temptation you end up giving in but find yourself repeatedly picking it up and putting it down. Finally, your mother comes in and breaks you away from the ritual by yelling, "You're going to be late for the bus." She rushes you along and gets you off to school.

Now you are sitting in math class and feeling very nervous. Mrs. Green is passing out the tests. As you look at your test paper, your heart is pounding, and you find that your mind goes blank. You seem to have forgotten all the material you tried to study. You begin to think, "What if I fail? Mom and Dad will be so angry and disappointed with me." Your breathing gets faster and you are beginning to sweat. Time is passing and you still can't remember how to do the problems. You look at your paper and you have only been able to write your name and the date. Other classmates are finishing the test and don't look worried to you at all. Mrs. Green is now collecting the tests; she asks for your paper and begins to pick it up off your desk. You can see the frown on her face as she notices that the test is blank. She is standing over you and you can tell she is getting angrier. Mrs. Green announces to the class that you are the only person to hand in a blank paper. You can hear the laughter and whispering of other students. You know they are laughing and whispering about you and how dumb they think you are.

You are arriving home now. You can tell by the look on your mother's face that Mrs. Green has called her and explained that you were the only person in her class to flunk. Your mother looks very angry and says, "Go to your room. Your father and I will talk with you when he gets home!"

Exposure in vivo is conducted during the second 45-minute segment of each session. Patients are confronted with the anxiety-evoking objects or situations in a gradual manner, starting with items evoking 50 Subjective Units of Discomfort (SUDs). The therapist models when necessary and encourages contact with the feared stimuli for the entire period. Each day a new item is added to the previous ones, until the highest item is introduced by the sixth day. All items combined are presented daily during the second and third weeks of treatment. A portion of the item hierarchy used in Steve's treatment is shown in Table 1.

The SUDs ratings were based on the understanding that no ritualistic behavior is allowed following the feared thought or action. The behaviors performed while having the above thoughts included repetition of actions such as brushing hair or teeth, dressing and undressing, tying shoes, or walking.

Response prevention consists of instructing the patient to refrain from engaging in any ritualistic behavior throughout the 3-week treatment period. For washers, contact with water or other cleaning agents is prohibited, with the exception of a 10-minute shower every fifth day. The exact nature of the response prevention procedures for checkers depends upon their rituals. In general, they are allowed to check items like doors and windows only once. Patients are supervised by designated relatives or friends who are often actively involved in the treatment process. At the least, they are contacted by the therapist daily to verify that response prevention instructions are followed by the patient. Patients are aware that their behavior is being observed and that violations are being reported

Table 1
Portion of Item Hierarchy

Item	SUDs rating
Thoughts of parents badly hurt in auto accident	100
Intentional failing of math exam	100
Thoughts of a dog being hit by car	80
Thoughts of failing a test	75
Intentional poor athletic performance	60

to the therapist. Whereas response prevention is not enforced by physical restraint, supervisors are instructed to try to encourage the patient to refrain from ritualizing.

All patients are required to complete the Self-Monitoring of Rituals Form throughout treatment. These forms are collected daily by the therapist, and the difficulties encountered by patients in adhering to treatment instructions are discussed. Any violations of response prevention instructions are reviewed daily by the therapist, the supervisor, and the patient. A sample of the Self-Monitoring Form completed by Steve is presented in Appendix B.

Daily homework consists of 45 minutes of listening to the taped imaginal scene presented in the preceding treatment session and 3 hours of *in vivo* exposure to items or situations to which patients were exposed during the previous sessions. Homework continues on the weekends.

As mentioned earlier, to facilitate generalization from treatment sessions to the patient's natural environment, 3 days after the last treatment session treatment is carried out at the patient's home. During these visits, the patient is exposed continuously to anxiety-provoking situations and is instructed to respond in a normal, unritualized manner. For washers, home treatment consists of contaminating their living environment (e.g., home, school) as well as their personal possessions. For washers, instructions for behavior at follow-up include three 10-second hand washings per day and one 10-minute shower per day. Checkers are exposed at home and school to situations that arouse their urge to check repeatedly. They are allowed to check once only, after which they are removed from that situation and are exposed to the next one (e.g., stoves, locks, faucets). During these 2 days, both washers and checkers are also exposed to situations outside their home (e.g., school, friends' homes) if indicated. All family members and relevant school personnel are asked to encourage the patient's compliance with the therapist's posttreatment instructions.

COURSE OF TREATMENT

As previously indicated, Steve's treatment was preceded by an extensive assessment to determine the specific thoughts, objects, and situations he feared. These items were then rated for the SUDs they produced when they occurred in his life. A hierarchy of items was then constructed. A treatment plan was developed as follows: First, Steve was confronted with an item that produced 50 SUDs. Over the next five treatment sessions, exposure progressed to increasingly uncomfortable situ-

Table 2
Rewards Used

Within session	
Computer games with therapist	100
Building of toy model	85
Going for a walk with therapist	75
Social attention from therapist	60
At home	
Favorite dessert	100
Playing soccer	90
Additional TV time (1/2 hr)	80
Going for walk with parent	75

ations. By the sixth session, Steve was exposed to the most difficult of the hierarchy items. For the remaining nine sessions, the top hierarchy items were used for in-session and homework exposures. Whereas treatment progressed fairly smoothly with Steve, considerable effort was required to keep him motivated to comply with the treatment program. Numerous within-session rewards were provided contingent upon compliance with the exposure demands. The reward structure at home was reengineered so that Steve was rewarded for efforts to comply with exposure homework and with response prevention. All parental attention and rewards were withdrawn when Steve was noncompliant. The rewards used in-session and at home were arranged in a graded hierarchy and were given on the basis of the difficulty of the assigned exposure and the degree of compliance evidenced by Steve. Examples of those used are shown in Table 2.

Steve's mother functioned as his primary supervisor during treatment and thus was involved in many treatment sessions. At first, she observed how the therapist worked with Steve, and later she functioned as a cotherapist during *in vivo* exposure. Such participation proved quite helpful since she was better able to understand Steve's symptoms and better able to refrain from inadvertently contributing to them. Given the relatively shortened attention span of children, she was helpful in keeping Steve focused on the exposure tasks.

Because some of Steve's rituals were performed to neutralize relatively unpleasant situations (e.g., test taking), it was essential to share information about treatment with school personnel directly involved with Steve. In particular, they were instructed in how to refrain from reinforcing his patterns of rituals. Once this had been instituted, a marked reduction in disruptions was reported school. It was also noted that Steve's performance at school improved such that he made the honor roll ,during the following school year.

In general, Steve's treatment program followed the format of exposure and response prevention used with adults. However, the following modifications were found necessary. It seems that in treating OC children, it is essential to involve the primary caregiver in treatment. The involvement of school personnel is often as important to ensure successful outcome. Reinforcement schedules in the home and school environment must be altered so that ritualistic behavior is not rewarded. Verbal refocusing is frequently needed during treatment sessions to keep the patient's attention on the exposure item at hand.

TERMINATION

The termination of treatment occurs following the home visit, at the point where the therapist, patient, and supervisor feel that the patient is capable of maintaining his/her treatment gains through the application of skills learned in therapy when urges to ritualize appear. Those maintenance skills are reviewed during the termination session. They include a clear understanding of how to determine the need for, and implementation of, exposure homework. For children, these considerations are discussed with the parents, and the implementation of homework is supervised by the caregiver.

The implementation of an exposure diary is useful in maximizing posttreatment compliance with a continued self-treatment program. Prior to treatment, the patient is asked to list about 20 *specific* feared items and to rate each of these items for the degree of pretreatment discomfort (0–100 SUDs) it produces. Following treatment the patient again rates each item every third day. A subsample of Steve's initial exposure diary is given in Table 3. All of the items in Table 3 were rated when the action was emitted while Steve was having fearful thoughts, but not ritualizing.

As is apparent, the diary proved helpful in evaluating progress. In addition, the diary is useful in monitoring compliance with homework assignments. The five highest items for each 3-day period are addressed in exposure homework for 1 to 2 hours daily following the end of the intensive treatment period. This procedure is continued until all diary items have dropped below a 15 SUDs rating. The diary/homework procedure can be reinstituted should any partial relapse occur. The diary also

Table 3
Subsample of Initial Exposure Diary

	Pretreatment	Posttreatment	3 days later	6 days later
1. Using toothbrush	85	0	0	0
2. Using hairbrush	82	0	0	0
3. Tying shoes	80	15	15	12
4. Dressing	85	0	10	5
5. Building models	80	0	0	0
6. Writing	90	10	20	15
7. Closing locker door	100	10	5	5
8. Taking tests	100	30	35	30

aids the patients and the supervisor to identify the nature of problems when they arise.

OVERALL EVALUATION

As indicated earlier, there are no controlled psychosocial treatment studies with OC children, although few single cases were reported. In light of the highly positive treatment outcome described here with Steve, and at least one other case report employing exposure and response prevention with an OC child (Foa, Steketee, & Milby, 1980), it seems justified to view childhood OCD as a distinct disorder that closely resembles that of adults. It is interesting to note that Steve was referred to our center following an unsuccessful treatment trial with clomipramine. Despite compliance and an adequate trial, the medication did not reduce his OC symptoms. Behavioral treatment started following a 2-week drug-free period. Thus, no drug was present in Steve's system during either the behavior therapy treatment or the follow-up assessments; the marked reduction in symptoms is therefore attributable to the behavioral therapy alone.

It is clear that systematic investigation of treatment for childhood OCD is badly needed. However, the rarity of this disorder in children renders such studies difficult to execute in any one site. Collaboration among centers as well as carefully designed single-case studies will help fill in the gap. Clomipramine was found effective with some OCD children (Rapaport, 1986), as was behavior therapy. A comparison between the two treatment modalities would yield important information.

APPENDIX A

Patient: Steve   Age: 14   Sex: Male

Assessor Ratings[a]

0	1	2	3	4	5	6	7	8
/	/	/	/	/	/	/	/	/
none		Mild		Moderate		Strong		Severe

	Pre-treatment	Post-treatment	3-month follow-up	1-year follow-up
Fear: Completing behaviors following "bad thoughts"	6	3	2	0
Global obsessions	6	3	3	0
Avoidance	0	0	0	0
Rituals				
1. Repeating	6	0	0	0
2. Head and hand gestures	6	0	0	0
Global compulsions	6	1	1	0
Urges to perform rituals	6	3	2	0
Interference of OC symptoms:				
At school	6	3	0	0
At home	6	3	0	0
With family relationships	2	1	1	0
With other social relationships	2	1	3	0
With personal leisure activities	4	3	1	0

[a] Ratings: none = 0, 1; mild = 2, 3; moderate = 4, 5; strong = 6, 7; severe = 8.

APPENDIX B

Self-Monitoring of Rituals

Name: Steve   Date: February 13, 1987
Ritual A: Repeating   Ritual B: Hand and head movements

In the second column of the table please describe the activity or thought that evokes rituals. In the third column record the anxiety/discomfort level (0–100). In the fourth column write the number of minutes you spend in performing rituals during the time stated in Column 1.

Time of day	Activity or thought which evokes the ritual	Discomfort (0–100)	Number of minutes spent on rituals: A	B
6:00–6:30 a.m.				
6:30–7:00				
7:00–7:30	Bad thoughts—Going to do bad on schoolwork	35	1	1
7:30–8:00				
8:00–8:30				
8:30–9:00	Bad thoughts—Dog was going to get bit by another dog	75	1	1
9:00–9:30				
9:30–10:00	Bad thought—Mom was going to get hurt	45	1	1
10:00–10:30				
10:30–11:00				
11:00–11:30				
11:30–12:00	Bad thought—Do bad on math	45	1	1
12:00–12:30 p.m.				

ACKNOWLEDGMENTS

The authors would like to thank Lisa Solomon for her help with this project. Support for the preparation of this chapter was provided in part by NIMH Grants MH 09349 and MH 31634 to the first and second authors, respectively.

REFERENCES

Achenbach, T. M., & Edelbrock, C. (1983). *Manual for the Child Behavior Checklist and Revised Child Behavior Profile.* Burlington: University of Vermont, Department of Psychiatry.

Clark, D. A., & Bolton, D. (1985). Obsessive–compulsive adolescents and their parents: A psychometric study. *Journal of Psychiatry, 26,* 267–276.

Dalton, P. (1983). Family treatment of an obsessive–compulsive child: A case report. *Family Process, 22,* 99–108.

Foa, E. B., Steketee, G., & Milby (1980). Differential effects of exposure and response prevention in obsessive–compulsive washers. *Journal of Consulting and Clinical Psychology, 48,* 71–79.

Freund, B. (1986). *Comparison of measures of obsessive–compulsive symptomatology. Rating scales of symptomatology and standardized assessor- and self-rated.* Unpublished doctoral dissertation, Southern Illinois University.

Hollingsworth, C. E., Tanguay, P. E., Grossman, L., & Pabst, P. (1980). Long-term outcome of obsessive–compulsive disorder in childhood. *Journal of the American Academy of Child Psychiatry, 19,* 134–144.

Kozak, M. J., Foa, E. B., & McCarthy, P. R. (in press). Assessment of obsessive–compulsive disorder. In C. G. Last & M. Hersen (Eds.), *Handbook of anxiety disorders.* New York: Pergamon Press.

Queiroz, L. O. D. S., Motta, M. A., Madi, M. B. B. P., Sossai, D. L., & Boren, J. J. (1981). A functional analysis of obsessive–compulsive problems with related therapeutic procedures. *Behaviour Research and Therapy, 19,* 377–388.

Rachman, S. & Hodgson, R. J. (1980). *Obsessions and Compulsions.* Englewood Cliffs, NJ: Prentice-Hall.

Rapoport, J. L. (1986). Childhood obsessive–compulsive disorder. *Journal of Child Psychology and Psychiatry, 27,* 289–295.

Rapoport, J., Elkins, R., Langer, D. H., Sceery, W., Buchsbaum, M. S., Gillin, J. C., Murphy, D. L., Zahn, T. P., Lake, R., Ludlow, C., & Mendelson, W. (1981). Childhood obsessive–compulsive disorder. *American Journal of Psychiatry, 138,* 1545–1554.

CHAPTER 7

Dysthymia

CYNTHIA L. FRAME, BRICK JOHNSTONE, and
MARKHAM S. GIBLIN

DESCRIPTION OF THE DISORDER

The *Diagnostic and Statistical Manual of Mental Disorders*, Third Edition (DSM-III; American Psychiatric Association, 1980) states that the essential feature of dysthymic disorder is "a chronic disturbance of mood involving either depressed mood or loss of interest or pleasure in all, or almost all, usual activities and pastimes, and associated symptoms, but not of sufficient severity and duration to meet the criteria for a major depressive episode" (pp. 220–221). For the reader's benefit, the specific DSM-III diagnostic criteria for dysthymic disorder are summarized below:

A. During the past year (for children and adolescents) the individual has been bothered most or all of the time by symptoms characteristic of the depressive syndrome, but that are not of sufficient severity and duration to meet the criteria for a major depressive episode.

B. The manifestations of the depressive syndrome may be relatively persistent or separated by periods of usual mood lasting a few days to a few weeks, but no more than a few months at a time.

C. During the depressive periods there is either prominent depressed mood (e.g. sad, blue, down in the dumps) or marked loss of interest or pleasure in all, or almost all, usual activities and pastimes.

CYNTHIA L. FRAME, BRICK JOHNSTONE, and MARKHAM S. GIBLIN • Department of Psychology, University of Georgia, Athens, Georgia 30602.

D. During the depressive periods at least three of the following symptoms are present:
   1. insomnia or hypersomnia
   2. low energy level or chronic tiredness
   3. feeling of inadequacy, loss of self-esteem, or self-deprecation
   4. decreased effectiveness or productivity at school or home
   5. decreased attention, concentration, or ability to think clearly
   6. social withdrawal
   7. loss of interest in or enjoyment of pleasurable activities
   8. irritability or excessive anger (in children usually expressed toward parents or caretakers)
   9. inability to respond with apparent pleasure to praise or rewards
   10. less active or talkative than usual, or feeling slowed down or restless
   11. pessimistic attitude toward the future, brooding about past events, or feeling sorry for self
   12. tearfulness or crying
   13. recurrent thoughts of death or suicide
E. There is an absence of psychotic features, such as delusions, hallucinations, incoherence, or loosening of associations.
F. If the disturbance is superimposed on a preexisting mental disorder, the depressed mood, by virtue of its intensity or effect on functioning, can be clearly distinguished from the individual's usual mood.

Although DSM-III is somewhat ambiguous in making the distinction between dysthymic disorder and major depression, it may be stated that dysthymic disorder represents a more chronic and long-standing, but less acute, form of depression. For example, while the duration of depressive symptoms need only be 2 weeks for a diagnosis of major depression, a duration of 1 year for children and adolescents and 2 years for adults is required for a diagnosis of dysthymic disorder.

Other features and complications that are often associated with dysthymic disorder in children and adolescents include feelings of anxiety, fear, irritability, brooding, excessive concern with physical health, somatic complaints, impaired peer relations, and decreased school performance. In prepubertal children, separation anxiety may develop, causing the child to cling to parents or to refuse to go to school. With boys, particularly adolescent boys, negativistic or antisocial behaviors may be exhibited.

In children and adolescents, predisposing factors include the presence of attention deficit disorder, conduct disorder, mental retardation, a severe specific developmental disorder, or an inadequate, disorganized, rejecting, or chaotic environment. The disorder may begin at any time during childhood or adolescence, and seems to occur with equal frequency in males and females. Dysthymic disorder typically begins without clear onset and has a chronic course.

CASE IDENTIFICATION

Jenny was a 9-year-old third-grader who was brought in for treatment by her mother. Jenny's parents were divorced when she was 7 years old. She lived with her mother, Mrs. Haley, who worked as a secretary, and her 12-year-old brother. She visited her father, who lived nearby, about twice a month. Prior to the divorce, Jenny's mother had not worked outside the house. Financial difficulties resulting from the divorce, however, led her mother to take a full-time job and move the family into an apartment when Jenny was 8. The move took place during the school year and resulted in Jenny's having to transfer to a new school midway through the school year. Shortly after the move, Jenny's mother began dating again. After approximately 6 months of dating one man (Jack) extensively, Jenny's mother announced that she was planning to marry him. It was about 2 months after announcing her engagement that Jenny's mother first brought Jenny in for treatment.

PRESENTING COMPLAINTS

During the initial interview session, Jenny offered little information and responded only when directly questioned. She spoke in a very subdued manner, made little eye contact with the therapist, and generally appeared to be apathetic. She did, however, state that she did not feel there was a need for her to talk with anyone. Jenny's mother did most of the talking and stated that gradually, over the past year and a half, Jenny had seemed to become generally unhappy. She further stated that Jenny was sluggish, didn't seem to enjoy herself anymore, and was beginning to do poorly in school in subjects where she previously had done well. She added that Jenny had had plenty of close friends in her old neighborhood and school but that she had not made friends in her new environment. The session was concluded by the mother's stating that the problems Jenny was experiencing were not severe but had been continuing on and off for such a lengthy period of time that she thought it best to have Jenny see someone.

HISTORY

Jenny was described by her mother as having been a fairly normal child. She did well in school, earning average to above-average grades, and she kept busy with occasional after-school activities. She had taken a gymnastics class yearly since the age of 5, actively participated in Brownies, and had had numerous friends with whom she played after school and on the weekends. She got along reasonably well with her older brother and had seemed to be relatively unaware of her parents' earlier marital problems.

Initially, her parents' divorce seemed to be hard for Jenny to accept, since she frequently asked when her parents would live together again, but she eventually seemed to adjust to the changes it brought to her life. She told her mother that she missed having her father around their home, and she looked forward to the weekends she saw him. At first she seemed to thoroughly enjoy the time she spent with her father, but she eventually appeared to grow tired of it, complaining that he would make derogatory remarks about her mother when she was with him.

Approximately a year after the divorce, Jenny's mother was forced to find full-time employment, which resulted in the family's moving approximately 20 miles to a neighboring town. This also involved a change in school for Jenny halfway through the school year. Jenny seemed to be sad to leave her familiar surroundings and all of her old friends, but she also seemed to enjoy the excitement of moving to a new apartment, fixing up her own bedroom, and the opportunity to make new friends in the larger school she would be attending.

At first she made a few acquaintances and performed well in her new classes, but she eventually began to withdraw and spend more time by herself in their new apartment. Part of this seemed to be her choice, since she declined invitations from neighborhood children to play, but it was also forbidden for her to have guests over when her mother was not home. Because of her new job, Mrs. Haley was no longer there when Jenny arrived home from school. Jenny did occasionally do things with her brother, but most of the time he was busy with his own friends. The move to the new town and her mother's demanding schedule did not allow for Jenny to continue her old gymnastics class, and she expressed no interest in the Brownie troop associated with her new school. As a result, Jenny would frequently spend time in her room alone or in front of the television until her mother came home at dinnertime.

Soon, the little time Jenny was able to spend with her mother was drastically reduced when her mother started to seriously date Jack, a man with whom she worked. It was at this time that Mrs. Haley was first informed of increasing problems in Jenny's performance at school. Her grades began to fall. She would frequently fail to turn in assignments, sometimes even when her mother knew she had completed them. Occasionally she would "act out" in class, either by teasing classmates or by being disrespectful to the teacher, behaviors in which she had never previously engaged.

Jenny did have brief periods in which she would do well in school and seem to be happy, especially when she was able to spend time with her old friends. In general, however, for the year and a half prior to coming to therapy Jenny seemed to have gradually changed into an unhappy, isolated young child who was not living up to what others believed to be her potential.

ASSESSMENT

The first session that Jenny and her mother spent with the therapist involved the mothers' stating the reasons she was bringing Jenny in for help. She also gave Jenny's developmental, medical, and psychiatric histories, all of which were normal. Mrs. Haley, Jenny, and the therapist agreed to meet for 1 hour per week, with a plan for the therapist to see Jenny individually at times, as well as seeing Jenny and her mother together.

Over the course of the next 3 weeks, several different facets of Jenny's life were assessed. Areas evaluated included the social, emotional, and behavioral dimensions of Jenny's life, using a structured interview schedule as a guide (Kiddie-SADS; Puig-Antich & Chambers, 1978). In addition, Jenny was asked to complete a self-report questionnaire about depressive symptoms, the Childrens Depression Inventory (CDI; Kovacs & Beck, 1977), and her mother rated her using the Child Behavior Checklist (CBCL; Achenbach & Edelbrock, 1978). A school visit was made by the therapist to obtain the teacher's observations of Jenny's functioning.

In assessing Jenny's current emotional state, the therapist first evaluated vegetative symptoms because depression seemed to be a plausible explanation for Jenny's behaviors and emotional state. When asked about how she had been feeling recently, Jenny initially stated that she felt fine, but when pressed she admitted to feeling down and "having the blahs" over the past year and a half. She added that she generally felt restless, as if something were bothering her, but she could rarely pinpoint anything that was causing her to feel bad. Neither she nor her mother could identify any one specific antecedent event that had appeared to precipitate the onset of the problem, although there were many happenings during the past several years that did bother Jenny. Both agreed there were a few periods, none exceeding a week, when Jenny appeared to feel as fine as she once had.

Jenny told the therapist that she didn't do as many things as she used to because she really didn't have the energy. She stated that she was content watching television and spending time by herself in her room, since none of the new neighborhood children enjoyed doing the things she enjoyed. When asked about her decreased school performance, Jenny stated she didn't complete her work because she just didn't feel like it. She was still passing, although only barely, and no longer cared about getting good grades. She said that they didn't seem to matter to anyone anymore.

Regarding her sleeping habits, both Jenny and her mother agreed that she was sleeping fine and always had. Occasionally she would have difficulty getting up in the morning, but Jenny's mother stated she did not believe this to be noteworthy since Jenny's brother had the same difficulties waking in the morning. She believed it to be normal for children of that age. No changes in her eating habits were noticed either, and her weight had stayed fairly constant for her size.

One of the biggest changes Jenny's mother had noted was her lack of interest in activities that she previously thoroughly enjoyed, such as gymnastics and Brownies. Although Jenny was unable to attend the gymnastic classes she had taken before her parents' divorce, she did not show any interest in continuing Brownies, despite there being a very active troop that met at her new school. Mrs. Haley also stated that whereas Jenny had been a self-starter and a leader before, she no longer initiated any activities and was becoming a very passive person.

Jenny could not identify many of the changes others saw in her over the past several years. She did, however, notice a change in the relationships she made and maintained. She stated that she no longer had any close friends, nor did she wish to, because she did not like "the kids in this town." She also stated that she no longer cared to spend time with her father, giving as a reason that he said only negative things about her mother when they were together. The only person Jenny seemed to enjoy spending time with was her mother, but even this had decreased recently because of Mrs. Haley's new boyfriend. Jenny confided to the therapist that she was afraid her mother no longer cared for her and that her mother might leave her if she married Jack.

The only other aspect of Jenny's life that had seemed to change slightly was her attention span. Although Jenny did not notice any differences, her mother reported that Jenny would become very preoccupied with her own thoughts at times and appear to be very distant. Mrs. Haley also said that Jenny's teachers had complained of inattention and lack of concentration on several occasions. She added that Jenny had never had these problems at her old school.

When investigating any precipitating events to changes in Jenny's behavior and emotional state, neither Jenny nor her mother could point to one specific event that led to her depressed state. Rather, several different factors, including her parents' divorce, her move to a new school, her social isolation, and the decreased amount of time she was able to spend with individuals close to her, all appeared to contribute gradually to her distressed state.

Regarding the consequences of Jenny's behaviors that may have contributed to maintaining these problems, no specific reinforcers could be identified. Mrs. Haley admitted that Jenny had more or less gotten "lost in the shuffle" with all of the changes in their life, and that she received little attention from her family no matter what she did.

During the assessment period, the therapist asked Jenny to keep a daily log of the number of pleasant activities in which she engaged, the contacts she had with friends, and her mood. Mrs. Haley was asked to keep a similar log independently. Jenny was also made responsible for bringing home a weekly report card from school. These data indicated that Jenny was experiencing only one or two minor pleasant events each day, had no contact with any friends, and felt her mood to be bad but not awful. Her weekly report card showed a need for significant improvement.

After the three assessment sessions, the therapist compiled his information. On both the self-report and mother-completed depression measures, Jenny received scores approximately 1 standard deviation above the mean. These scores were indicating some distress, but they were not above the typically used cutoff score for major depression of 2 standard deviations above the mean. The therapist considered this in conjunction with the data from the daily report card, from Jenny's and her mother's logs, and from his interviews. He decided on a diagnosis of dysthymic disorder. Jenny's behaviors and emotional state were not severe enough to meet the criterion for major depression, but they clearly did meet the criteria necessary to be considered dysthymic disorder.

SELECTION OF TREATMENT

Given the diagnosis of dysthymia, a treatment plan was developed that followed general behavioral treatment techniques commonly utilized for the treatment of major depression. These included (1) increasing the number of pleasant activities Jenny was engaging in, (2) parent training to demonstrate to Jenny's mother how to reinforce Jenny for any positive social interactions or other desired behaviors, (3) a positive reinforcement program for Jenny's school performance, and (4) social skills training to assist Jenny in developing friendships in her new school.

COURSE OF TREATMENT

Determining that Jenny's lack of interest in doing things she once enjoyed was the most prominent feature of her dysthymia, the therapist initially stressed the importance of identifying activities Jenny might again enjoy doing and encouraging her to engage in them. Since Jenny seemed to enjoy most spending time with her mother, it was agreed that Jenny and her mother were to spend at least 1 half hour a day together during the weekdays and at least 3 hours together during the weekends. Jenny was to determine how her time was to be spent with her mother, with possibilities including working on her homework, going for a walk, playing a game, or whatever Jenny wished at the time. Furthermore, it was arranged for Jenny to visit her old friends once per month on weekends in place of a 3-hour period with her mother.

During the first treatment session the therapist also met individually with Jenny's mother to discuss ways in which she could reinforce Jenny for what was considered to be any positive behavior, particularily for any contact she had with the neighborhood children. It was agreed that Mrs. Haley would verbally reinforce Jenny for being in a good mood with statements such as "It sure is nice to see you acting so happy" or "I'm glad you're enjoying yourself doing. . . ." Furthermore, Jenny was to be gently encouraged, but not pushed, to play with the neighborhood children and to get out of the house and away from the television, and to be praised any time she did so. During treatment both Jenny and her mother were instructed to continue the weekly report card and daily logs as before.

Jenny began to improve during the next 2 weeks. Both logs indicated that rate of pleasant events had increased somewhat, as had Jenny's mood. On the other hand, there were still no contacts with friends, and the weekly report cards were poor. The following dialogue highlights Jenny's progress:

THERAPIST: Have you noticed any changes in how you've been feeling lately?

JENNY: I've been feeling pretty happy at home—Mom and I have been having lots of fun together.

THERAPIST: How about school and your new friends?

JENNY; School's still a bummer. Schoolwork is boring and the kids aren't like my old friends. They don't act like my old friends so I play by myself and with Mom.

Jenny's lack of progress regarding school performance resulted in the implementation of the school-based positive reinforcement program. In an attempt to improve her school performance, Jenny and her mother agreed that Jenny was to receive 40 cents for each C she received, 60 cents for every B, and 80 cents for every A that occurred on the weekly report card. Jenny stated that she wished to be paid every Saturady morning so that she could possibly go shopping with her mother for their weekend activity.

For the next several weeks Jenny was also given basic social skills training to assist her in making new friendships. Specific social skills addressed included how to enter a group, how to maintain a conversation, how to ask questions about others, and how to ignore unpleasant comments from her peers. Therapy included discussion of real-life encounters that had occurred since the last session, modeling, extensive role-playing, and homework, which stipulated that Jenny attempt to enter a peer group once a day during school and invite a peer over for dinner once during the week. She was to keep a record in her log describing every time she did this so that she could review these encounters with the therapist. She was further discouraged from discussing her old friends with her new peers. Increasing pleasurable experiences was still stressed, and Jenny and her mother continued to spend the specified time together on each day.

Jenny initially made little progress in improving her grades after the school performance contingency program was initiated. However, after the second week she seemed to enjoy earning money, and her grades eventually began to improve. Within a month her grades had improved so much that it was necessary to change the contingencies of her reinforcement program. It was agreed that Jenny would now earn money only for A's and B's, but that if she earned nothing lower than C's and at least three B's, then she would be allowed to bake, a new hobby she was beginning to develop.

Regarding the attempts to increase Jenny's interactions with her peers, only slight progress was being made. According to both logs, Jenny continued to enjoy seeing her old friends but still had little success making new friends. Her progress was described by her mother in the following dialogue:

THERAPIST;   How about Jenny's interactions with other children—has she made many new friends?

MOTHER: No, this is one area where Jenny hasn't changed much that still worries me. She does her homework by talking with new children, but she seems to do so just to please me. She likes seeing her old friends and seems to be content just seeing them occasionally.

THERAPIST: Has she made any new friends at all?

MOTHER: Just one, Debbie. But Jenny will play with her only when it's just those two— she refuses to do anything when there's a group of children.

After considering numerous options, Jenny's mother and the therapist decided that Jenny would be required to take her new friend Debbie with her when she visited her old friends, or she would not be permitted to go. In this manner they attempted to have the new friendship benefit from association with the positive aspects of the old friendships.

At this point in therapy Jenny's mother started to complain that she was having difficulty spending time with Jenny every night, stating that she was very tired from work when she got home, and she believed she needed to spend more time with her fiance. These concerns were discussed with Jenny, and it was agreed that they would spend a half hour together on only 3 nights instead of 5, in addition to the time they spent together on the weekends. In order to encourage more social contacts for Jenny to compensate for the decreased amount of time she would be spending with her mother, she was strongly encouraged to attend Brownies or enroll in a new gymnastics program, or any other program associated with her school. Jenny refused to attend gymnastics but stated she would not mind attending a baking class offered after school. This was strongly encouraged since Jenny had suggested the class herself. Jenny also agreed to try the Brownie troop, but only because Debbie was in it.

Over the next several weeks Jenny's mood ratings continued to improve. Both her own and her mother's logs showed that she had not spent as much time alone. Her grades were consistently above average, and she no longer demanded as much time from her mother. Most important, Jenny's relationship with Debbie began to develop, and she began to make additional friends through her activities with Debbie. She became very involved with her baking class and eventually came to invite some girls she met there over to her home. Jenny's involvement in Brownies followed the same course—she began to make new friends with the help of Debbie and became a very active member of her troop. As Jenny became increasingly busy, she herself suggested that her special time with her mother be decreased to 2 nights per week.

At this point, therapy focused on phasing out the material reinforcers involved in her contingency program. Jenny was no longer required to bring home a weekly report card, but her mother was strongly encouraged to continue to show interest in her work and to verbally reinforce her whenever she did well. Instead of withdrawing all monetary rewards, since Jenny had responded so well to them, Jenny and her mother agreed that Jenny was to be able to earn an allowance for performing chores in their home. At this point, social skills training was terminated; Jenny was forming adequate peer relationships.

At first Jenny did not respond well to having the school performance contingent reinforcers phased out. Her teacher phoned Mrs. Haley to report that her school work deteriorated for about a week, but this improved after she was able to earn money by performing household responsibilities. Her mood ratings continued to be good, and the logs indicated that she continued to have numerous pleasant activities and contacts with friends. The following sessions were structured to prepare Jenny and her mother for the termination of treatment.

TERMINATION

It was finally determined that therapy was to be concluded. Jenny had made substantial improvements over the past 10 weeks in all areas of concern. She had begun to show interest in several activities and become very involved with them, had developed numerous new friendships, had improved her school performance to levels commensurate with her abilities, and generally seemed to be a happier individual.

During the last session, important issues were reviewed, suggestions were made, and potential problems were discussed. Jenny was strongly encouraged to stay involved with her new interests and to maintain her new friendships. Her mother was directed to continue to show interest in Jenny and her activities, verbally reinforcing her whenever appropriate. All agreed that Jenny should continue to be allowed to earn an allowance. It was suggested that Jenny continue to spend some special time with just her mother each week, and that she begin to spend more time with her mother and her fiance together. This was to let Jenny know that she was still special to her mother but also to help Jenny become accustomed to having a new family member. Finally, it was acknowledged that Jenny might experience periods of mild depression at some time again in the future, and if so, they should feel free to contact the clinic at any time.

Jenny completed the CDI again, and her mother filled out the CBCL. Jenny's scores on both measures were in the normal range.

FOLLOW-UP

At the request of the therapist, Jenny and her mother returned 6 months later to assess Jenny's progress. Both had been asked to keep a daily log of Jenny's pleasant events, contacts with friends, and mood ratings for the week preceding the appointment. These measures demonstrated maintenance of treatment gains. Jenny appeared to be very pleased with her life and told of the various activities she was involved in. She had become very active in Brownies, winning several achievement awards, had "graduated" from her baking class, and had started to participate in gymnastics again. She reported four new friendships and said that sometimes she was now too busy to see her old friends. Her grades were all A's and B's. Jenny's mother reported that Jenny had appeared mildly depressed immediately after the mother's marriage to Jack 3 months previously, but that her emotional state gradually improved over the first month of family life as she became used to her new stepfather. When the CDI and CBCL were readministered, Jenny continued to score in the normal range.

This assessment procedure was repeated at 1-year follow-up. Jenny was found to be performing well in school, remaining active in Brownies, excelling at gymnastics, and feeling fairly happy at school and at home. Again, CDI and CBCL scores were within the normal range.

OVERALL EVALUATION

In this case of dysthymic disorder, multimodal treatment resulted in noticeable improvement in the child's mood and behavior within 10 weeks. Careful assessment indicated the need to consider several elements of the client's behaviors related to the diagnosis. Basically, it was determined that she had been failing to receive enough positive reinforcement for any of her behaviors. A secondary consideration was Jenny's lack of knowledge and skill in forming new friendships. Thus, treatment consisted of increasing pleasant activities, increasing positive reinforcement, and training specific social skills related to peer group entry. Progress in these areas, as well as change in mood, was monitored via daily logs kept by the client and her mother. Level of distress was also evaluated pre- and posttreatment via standard questionnaires for depression. All measures, as well as personal reports by the child and her mother, demonstrated that following treatment Jenny was no longer evidencing any significant psychological problems.

REFERENCES

American Psychiatric Association. (1980). *Diagnostic and statistical manual of mental disorders* (3rd ed.). Washington, D.C.: Author.

Achenbach, T. M., & Edelbrock, C. S. (1978). The classification of child psychopathology: A review and analysis of empirical efforts. *Psychological Bulletin, 85,* 1275–1301.

Kovacs, M., & Beck, A. T. (1977). An empirical-clinical approach toward a definition of childhood depression. In J. G. Schulterbrandt & A. Raskin (Eds.), *Depression in childhood: Diagnosis, treatment, and conceptual models.* New York: Raven Press.

Puig-Antich, J., & Chambers, W. (1978). *Schedule for affective disorders and schizophrenia for school-age children (6–16 years)—Kiddie-SADS.* New York: New York State Psychiatric Institute.

CHAPTER 8

Major Depression

WILLIAM M. REYNOLDS

For decades, children who were characterized as sad, introverted, and melancholic, and adolescents who were viewed as brooding, detached, and lethargic were considered to be going through a difficult, although relatively normal, stage of development or, in extreme cases, a reaction disorder of childhood. Depression in children and adolescents is now accepted by psychologists and psychiatrists as a valid syndromal disorder, similar in most aspects of clinical symptomatology and course to major depression in adults.

Since the late 1970s, a growing body of research on depression in youngsters has emerged, with investigations describing epidemiology, psychosocial and biological correlates, individual differences, classification, diagnosis, and assessment (Reynolds, 1985). However, unlike the study of depression in adults, which includes numerous experimental investigations of psychological intervention procedures as well as studies comparing psychotherapy and pharmacotherapy outcomes, there have been few experimental studies of psychological treatments for depression in children and adolescents. To date, there are more investigations related to the dexamethasone suppression test, an episode-specific neuroendocrine (biological) marker for endogenous depression with limited specificity (see Reynolds, 1985 for a description of this procedure), with children and adolescents than there are psychological treatment studies of depression in youngsters.

Over the past few years, the author and colleagues have investigated the efficacy of a number of therapeutic procedures for the amelioration

WILLIAM M. REYNOLDS • Department of Educational Psychology, University of Wisconsin, 1025 West Johnson, Madison, Wisconsin 53706.

and reduction of depressive symptomatology in affected youngsters (Reynolds & Coats, 1986; Stark, Reynolds, & Kaslow, 1987). The intervention procedures utilized in these clinical investigations may be viewed as falling under the general rubric of "cognitive–behavioral" therapies. To a large extent treatments are adapted from contemporary cognitive and behavioral theories of depression, and from treatment packages designed for use with adults. The author has found that in clinical practice it is useful to go beyond the application of a treatment based on a single theoretical model, such as self-control or cognitive therapy. This allows for the greatest broad-spectrum treatment of depressive symptoms and modification of dysfunctional cognitive and behavioral mechanisms.

DESCRIPTION OF THE DISORDER

Major depression is a diagnostic classification utilized in the third edition of the *Diagnostic and Statistical Manual of Mental Disorders* (DSM-III; American Psychiatric Association, 1980). Major depression as a DSM-III diagnostic syndrome is included under the general domain of affective disorders and is defined by the following criteria and symptomatology: (a) the presence of *either* dysphoric mood or anhedonia, and (b) at least *four* of the following eight symptoms (with at least three of symptoms 1, 3, 5, and 6 present in children under 6 years of age): (1) sleep problems as indicated by insomnia or hypersomnia; (2) complaints or other evidence of diminished ability to think or difficulty concentrating; (3) loss of energy and general fatigue; (4) eating problems as manifested by decreased or increased appetite or significant weight loss or gain (in young children below the age of 6 years failure to make expected weight gains is symptomatic); (5) psychomotor retardation or agitation (hypoactivity in children under 6 years of age); (6) loss of interest or pleasure in usual activities (evidence of apathy in children under 6 years); (7) suicidal or morbid ideation, death wishes, or suicide attempts; and (8) feelings of self-reproach, worthlessness, or excessive or inappropriate guilt (which may be delusional). Duration criteria specify that the symptoms need to be present nearly every day for a period of at least 2 weeks. In addition to the inclusion criteria noted above, a number of exclusion criteria are specified that preclude a number of other pathologies, such as organic mental disorder, as concomitant problems, in order to make a diagnosis of major depression.

It should be noted that the criteria specified above are those delineated by DSM-III for major depression. Quite frequently, other symptoms of depression are found in youngsters as well as in adults. These may include crying, anxiety or worry, social withdrawal, and other symptoms associated with depression, but they are not viewed as specific diagnostic criteria for major depression according to the American Psychiatric Association. Nevertheless, the clinician should be observant for these and other associated symptoms in children and adolescents.

Presented below is a prototypic case study of a 16-year-old youngster. This case represents an amalgamation of cases from therapeutic studies of depression in children and adolescents, and it is utilized here to illustrate these procedures for clinicians and researchers. Although not an actual case, in that "Henry" is drawn from a number of children, the complaints, history, and treatment procedures are drawn from actual clinical cases.

The author's orientation to the treatment of major depression in children and adolescents is a systematic integration of therapeutic components derived from various contemporary models of depression (e.g., behavioral, cognitive, learned helplessness, self-control), as well as the addition of ancillary procedures, such as relaxation training. This approach to therapy results in a broad-spectrum intervention program for treating depression in children and adolescents. Although it is presented as a semistructured treatment package, clinical observations and judgment should be utilized as treatment progresses, noting specific cognitive or behavioral distortions or deficits that may be targeted for additional intervention.

CASE IDENTIFICATION AND PRESENTING COMPLAINTS

The prototypic case is that of Henry, a 16-year-old youngster, first identified in school through a schoolwide multiple-stage screening procedure (Reynolds, 1986) that was conducted as an annual activity for the identification of depressed youth. The identification of depressed children and adolescents is fraught with problems if one depends on self- or parent referral for the identification of depressed youngsters. The school-based depression screening procedure utilized is designed to overcome the problems inherent in the passive dependence on self-referral or in unreliable reports by untrained teachers or parents. The general consensus among researchers is that if one wishes to know if a child or adolescent is depressed, the best method to obtain such information is to directly ask the youngster.

The depression screening procedure implemented by the school as an annual mental health activity consists of three assessment stages. The first stage involves the schoolwide administration of a self-report depression measure shown to be a reliable and valid measure for adolescents (Reynolds, 1986). Students identified as at risk (above a critical cutoff score) for clinical levels of depression at the initial assessment stage of the screening program are then retested on the same depression measure approximately 1 to 2 weeks later. At the initial testing, approximately 10% of the youngsters in the school were identified as scoring at or above the critical cutoff score. These students were then reassessed in small groups of 20 to 25. Youngsters who upon retesting continued to demonstrate a clinical level of depressive symptomatology were then individually interviewed with a semistructured clinical interview for depression.

Henry manifested a significant level of depressive symptomatology across all assessment points and measures. Around the same time as the mental health screening, Henry was referred to the school psychologist by a teacher who noted a rapid decrease in his school performance, and who had observed lethargy and an overt appearance of sadness in the classroom. Henry was then referred for further evaluation to an experimental program conducted in the school for the treatment of depression.

HISTORY AND ASSESSMENT

A comprehensive evaluation of the depressed youngster is a necessary initial step, once permission for treatment has been provided by parents, and the child or adolescent understands the nature of the upcoming treatment and consents to therapy. As noted above, a three-stage assessment procedure for the identification of depressed youngsters was implemented in the high school Henry was attending. On the basis of a critical level of self-reported depressive symptomatology on a depression questionnaire that was group-administered on two successive occasions, Henry was identified for an individual evaluation. This evaluation consisted of a semistructured clinical interview that constituted the third stage of the multiple-stage screening procedure. In addition to the formal interview, a current life history was taken, focusing on current family situation, major life events, daily hassles, and the determination of available social supports. As a further evaluation, Henry's cognitive appraisal of events and situations was examined. By assessing Henry's perceptions of the cause of problems, his perceived ability to deal with them, and his cognitions of responsibility or blame, the clinician is able to judge the adequacy of Henry's self-control (self-regulatory) skills, evaluate his attribution system, and identify potential cognitive distortions and/or deficits.

Henry appeared at the initial interview with a distinctly sad and downcast appearance. His movements were slow, and he communicated in a soft, slow monotone, suggestive of significant psychomotor retardation. The author introduced himself to Henry and indicated that his mother had provided permission for the interview and subsequent sessions. Henry nodded and recalled his mother's telling him that he might be seeing someone in school. The interview started with a brief assessment of his current family, school, and extracurricular situations. Henry, in describing his current family situation, explained that he was living with his mother, who was an alcoholic and required a significant amount of his attention. He also had a paper route after school to help support them. Henry indicated that he had few friends and engaged in few social activities. When asked if anything bad had happened to him in the past few months, Henry related to the author how 3 weeks prior to the interview he had hit a hitchhiker with the family car when attempting to get onto the highway. He then told how the hitchhiker was currently in a coma in the hospital. This event was unknown to the school, and Henry had accepted this as another indication of the hopelessness of his life situation. During the clinical interview, it was determined that Henry was not suicidal, although he admitted to thoughts of death and morbid ideational themes. These latter cognitions seemed somewhat specific to the individual whom Henry had accidentally injured. Henry indicated that his life generally seemed quite worthless, and his view of the future suggested a hopeless perspective. However, at the present time he had no specific thoughts or intentions toward taking his own life. When asked, he reported that he had never made a suicide attempt, although about a year or so before he had been thinking about it, and had been troubled that he had such thoughts.

An examination of specific symptoms and symptom clusters suggested pervasive anhedonia, as indicated by his lack of pleasure and enjoyment of activities that he usually engaged in and found pleasurable. In addition to anhedonia, Henry indicated extensive self-deprecatory ideation, and associated thoughts of worthlessness and helplessness. Given his sad appearance and very low mood, Henry demonstrated a distinctly dysphoric mood. When queried, Henry indicated that he had been feeling this way for about 2 months, and that his low mood had been going on even before the automobile accident occurred. He indicated that he had been feeling depressed for some time and generally felt that things were pretty bad and unlikely to get better. Henry also complained of general fatigue and difficulty concentrating on school. Going to school required a significant amount of effort and, according to Henry, was getting more and more difficult. Additional symptoms included occasional tearfulness and difficulty falling asleep at night (initial insomnia). A diagnosis of major depression without melancholia was made, with the possibility that a previous episode had occurred approximately 1 year previously.

SELECTION OF TREATMENT

The treatment approach utilized was a multimodal procedure that can be characterized as a cognitive–behavioral intervention. Cognitive–behavioral programs have been used in the treatment of depression in adults and, with appropriate modifications, have been shown to be effective with children (Stark *et al.,* 1987) and adolescents (Reynolds & Coats, 1986). The author and colleagues have developed structured treatment manuals for the application of these therapeutic procedures with depressed youngsters. For the most part, these procedures draw from a number of theoretical models of depression, including self-control, cognitive, social reinforcement, and learned helplessness. Therapeutic components based on these models are integrated into a logical sequence of skill-building activities and homework assignments.

Therapy was brief and intense, administered in 10 50-minute sessions twice a week, over a 5-week period. This short-term approach to psychotherapy is consistent with many contemporary psychotherapeutic procedures used with adults. In youngsters, relatively brief, structured psychotherapies designed to be administered over a 5- to 10-week period are advisable because they quickly demonstrate to the youngster that a change in their affect can occur if they maintain compliance to the therapeutic regime.

Treatment compliance is a major concern in the treatment of depressed youngsters. Depressive symptoms of fatigue, withdrawal, feelings of worthlessness, and generalized anhedonia contribute to the difficulty often experienced by the therapist when treating depressed youngsters. Further, many of the depressive cognitions experienced by children and adolescents suggest to them that nothing they do helps, and that the future is hopeless. These factors, combined with the developmentally normal perspective of children and some adolescents that curing a hurt means making it go away quickly, support the application of effective brief psychotherapies. Without the relatively quick demonstration that change is possible, negative, dysfunctional cognitions, such as hopelessness, become even more entrenched because there was an initial promise of symptom relief. Children seem especially in need of proof that therapeutic relief will be forthcoming if they do as the therapist asks.

In conducting therapy for depression with children, it is advisable to incorporate enjoyable "fun" activities within the therapy session and, whenever possible, to utilize such activities in teaching of skills and concepts. Incorporating enjoyable activities, such as role playing, within a friendly, relaxed, "fun" therapeutic atmosphere will assist in engaging the youngster in therapy and complying with treatment requirements. Such activities, used in conjunction with reinforcement, and applied contingent upon treatment compliance and involvement, assist in the youngster's acceptance of therapy.

The short-term nature of the therapy described below allows for the youngster to quickly build self-help and social problem-solving skills and, with the guidance of the therapist, to apply these skills that they have mastered to real-life situations. The basic tenets of the treatment focused on the training of self-control skills, including self-monitoring, self-evaluation, and self-reinforcement. These components were introduced within a framework that emphasized the learning and application of these skills within a self-change plan.

Reinforcement was provided during and at the completion of the treatment program contingent on involvement in therapy (attending sessions, completing homework assignments). The treatment program utilized a structured treatment manual, with sessions and their rationale clearly delineated. The basic focus of the program involved the teaching of specific self-help skills, within what might be called a psychoeducational model. Like depression in adults, depression in children and adolescents is often characterized by behavioral and cognitive deficits and/or distortions. Therefore, a major emphasis of therapy was the modification of cognitive distortions and development of cognitive strategies where deficits are evidenced.

COURSE OF TREATMENT

As noted above, the treatment selected was a short-term psychotherapy, relatively structured in presentation and originally designed to be completed in a 5- to 6-week period. The time and length of treatment is not a set requirement, and it should be considered quite flexible in that it may be extended in duration of sessions (i.e., some sessions may go to 75 minutes or more) and in number of sessions. The latter is recommended, especially with younger children, because it allows for therapeutic components to be presented with greater specifications and examples, as well as providing the youngster with more opportunities to practice the homework exercises and receive and act upon therapist-provided feedback. It should also be noted that treatment was administered within a group format, with four depressed youngsters, including Henry, in the group. In using the group format, we have found that it works quite well as a means of providing therapy, as well as allowing youngsters to see that their problems are not unique only to them. Furthermore, it provides a mechanism for developing social skills and often results in a time-limited social support network. Each therapy session is described in summary form below, along with a delineation of specific therapeutic goals and examples of treatment elements.

Session 1. The first session began with a general introduction to the goals of therapy and discussion of some general problems manifested by depressed persons. A rationale for the treatment was presented with examples specific to depressed youngsters. This included a discussion of how mood is related to activity and how in order to overcome depression it is necessary to understand the relationship between mood and activity. It was discussed how people who are depressed tend to focus on unpleasant events to the exclusion of positive activities, such that the therapist would say, "For example, if you were complimented by a friend during the day or did well on a difficult exam, but later lost in a game of tennis or had to stay with your mother instead of see your friends, you might be likely to think of the negative events rather than the compliment or doing well on the test." During this session, it was explained how people who are depressed focus on immediate rather than delayed outcomes, especially delayed rewards. These points were related to an explanation of self-monitoring and the importance of making accurate self-observations for influencing mood. Henry was provided with a logbook for use in self-monitoring positive activities, as well as recording his mood at the end of each day. The logbook also included a list of pleasant activities that had been generated to assist Henry by providing examples of pleasant events to self-monitor. Henry was instructed to use a new log sheet for each day, and to bring his logbook to each session. As a homework assignment, Henry was directed to record his daily mood and positive activities in the self-monitoring log.

Session 2. The second session focused on teaching Henry the relationship between mood and activity, and how mood can be changed by changing activity. The self-monitoring logs for several days were examined to see how the number of pleasant activities engaged in related to the mood of the day. Praise for completing the homework assignment was given, with an emphasis on the effort taken and a discussion of the aspects that were completed correctly. In this session, as in all others, very little attention on the part of the therapist was spent in attending to complaints or negative statements.

As a specific activity, Henry was asked to graph the number of positive activities along with the associated mood for each day for a week. Using his self-monitoring logs for the past few days, Henry graphed the number of positive activities along with his mood, on a 1 (low)- to 10 (positive)-point scale, on a specially prepared graph that the therapist provided. In this exercise, Henry was told, "Look at the one or two days on which your mood was the most positive and figure out the number of positive activities or pleasant events for those days. Now do the same for the days that your mood was the lowest. Is the number of activities higher for the days when your mood was good?" Further explanation on the connection between mood and activities was presented, with Henry encouraged to identify those activities that were consistently associated with a positive mood. He was also told to try and increase those activities related to positive mood, and to continue to self-monitor both positive activities and daily mood.

Session 3. In this session, the tendency of depressed persons to attend to immediate rather than long-term, delayed outcomes of their behavior and events was noted. Cognitive distortions and the tendency to view the world in a negative manner were presented as a way depressed persons maintain their low affect. Henry was given an Immediate vs. Delayed Effects Worksheet and was told to choose four different activities from his self-monitoring logs during the past week and to indicate the effects for each activity. Effects can be viewed as either positive or negative, and have immediate or delayed consequences. As an example, Henry was told that the activity of eating an ice cream sundae might be viewed as having the immediate positive effect of tasting good, and the delayed positive effect associated with getting more done if one takes a break every now and then. Conversely, it might be viewed as having the immediate negative effect of costing too much money, and the delayed negative effect of gaining weight. All of these are potential outcomes and Henry was asked: "Which are easier to think of, immediate or long-term effects? Positive or negative effects? Which are you more likely to think of when you are doing something?"

Henry was then instructed to fill in the effects from four activities selected from his self-monitoring logs. The tendency to selectively attend to immediate negative events, often to the exclusion of delayed positive outcomes, was noted as a characteristic of depressed persons. In this activity, Henry was told to attend more closely to the delayed positive outcomes of this behavior and events, and to fill in a positive delayed effect of at least one positive activity each day on his self-monitoring log.

Session 4.   During this session, the focus of therapy was in the initial development of self-evaluation skills and in attribution retraining. The emphasis of this session was on making accurate self-evaluations for success and failure, and on setting realistic, obtainable goals. A rationale was presented that depressed individuals often make inaccurate evaluations, particularly for their successes and failures. Thus, depressed persons hold faulty beliefs about their responsibility for events. This session explored the assumptions people make in assigning responsibility for events, and how accurate self-evaluations for the outcome of events can assist in reducing depression. The focus was on teaching Henry to accurately evaluate the extent to which his own effort, skill, and ability (or lack of these) were responsible for the occurrence of positive and negative events, as well as the extent to which other people, chance, or luck were responsible. The goal was for Henry to maake realistic and adaptive attributions (attribute failure to more external, unstable, and specific factors and success to internal, stable, global factors) for his behavior and events.

An Attribution of Responsibility exercise was presented to illustrate the assumptions people make in assigning credit, blame, or responsibility for various events, and how depressed individuals often make faulty assumptions about responsibility for both positive and negative events. Using the self-monitoring logs to identify several fairly important events, Henry was directed through an exercise designed to show how he had considerable responsibility for the positive events in his life, and how he was able to influence or increase these events. Likewise, examples of unpleasant events were used to illustrate to Henry that he was not solely responsible for their occurrence, and that in most cases these latter events could be attributed to external factors, such as others or chance. As a homework assignment, Henry was asked to continue to self-monitor on his daily log, and to record the percent to which he was responsible for each of the positive activities.

Session 5.   This session introduced the basic skills necessary for developing a self-change plan. The bases for a self-change plan were presented as (1) the belief that you can change, (2) knowing that self-change, like self-control, is a skill that can be learned, and (3) awareness that to change, one has to develop a self-change plan. Most of the session involved teaching how to make a self-change plan. This included how to specify a problem and decide what to change; how to collect baseline information and keep track of progress; discovering antecedents (events or conditions such as social situation, own feelings/behaviors, physical setting, behavior of other people) related to the problem and how to control these antecedents; discovering consequences of engaging in specific behaviors, with the understanding that we wish to increase behavior that is followed by positive consequences and decrease a behavior that is not followed by a positive behavior.

This session also assisted in helping Henry feel that the problems he faced could be overcome, and that he could have an active role in changing things for the better. The emphasis on skill building and positive change due to his own actions, effort, and ability was designed to promote a sense of self-efficacy or self-mastery. Henry was told that the next session would involve instruction in setting goals and contracting. As a homework assignment, Henry was requested to identify a specific problem to work on, and to begin to collect baseline information using a tally sheet. Included in this assignment were instructions to attend to antecedents and consequences of his behavior and events.

Session 6. This session continued training in self-change skills, with the focus in this session on setting realistic, obtainable goals and subgoals; contracting; and obtaining reinforcement. It was presented that depressed persons set unrealistically high goals for themselves, often setting themselves up for failure, and have poor self-evaluations. Henry was taught to select a realistic goal that was within his control, and to break this goal down into small subgoals. Goals should be modest and attainable, goals might be changed, and increasing goals should be done slowly, and only after a previous goal has been reached. It was stressed that Henry should make a contract or a specific agreement to reward himself if he accomplished a subgoal, with the specific reward determined in advance and awarded as close to the achievement of the goal as possible. Furthermore, the reward (reinforcer) should be one that made him feel good, was accessible, fit the effort expended in reaching the goal, and was under his control. (Note: With young children, the participation of parents in providing reinforcers is important.) A Goal-Setting Worksheet was passed out for Henry to develop a long-range goal and subgoals based on the problem he had identified in the previous session, and to begin collecting baseline information. The therapist provided feedback and praise for Henry's efforts to construct subgoals. As homework, Henry was told to further examine his goal and subgoals, making revisions to ensure that they were realistic, in his control, and specific.

Training in progressive relaxation techniques was introduced in this session. A rationale was presented highlighting the relationship between stress-related problems and depression. It was explained to Henry that the goal of muscle relaxation training was to reduce tension resulting from stress, and to allow for more accurate self-monitoring of mood, events, and the outcome of behavior. A standard program of progressive muscle relaxation exercises was provided, along with relaxation homework assignment log sheets.

Session 7. Once Henry had learned procedures for goal setting in Session 6 and had practiced these procedures, the process of self-reinforcement was presented in Session 7. The case was presented that depressed individuals do not self-reinforce sufficiently, and in fact may punish themselves too much. It was shown how systematic errors in thinking could lead to negative interpretations and self-evaluation, resulting in self-punishment. The emphasis of this session was to learn how to self-reward rather than self-punish by learning some basics of self-reinforcement. This was done in part through the development of a reward menu, which is a list of many enjoyable rewards, ranging in magnitude from large to small, and relatively obtainable.

Henry was instructed to develop a self-reward program, to assist in increasing his goal-related activities. It was pointed out that self-reward was a more effective way of producing desired long-range change, and that one goal should be to replace self-punishment with self-reward in his life. A sheet for developing a Reward Menu was passed out with the directions that rewards should be truly enjoyable, varying in magnitude from large to small, and relatively open to when he might obtain them. Rewards might be material things, such as clothes, or things to play with (i.e., electronic games or puzzles), of even activities, such as going to a movie, taking a hike, or eating out. Each reward on the menu was then assigned a point value from 1 to 10, depending on the magnitude of the reward. After Henry had done this, he was instructed to assign points (1 to 10) to the subgoals he had established earlier. He was then told to consider the points earned in carrying out his subgoals as applicable toward spending on the rewards on the menu, and to use the self-monitoring logs to keep track of points earned and spent. It was explained that it was important to cash points in as soon as possible so that the reward was contingent on performing and achieving the subgoal.

Session 8. In previous sessions, activities were focused on the increase of overt self-reinforcement and the decrease of over-self-punishment. In this session, Henry was taught procedures (similar in many respects to components of self-instruction training) for covert self-reinforcement. The rationale was presented that rewards or punishment might be overt (having or denying oneself a piece of cake) or covert (praising oneself or thinking about one's failures), and that people who were depressed tended to engage in extensive covert self-punishment, often to the exclusion of covert self-reward. To counteract this tendency, an exercise for increasing covert self-reinforcement was presented. Henry was first asked to make a list of positive self-statements that described his best qualities, assets, and achievements. He was then instructed to repeat this list of positive attributes to himself for 30 seconds. It was noted how difficult it often was for people to talk well of themselves to themselves. Henry was told to say something positive about himself to himself (covertly) every time he undertook one of his subgoals. For example, he might say to himself, "That was good, I'm making progress," or "I finished this just like I had planned to; I must be doing well."

Session 9. This session functioned as a check, review, and practice session. Of primary importance was checking Henry's compliance with the treatment components and instructions. This involved a check of how well he had monitored and increased his performance of positive activities or engagement in pleasant events, as shown by his self-monitoring logs. Henry was told that in addition to overt pleasant activities and events, such as going to a movie or to a party, pleasant thoughts could also be viewed as a positive activity to engage in, and as such were fairly covert and readily attainable.

In this session, the therapist checked on Henry's selection and revision of goals and subgoals and how well these goals met the criteria of controllability, attainability, and operationalization. The therapist provided praise and feedback for Henry's assignment of points to the subgoals and the creation of a reward menu for use in reinforcing the attainment of the subgoals, as well as for his list of positive self-statements for use as covert reinforcers for each subgoal achieved.

Session 10. This last session was a review of the basic principles that were presented relevant to the reduction of depression and the associated activities for instituting change. The therapist provided extensive praise and encouragement for Henry's compliance and therapeutic gains. It was important that Henry have a firm understanding of what he had learned, and that these skills should be maintained and practiced after the conclusion of therapy. This session focused on providing a sense of hopefulness and optimism about Henry's current level of affective functioning and his ability in the future to reduce his depression if it affected him again. At the beginning of the session, Henry completed a self-report depression questionnaire as well as a semistructured clinical interview. At this time, there were very few symptoms of depression evident. Upon recalling his previous response to the questions, the level and magnitude of change became evident to Henry. Henry could now accurately see the progress he had made. Nearly all of the major symptoms of depression were gone. He had no difficulty falling asleep, enjoyed engaging in activities, and showed an interest in school and being with his friends. Although his mother was still a problem, Henry felt capable of dealing with it and did not dwell on the negative aspects of this situation.

Additional Therapeutic Considerations

In the treatment for major depression described above, the depressed youngster was an adolescent. When treating children, it is advisable to increase the number of therapy sessions and to incorporate greater parental participation during treatment. This is especially necessary for increasing pleasant events, as well as in operationalizing a reinforcement schedule, where parents need to be involved in carrying out activities, providing transportation, and taking care of monetary costs.

The clinician should be aware that it is not unusual to find affective disorders in parents of children who are also depressed. The nature of this relationship is complicated by potential biological, psychosocial, environmental, and social learning causal links. For whatever the reason, depression (as well as many other psychopathologies) in one or both parents is a complicating factor in the treatment of depression in children and adolescents. Depression in parents is sometimes a difficult diagnosis to make since the primary client is the youngster, although a brief talk with both parents, individually and together, usually provides opportunity to determine the parents' affective status. Moreover, a depressed parent, especially one who is reluctant to seek treatment, may reinforce depressive cognitions and behaviors in the youngster. In this way, treatment may be compromised unless an effective therapeutic relationship can be developed with the parent for the good of the child. In our research, we have also found that marital discord is strongly related to depression in youngsters, especially in girls. Educating parents who are in conflict situations that any constructive actions they may take toward resolving their own conflict in an amicable manner should assist in the mental well-being of their youngster is a useful tactic, although not always effective with resistant families.

TERMINATION AND FOLLOW-UP

The treatment program utilized may be considered a brief psychotherapeutic procedure that is time-limited in structure. At the beginning of therapy, the program was described to Henry and a contract drawn, with reinforcement to be received contingent upon attendance and completion of homework assignments throughout the course of treatment as well as at the conclusion of the program.

At the completion of the primary treatment program, Henry was provided with additional therapeutic exercise forms and told to continue to self-monitor and engage in the therapy activities that were used as homework assignments. He was also allowed to select a major reward from a list prepared by the therapist (in conjunction with his mother). A 5-week follow-up evaluation was conducted with self-report depression measures and a clinical interview. At this time, Henry reported no significant depressive symptoms, and seemed fairly optimistic about the future. He was reminded to continue to utilize the procedures learned in therapy and to be observant for any reoccurrence of depression. Henry was reevaluated 1 year after therapy as part of the school's annual mental health screening, and he scored in a nondepressed range on the screening measure.

OVERALL EVALUATION

The cognitive–behavioral treatment for major depression described above has proven to be effective in treating children and adolescents. Modifications should be made for younger children, with extensive use of role-play and social problem-solving activities. In addition, the use of family involvement and family therapy as components of a broad-based intervention is recommended. Our knowledge to date on the treatment of depression in children and adolescents is predicated on modifications of treatment approaches for adults, as well as the melding of techniques, such as self-instructional training, that have been developed for use as components in the treatment of other disorders (i.e., impulsivity). The author and colleagues have found that cognitive—behavioral interventions with children and adolescents work quite well in a small-group format, with between three and five children who are relatively matched with regard to maturity level.

The treatment of major depression in children and adolescents must be undertaken with caution. A number of considerations should be noted prior to a therapist's beginning treatment. These include the determination of suicide potential, and whether the depression is concomitant to other pathology, such as conduct disorders, that may create a less than optimal therapeutic situation.

One additional clinical *caveat* should be made regarding the use of psychotherapy to treat major depression in children and adolescents. In the clinical case study presented here, the sole therapeutic technique was psychological in nature. The utilization of pharmacotherapy in conjunction with psychotherapy should be viewed as a recommended procedure for use with some depressed children and adolescents. Pharmacological treatment outcome studies with tricyclic antidepressants, such as imipramine, are somewhat mixed when comparisons are made with placebo conditions. However, the utility of antidepressants as an adjunct to producing a more receptive mood for the learning and development of skills and procedures taught within the psychotherapeutic milieu described above should not be overlooked. This latter recommendation may be particularly appropriate when dealing with extremely despondent youngsters who are unresponsive to engagement in therapy owing to their depressed condition.

In summary, the case study presented here represents an illustration of the treatment of major depression in youngsters that is predicated on our early experiences with psychologically based therapies for this purpose. It is anticipated that the treatment technology will advance from these beginnings. However, we do now know that efficacious treatment of depression in youngsters is possible.

REFERENCES

American Psychiatric Association. (1980). *Diagnostic and statistical manual of mental disorders* (3rd ed.). Washington, DC: Author.

Reynolds, W. M. (1985). Depression in childhood and adolescence: Diagnosis, assessment, intervention strategies and research. In T. R. Kratochwill (Ed.), *Advances in school psychology* (Vol. 4, pp. 133–189). Hillsdale, NJ: Erlbaum.

Reynolds, W. M. (1986). A model for the screening and identification of depressed children and adolescents in school settings. *Professional School Psychology, 1,* 117–129.

Reynolds, W. M., & Coats, K. I. (1986). A comparison of cognitive-behavioral therapy and relaxation training for the treatment of depression in adolescents. *Journal of Consulting and Clinical Psychology, 54,* 653–660.

Stark, K. D., Reynolds, W. M., & Kaslow, N. J. (1987). A comparison of the relative efficacy of self-control therapy and a behavioral problem-solving therapy for depression in children. *Journal of Abnormal Child Psychology, 15,* 91–113.

CHAPTER 9

Mild Developmental Retardation

JOHN T. NEISWORTH and RONALD A. MADLE

DESCRIPTION OF THE DISORDER

By definition, mental retardation (MR) involves deficits in learning and adapting to new situations. It is, however, a multifacted disorder that often includes additional problems.

Various diagnostic manuals define mental retardation as a condition with three components. The first is a level of measured intellectual functioning that is 2 or more standard deviations below the mean. On most standardized tests (with a standard deviation of 15 or 16), this means an IQ of 69 or lower. Second, the individual must exhibit delays in the development of various adaptive behaviors: that is, day-to-day skills needed to adapt to the world. These skills are, of course, the primary domain of the behavior therapist in working with the retarded (Neisworth & Madle, 1982). The last criterion for MR is occurrence of deficits before age 18, thus excluding intellectual impairment acquired throughout adulthood and the cognitive deficits associated with senility. Given these criteria, the term *developmental* retardation is preferred by the authors and is used throughout this chapter.

"Mildly developmentally retarded" refers to individuals who present measured IQs in the range of 55 to 69 on the Wechsler Intelligence Scales. Some diagnostic systems, especially the educational one, consider indi-

JOHN T. NEISWORTH • Department of Special Education, Pennsylvania State University, Moore Building, University Park, Pennsylvania 16802.   RONALD A. MADLE • Laurelton Center, Laurelton, Pennsylvania 17835.

viduals as mildly retarded with IQs as low as 50 and as high as 80. In the educational system the group is often referred to as "educable." The adaptive behavior deficits of this group, while minimal, are often numerous. Many of these, such as fears and social interaction problems, are the same as in the intellectually average. The most common deficits are in academic and social areas.

Mildly retarded individuals usually go undetected during infancy and early childhood since the deviation from normal children is minimal. By school age, however, they show accumulated and, thus, noticeable learning and associated socioemotional delays. Mildly retarded youngsters tend to learn slowly and have poor language and communication skills, resulting in academic delays. Academically, their achievement is noticeably below the norm. Learning tasks requiring abstraction, reasoning, and concept formation are especially difficult for them. They tend to have counterproductive work and study habits, inefficient learning styles, and poor time-on-task behavior. This often leads to problems such as absenteeism, immature and impulsive behavior, lack of motivation, and a variety of other emotional disturbances that stem from coping with academic demands. Socially, they usually adapt poorly to school, show little interest in academic activities, and engage in uncooperative, disruptive, and sometimes aggressive classroom behavior. Most mildly retarded youngsters will not display any serious sensory or motor involvement. In contrast to the biological causes of more severe forms of developmental retardation, mild retardation is usually thought to result from psychosocial factors, such as low socioeconomic status, poor education, and family disorganization.

CASE IDENTIFICATION

Billy S. is a 13-year-old white male of average height and weight, muscular, with brown hair and dark complexion. He attended sixth-grade classes in school for subjects such as social studies, industrial arts, and gym. He was placed in a noncategorical resource room at school for his core subjects (math, reading, spelling, and English) owing to his academic problems.

Billy lived with his mother, his stepfather, and his younger half-sister, Beth, age 6, in a small, rural town. Mr. S. was employed as an auto mechanic; Mrs. S. was a homemaker. They had been married for 7 years. While slightly below the intellectual norm, they did not appear to be retarded. Mrs. S. had dropped out of school in the 11th grade, while Mr. S. completed a vocational–technical curriculum in auto repair and was graduated from high school. The couple had few marital problems, except for occasional conflicts as to how the children should be disciplined.

PRESENTING COMPLAINTS

Billy had been referred for behavioral treatment by his parents at the suggestion of the school psychologist, primarily because of poor academic performance in school and because he was also becoming more difficult to control in the school setting. He increasingly refused to comply with his teachers' requests and occasionally was openly disobedient and defiant. He frequently arrived late at school and on occasion was truant. When Billy was in school he invested little effort in trying to learn. He often was off task or appeared to be daydreaming. When he did complete his schoolwork, it was done impulsively and incompletely. While he was not diagnosed as "hyperactive" in the classic sense, he was impulsive and "got into things" at school. He was involved in frequent fights and arguments with his peers. Recently, he was caught stealing items from another student.

Billy's parents reported that many of the same problems—in particular, noncompliance and arguing—were problems at home. Billy also was getting into more and more fights with other youths at a video game parlor, which was the local hangout. On one occasion of fighting he was brought home by the police.

HISTORY

Billy was born to a couple living in a small town in a predominantly rural state. His birth was unremarkable, although he was almost 1 month premature. The biological father deserted Billy and the mother when Billy was $1\frac{1}{2}$; Billy does not remember his father. After her husband left, Billy's mother went on and off welfare until she married an auto mechanic when Billy was 6. The family had difficult times during Billy's preschool years. Billy was cared for by numerous part-time sitters while his mother had part-time jobs in knitting mills and as a cleaning woman. There was little unusual about Billy's early physical development, although there were some minor delays in developmental milestones such as toileting, dressing, and language. The mother was an authoritarian, quick-tempered woman who frequently yelled at the slightest provocation. She would often spank or hit Billy when she disapproved of his behavior. Billy spent as little time at home as possible as he grew older, possibly an under-standable adaptive escape/avoidance pattern.

Billy's first-grade teacher was also strict and used aversive methods of discipline. Billy spent most of his time in school trying to avoid doing schoolwork. He was reported to have great difficulty sitting still for any length of time. When promoted to second grade, Billy was placed in a special section for slow learners, where he continued his pattern of avoiding schoolwork. With some remediation in this class, however, he learned all his letters and began to read simple words. In the third grade he was held back a year. Billy continued in special sections until he reached middle school. There, he was placed in regular classes with enrollment in a noncategorical resource room for his core subjects. Throughout school he increasingly got into fights and arguments with his classmates. It seemed that, as in the case of his mother, the slightest provocations would result in strong and impulsive reactions. In middle school he occasionally was seen by the school counselor, who attempted to help him control his chronic fighting.

About 1½ years ago he began helping his stepfather at the auto repair shop on weekends. He had already learned a good deal about repairing cars and really seemed to enjoy working on them. At this point Billy spends most of his spare time either at the local video game parlor or helping out at the auto repair shop.

ASSESSMENT

A comprehensive developmental and behavioral assessment was used, as recommended by most current literature (Neisworth & Bagnato, in press). This process included direct testing, interviews and reports, and, when possible, observational measures. Regardless of the mode employed, the emphasis of the assessment was on behavioral description rather than on diagnosis. Billy's status on the dimensions of concern were described in order to prescribe a comprehensive treatment program.

Standardized Measures

Several standardized measures were administered in order to determine overall intellectual and adaptive skill levels. The Wechsler Intelligence Scale for Children (WISC-R), used with 6- to 16-year-olds, was administered. Billy obtained a full scale IQ of 63. This placed him well within the range for mild developmental retardation. His verbal and performance IQs were 62 and 69, respectively, indicating somewhat stronger functioning in the performance areas, as is often the case in mild retardation. The results on the Peabody Individual Achievement Test Provided by the school indicated that Billy was functioning at 1.5 to 3 years below grade level in the areas measured (mathematics, reading recognition, reading comprehension, spelling, and general information).

As a measure of his overall adaptive behavior, the Public School Version of the AAMD Adaptive Behavior Scale was completed by Billy's resource room teacher. This scale measures both adaptive and maladaptive behavior domains. The scores Billy obtained on this scale generally were typical of those obtained by mildly retarded children. Several areas were, however, particularly low. In Part I he showed weak functioning on the self-directed and socialization sections. In Part II, which measures maladaptive behaviors, he manifested problems on the inappropriate interpersonal manners section.

Behavioral Assessment

In order to conduct a more detailed behavioral assessment, the school psychologist assisted in scheduling a meeting at the school between the behavior therapist, resource room teacher (Mrs. K.), and Billy's parents. Prior to this meeting, Billy's psychological evaluations and reports from teachers were reviewed for areas of concern. At the meeting, the overall picture of the presenting problems was discussed. From this discussion the parents and the teacher helped the therapist to develop a list of Billy's discrete behavioral excesses and deficits, as well as behaviors that occurred in inappropriate situations. The teacher and the parents then rank-ordered the problems to identify those most in need of modification.

Finally, the behavior therapist discussed with the parents and the teacher the conditions under which the behaviors occurred or did not occur, as well as the existing consequences for the behaviors. This resulted in the behavioral specification list shown in Table 1. From this list, several specific target behaviors were selected for change in both the school and the home setting.

At the end of the session both parents and Mrs. K. were given data collection sheets (with an explanation of their use) for collecting data on the problem behaviors for the week.

The following week, Billy was interviewed by the behavior therapist to obtain his input about the problems. At first, Billy had some difficulty understanding what the problems were. From his perspective, the fighting and arguing were simply the way he "had to be" to deal with others who

Table 1
Problems, Settings, and Consequences for Billy

Problem behavior	Consequences
	School problems
Arguing and fighting with classmates	Talks with school counselor, being placed in detention
Daydreaming and off task	Prompting by teacher, occasional criticism
Incomplete and sloppy assignments	Low grades, teacher disapproval
Noncompliance	Prompting by teacher, occasional criticism
Arriving for school late	Teacher disapproval, scolding by mother
Being truant from school	Talks with school counselor, detention
	Home problems
Arguing and fighting at the video game parlor	Scolding by parents
Talking back to his mother	Screaming by mother, spankings when younger

bothered him. After all, his mother was doing the same thing with him. The interview showed that Billy was highly motivated to learn when it came to repairing cars, but in school he avoided trying to learn whenever possible. He had a long history of failing and, as with many mildly retarded individuals, seemed to be less upset by not trying than by actively trying and being punished by failing. That is, he received little positive reinforcement (ratio strain) for trying but considerable punishment whenever he failed. The only exception to this was when he worked on cars with his stepfather. Mr. S. was patient, and he carefully and positively corrected Billy's mistakes, lavishing much praise on him when he did well. Included in this session was an assessment of what behaviors Billy saw as problems. These included the way his mother and his teachers reacted to his learning problems and the difficulty he had in handling the teasing of other children.

SELECTION OF TREATMENT

Billy's behavior and the surrounding conditions suggested that several factors were operating. First, Billy found that achievement situations, especially in school tasks, were followed by punishing consequences. While initially he was described as "unmotivated to learn," this was an apt description only at school and quite understandable, given the irrelevant and aversive school circumstances. At the auto repair shop Billy learned tasks rapidly and was excited about learning more. This situation is not uncommon among children with learning problems; they have experienced so much past failure that school situations are actively avoided. Many of his social/interpersonal problems appeared to be manifestations of such avoidance. Noncompliance, lateness, truancy, daydreaming, and being off task were all effective methods of avoiding schoolwork. Even the impulsive, sloppy schoolwork seemed to be an aspect of avoidance.

The treatment component selected for dealing with the motivational and failure problems consisted of standard operant techniques. A plan was developed that involved a consistent, positive approach to learning, with clear, graded tasks (task analysis/shaping) that would lead to success and liberal positive reinforcement of learning. Since the problem was broad-based, his parents and teachers all were involved in program implementation using a mediated, *in situ* approach. Given his mother's use of aversive procedures, both parents were also trained in the use of basic positive reinforcement methods. While the mother never really changed her fundamentally aversive approach, she did begin to employ some positive remarks, which seemed to surprise and influence Billy. Regular consultation with the teachers was also incorporated with the resource room teacher, who was the in-school coordinator of the program.

The second major problem area tackled was the fighting and arguing with peers, teachers, and parents. Billy's early history involved primarily aversive control of his behavior, with little opportunity to learn appropriate, adaptive social interaction. As a consequence, he fought and argued, since he did not have the requisite social skills to deal with teasing and other strained social situations. For the social skills deficits, a clinic-based social skills program was used (Goldstein, Sprafkin, Gershaw, & Klein, 1980). Billy was seen weekly in structured social skills training sessions conducted by the behavior therapist.

An overall motivational program was also established for Billy during a session with him, his parents, and the resource room teacher. The program consisted of a contingency contract specifying the behaviors to be changed, the consequences for the behaviors, and the individuals responsible for implementation of consequences.

COURSE OF TREATMENT

Treatment proceeded in three related but separate components: contingency contracting, parent/teacher training and consultation, and social skills training sessions.

Contingency Contracting

In the first actual treatment session following the assessment phase, the contingency contract to be used was developed jointly with Billy, Mrs. K., and his parents. As with most joint meetings, it was held at the end of the school day. The list of target behaviors previously established was reviewed and behaviors to be exhibited or not exhibited were identified for both home and school settings. Billy's teacher and parents, with the assistance of the behavior therapist, then identified consequences and conditions that could be used for each objective. As part of this process, the therapist explained the Premack Principle to the teacher and parents and how Billy's interest in cars and video games might be used as preferred activities to follow the desired target behaviors. While several consequences were built into the contract, the primary one was that Premacking (e.g., a "good" report from school) allowed Billy to work at the auto repair shop on the weekend. A specific allowance was also built into the contract that was used as a consequence for completing homework assignments. Some behaviors, such as truancy, lateness for school, and fighting, resulted in restriction from the video game parlor for 1 to 3 days. Additional data collection sheets were also provided and were used to collect daily data on Billy's target behaviors.

The contingency contract was explained to Billy. Initially, he had some difficulty understanding the conditions of the contract; with adaptation of the language and appropriate paraphrasing, Billy was pleased with the contract. He said it was one of the first times in his life that he felt he was being treated more like an adult (showing responsibility for his behavior) than like a little child. The use of training sessions for the social skills deficits was also presented to Billy at this session.

Parent Training

Billy's parents attended the initial parent training session the week after the contingency contract session. They were given a short quiz (O'Dell, Tarler-Benlolo, & Flynn, 1979) to test their knowledge of parenting skills and behavior modification. This was followed by a discussion of the importance of positive reinforcement and guidance/prompting in helping Billy achieve increased success. At the end of the session they were given a copy of *Families* (Patterson, 1971). They were to read this and, the following week, attend a session to discuss the book and to retake the quiz. Any questions they had about the methods were answered, and several situations were role-played to help apply the procedures. Both parents were enthusiastic about the methods, although the mother continued to have some problems in using positive consequences for Billy's behavior.

The parents were instructed to call the therapist at any time during the week to discuss situations that they had difficulty in handling. Weekly meetings were established to discuss and reinforce use of the procedures, as well as to review the data on Billy's behaviors.

Parent/Teacher Consultation

The weekly meetings with the parents and the teacher were held for the first month following program implementation to review Billy's progress, to offer suggestions, and to adjust the techniques being used.

At even the first review session, the data looked promising. Billy was not late for school at all and had improved his compliance at school. The data showed that he was off task about 37% of the time, as compared with a baseline of 73%. He was still having difficulty with arguments and not complying with his mother's requests. To help with this issue, the contingency contract was amended to include time playing a home video game if there were no instances of noncompliance at home each day.

By the fourth review session, Billy was on task 87% of the time, had been late only once, and was beginning to show a decline in his frequency of arguments with classmates and peers at the video game parlor. Eight weeks into the program, the data showed continuing improvements in all target behaviors.

Social Skills Training

Social skills training with Billy was begun the week after the contracting session. The skill areas included were from three areas of the Goldstein *et al.* (1980) program, but these were modified for an individual rather than a group approach. The specific skills taught were expressing your feelings, understanding the feelings of others, using self-control, responding to teasing, avoiding trouble with others, keeping out of fights, dealing with being left out, and responding to failure. They were covered in four weekly sessions, with two skills per session.

The format for each session consisted of reviewing the use of the skills taught the previous week and then discussing the steps involved in the new skill to be learned. For example, in responding to teasing, Billy was told you need to first decide if you are being teased (are others making jokes about you? whispering about you?). Then you think about ways of dealing with the teasing (gracefully accept it, make a joke of it, ignore it, or leave the situation). Last, you have to choose what you will do and then do it. Following this component, the therapist role-played an appropriate situation from the school or neighborhood and guided Billy through the specified steps. This was done two or three times for each skill with progressively less therapist assistance. Finally, the therapist provided systematic performance feedback for behavior improvement.

Billy responded well to this instruction and gradually began to use the skills in the natural setting. Throughout the sessions he was increasingly pleased with the responses he was getting from the other youths, both at school and in the neighborhood. The data received from home and school also indicated that fighting and arguing had become much less frequent. In fact, by the sixth week of the social skills training, the fights had stopped completely, although there was still an occasional argument.

TERMINATION

Given a standard (nontherapeutic or prosthetic) environment, developmental retardation is a lifelong disability. Thus, there is no real termination of treatment, only the termination of a specific intervention episode. In this case, the treatment for the presenting problems that brought Billy to the behavior therapist began to be withdrawn 12 weeks after treatment was begun. The social skills sessions were terminated completely and the frequency of review sessions was reduced from weekly to monthly for a 3-month period. The contingency contract and continued data collection by the parents and school remained in force and an essential part of the program. The parents were cautioned that Billy would possibly need additional assistance when new situations arose, since developmentally retarded youth are not as likely to adapt previously learned skills to novel situations. They were told to contact the therapist for additional work if new behaviors occurred or if the old ones reappeared.

FOLLOW-UP

Monthly follow-up telephone calls were made to both the parents and the resource room teacher for a period of 3 months after the treatment sessions had been terminated. During these calls, the data recorded on the target behaviors were reviewed and the parents and teacher were given suggestions for dealing with any problems that arose. The calls indicated that Billy had shown some minimal backsliding during this interval but did not require additional treatment sessions.

OVERALL EVALUATION

The case described was a composite but typical case of a mildly developmentally retarded youngster who displayed school avoidance and social skills problems. The problems were dealt with through a combination of *in situ* contingency contracting, parent training, consultation, and individual skill-based therapy sessions over a period of 3 months, followed by several months of follow-up. Of particular concern in this type of case was the reliance on a model of home–school cooperation. Too frequently, attempts are made to deal with these problems in only one setting. Overall, the treatment program was successful even though there was some mild recurrence of problems by the end of the follow-up period.

Throughout the case study, there was an emphasis on use of a multisource and multicomponent approach for both assessment and treatment; several sources (parents, teacher, psychologist) and assessment devices (observational systems, standardized devices, interviews) were employed. Further, treatment was ecological (rather than "clinic"-centered) and involved several settings and change agents. Conceptually, Billy's problems were seen as behaviors rather than traits, and intervention consisted primarily of behavior therapy (social/instructional engineering) rather than "personality adjustment" or "psychotherapy."

REFERENCES

Goldstein, A. P., Sprafkin, R. P., Gershaw, N. J., & Klein, P. (1980). *Skillstreaming the adolescent: A structured learning approach to teaching prosocial skills.* Champaign, IL: Research Press.

Neisworth, J. T., & Bagnato, S. J. (in press). Diagnosis and assessment of developmental retardation. In V. B. Van Hasselt & M. Hersen (Eds.), New York: Plenum Press.

Neisworth, J. T., & Madle, R. A. (1982). Retardation. In A. S. Bellack, M. Hersen, & A. E. Kazdin (Eds.), *International handbook of behavior modification and behavior therapy* (pp. 853–890). New York: Plenum Press.

O'Dell, S. L., Tarler-Benlolo, L., & Flynn, J. M. (1979). An instrument to measure knowledge of behavioral principles as applied to children. *Journal of Behavior Therapy and Experimental Psychiatry, 10,* 29–34.

Patterson, G. R. (1971). *Families.* Champaign, IL: Research Press.

CHAPTER 10

Severe and Profound Mental Retardation

JOHNNY L. MATSON and LARRY R. FRIEDT

DESCRIPTION OF THE DISORDER

Severely and profoundly mentally retarded persons present a challenge to service providers because multiple physical and emotional problems are often present. Conceptions of this group of individuals have changed dramatically for the better in the past few decades. Severely and profoundly mentally retarded persons were once considered hopeless and untrainable (Berkson & Landesman-Dwyer, 1977). This situation is no longer accepted because research has shown that progress can be made when training these persons. Today, service providers are focusing on "active" treatment, when in the past the standard of service delivery emphasized primarily custodial care and medical services. However, not all service providers have adopted this more optimistic view. Consequently, not all of the severely and profoundly retarded persons are given the treatment needed to improve in overall behavior and independent living. On the other hand, litigation, social policy, and great advancements in assessment and treatment have made the rehabilitation movement national, and one that is accelerating in scope and sophistication (Matson & Mulick, 1983). In our chapter we will attempt to outline some of the major issues and characteristics of severely and profoundly retarded persons. Also, a description of some recent innovative approaches to be-

JOHNNY L. MATSON and LARRY R. FRIEDT • Department of Psychology, Louisiana State University, Baton Rouge, Louisiana 70803-5501.

havior therapy will be provided. It is hoped that more providers will adopt an "active" treatment model in the future.

Persons with severe and profound mental retardation represent a heterogeneous group of individuals that constitute 8% of all mentally retarded persons (Whitman, Scibak, & Reid, 1983). It has been estimated that there are approximately 250,000 severely and 100,000 profoundly mentally retarded persons in the United States. There is considerable variability among individuals with severe and profound mental retardation. In general, the profoundly retarded individual functions intellectually at a level of up to approximately 2 to $2\frac{1}{2}$ years in mental age, whereas the severely retarded individual functions intellectually at a level of up to approximately 4 years in mental age (Cleland, 1979). To contrast the differences between these groups, persons with profound mental retardation generally exhibit less speech, have more sensory, skeletal, and physical abnormalities, and are more destructive. Cleland (1979) states that profoundly mentally retarded individuals are the most "fragile" of all human beings. He further suggests that persons with profound mental retardation have a high threshold for pain, although this hypothesis has not been demonstrated empirically. Such high thresholds for pain could help explain why self-injury is a relatively common disorder in this group of individuals as well as in the severely mentally retarded group.

Severely and profoundly retarded individuals have in the past been placed in institutions and therefore represent a large percentage of all retarded persons who are institutionalized. One issue that remains unresolved is whether severely and profoundly mentally retarded individuals are a qualitatively distinct group or if they are merely functioning at a lower level than other mentally retarded individuals (Berkson & Landesman-Dwyer, 1977). No resolution to this issue is possible at this time. However, whether these persons are qualitatively different or not, their lower level of functioning does influence how much effort is required in caring for them. For this reason, it often becomes necessary for the family to seek outside assistance.

Most severely and profoundly mentally retarded individuals live with their natural families during their early years. However, on average these individuals are more likely to be referred out of their homes for professional assistance at a younger age than either the mildly or moderately mentally retarded groups (Berkson & Landesman-Dwyer, 1977). Consequently, for those who are placed in institutions, there is often little, if any, contact with family members. This situation has come under increasing criticism in recent years, leading to greater efforts at community placement and parental support. Residential placements may be the most appropriate in some of these cases. However, in many situations little has been done to improve the quality of life for severely and profoundly mentally retarded individuals.

Problem Areas

Many problems are common to this group of individuals. One of the greatest difficulties to resolve is the limited communication between the mentally retarded person and others. Often, little if any speech is present, consisting only of short simple statements ("yes" or "no") or gestures. Because of such limited speech, one cannot be sure if the individual is hungry or in pain, or has some other need to be met. The lack of social interaction skills and abilities leads to greater isolation of the severely and profoundly retarded person and more frustration for staff designated to deal with these problems.

Medical difficulties are a second major problem area common in persons with severe and profound mental retardation. Mori and Masters (1980) concluded that the more severe the mental retardation, the greater the probability of physically handicapping conditions. These conditions often interfere with habilitative programming designed to improve quality of life. Therefore, in addition to limited intellectual functioning, severely and profoundly retarded individuals are often ill and unable to participate in their habilatative programming. Such confounding variables can slow progress dramatically. Some of the medical disturbances common in these individuals are metabolic disorders, seizures, diabetes, heart disease, respiratory disease, and gastrointestinal disorders. Also, many behavior problems are especially common in this group. Among the most serious are self-injury, stereotypies, pica, agitation, and poor impulse control.

The most current thinking is that it is important to focus on what these persons can do and not on what they cannot do. Many of these individuals have been neglected for years. Therefore, any attempts to train severely and profoundly retarded individuals can help to improve their lives. Behavior therapy has been perhaps the single most important therapeutic modality in assisting such individuals.

CASE IDENTIFICATION AND PRESENTING COMPLAINTS

Since self-injurious behavior is a severe problem that occurs frequently in severely and profoundly mentally retarded individuals, the following case of self-injury was chosen as an example of their behavioral treatment.

Susan is a profoundly mentally retarded black female resident at a large intermediate care facility for mentally retarded individuals. Currently, she lives on a large open ward with 29 other severely and profoundly mentally retarded individuals. Susan has been in an institution for 19 years and is 38 years old. Her physical appearance is striking, since she is 4 feet 6 inches tall and weighs 95 pounds. Moreover, she has a large red swollen area on the left side of her face next to her eye. Several chronic physical problems are also present, including a large decubitus ulcer on her left buttock, multiple ulcers on the skin surrounding her bladder, and recurrent bladder infections. These physical problems frequently interfere with her progress, since she will not cooperate when they are acute. Furthermore, her physician frequently restricts her to the ward area or to bed until she recovers. Thus, she is often unable to participate in recreational and other activities that require her ability to move about.

Susan has several other limitations. One critical limitation is that she is nonverbal, communicating only with moans and gestures. She also lacks several self-help skills. For example, she has limited dressing and toileting skills. She does have some abilities, however, such as feeding skills and ambulation (although she walks awkwardly with a broad-based heel–toe gait).

Self-injurious behavior in many cases could be viewed as a type of stereotypy, because it is highly repetitive and occurs at harm to the client. In contrast, self-injury often results in serious physical harm. Typical of Susan's self-injurious behaviors are head hitting, eye gouging, hand biting, and head banging. (See Gorman-Smith & Matson, 1985, for a review of this topic.)

In Susan's case, the target behaviors include face and body hitting as well as finger biting. These responses are ritualistic and repetitive, and seem to increase in rate when she is agitated. This sequence begins with Susan hitting her elbow on her knee, then using her fist to hit the back of her neck, followed by hitting the side of her face beside her left eye. This entire sequence takes about 5 seconds. Susan's behavior has resulted in large reddened sores in each of the three areas where physical contact is made. These areas become infected frequently and pose a constant medical problem. In addition to the medical difficulty, such ritualistic behavior interferes with the programming to teach her self-help skills. The direct-care staff interact with Susan by trying to make her stop hitting herself instead of devoting the time to teaching adaptive skills. This behavior has led to frustration of her direct-care workers and their decreased interaction with other clients because Susan requires frequent attention. The supervisor on Susan's unit asked for help in dealing with this problem because she stated that the behavior was "getting worse."

HISTORY

Susan was the 9th of 14 children born to a poor rural family. Prenatal development included many complications. Early in the pregnancy her mother had frequent occurrences of nausea and vomiting that lasted throughout the day, which was followed later by toxemia and several close calls with miscarriage. Birth was preceded by 72 hours of difficult labor, which ended with a breech presentation of the infant. Spina bifida was present at birth, and the child underwent surgery before her first birthday to correct meningomyelocele (this condition is a protrusion of the membranes and spinal cord through a defect in the vertebral column). Surgery was successful and the child returned home after 2 weeks. At 7 months of age the child developed bronchial pneumonia and was again hospitalized. Yet another medical problem (hydrocephalus) was discovered when Susan was 3 years of age. These numerous and severe complications proved to be overwhelming to the family.

In general, Susan's development was extremely delayed, and some very rudimentary developmental milestones have never been achieved. She began walking at $2\frac{1}{2}$ years of age, no comprehensive language has developed, and toileting skills are impaired.

Susan lived at home in a small three-bedroom house with 13 siblings before she was institutionalized. The family was, and remains, very poor. Her father was a hardworking man with limited education and a low-paying job. He was simultaneously employed in two jobs as a janitor and grounds keeper. His employment kept him away from home much of the time, which left the mother with the 14 children. The mother sewed and baked to supplement her husband's income. With a large number of children there was never sufficient income, resulting at times in malnutrition in the children. Neighbors often brought food to the family and helped the mother with the feeding and bathing of her children.

The parents reported that the children were frequently in conflict with one another. As the children reached adolescence, they became discontented with their family's poverty. Few of the children completed school past the sixth grade. Some of the boys quit school to find jobs and made efforts to help support the family.

While in school, three of the brothers and one sister were classified as "slow learners," which led to frequent contact between the mother and the school. Susan's mother believed that school was important, but with her many responsibilities she was not able to help the children with their schoolwork. Furthermore, one of Susan's younger sister's had epilepsy, which placed additional strain on the family.

It is evident that this family was very severely stressed on a number of levels. With limited resources and the large number of children, problems were constantly presented to the parents. Therefore, after 19 years of trying to care for Susan in the home, the family decided it was best to institutionalize her.

ASSESSMENT

For a complete assessment, the level of intellectual functioning, adaptive functioning, and behavioral evaluation of the target behaviors should be examined. In the following three sections assessment is described and results from Susan's case study are given.

Intellectual Functioning. This part of the assessment involves the administration of a standardized intelligence test that delineates how the individual compares with other individuals. When assessing severely and profoundly mentally retarded persons, it becomes necessary to use an instrument that is sensitive to the population. Tests such as the Stanford-Binet Intelligence Scale and the Wechsler Intelligence Scales do not have the discriminative ability with persons functioning below an IQ of approximately 40. Thus, little is known about the individual other than that he or she is at least severely mentally retarded. Two appropriate scales to differentiate intellectual functioning below the level of the above described scales are the Bayley Mental Scale of Infant Development and the Cattell Infant Intelligence Scale. Both of these scales provide the level of functioning in months, and the Cattell Scale provides an IQ. The intelligence level of Susan was assessed with the Cattell Infant Intelligence Scale. She obtained a mental age of 13 months and an IQ of 11.

Adaptive Functioning. Instruments that are used to assess adaptive behavior do not require a standardized testing situation. They rely on an evaluation by individuals who are familiar with the client (family or direct care staff) and on direct observation. Several areas of adaptive behavior can be examined using this type of instrument. Some of these areas include ambulation, self-feeding, toileting, dressing, grooming, communication, and stereotyped and self-destructive behaviors. This portion of the assessment is aimed at identifying areas for training the individual. The Vineland Adaptive Behavior Scale is one instrument that is useful in this area. On this instrument, Susan obtained an Adaptive Behavior Composite of 11 months. Some of the domains assessed were communication (11 months), daily living skills (16 months), and socialization (5 months).

Particular strengths were receptive language (she attends to others) and personal skills (feeding).

Behavioral Assessment. Before conducting an elaborate assessment of the behaviors, there are several factors that need to be addressed. First, it is important to determine if the behavior is socially significant or not. In an institutional setting a referral is sometimes made when the behavior, in fact, is not really a major problem. Second, medical problems that may be contributing to the problem behavior should be ruled out. Third, an examination of all possible resources for dealing with the behavior should be conducted. It is useless to have an ideal treatment regimen with no possible means of implementation. Such factors as staff availability, materials, staff cooperation, and administrative support are among the issues to be considered.

The first step in assessment is to operationally define the target behaviors (Barlow & Hersen, 1984). Next, a functional analysis can be carried out to identify antecedents and consequences of the behavior, which may reveal relatively simple environmental manipulations that can be implemented. During the baseline phase, data should be collected until the performance level is stable or a trend in the data is evident in the opposite direction of the desirable effect (Bates & Hanson, 1983). Furthermore, all chemical restraints and/or physical restraints should be removed during this time.

Susan was referred to the unit psychologist for her self-injury. Her behavior was deemed socially significant (with no apparent medical contribution) after the staff physician ordered and reviewed several laboratory tests. No chemical or physical restraints were being used to control Susan's behavior at the time of referral, but they had been attempted in the past. The target behaviors identified were hitting and biting. Hitting was defined as either hitting or slapping any part of her body with her hand or elbow. Biting was defined as placing any of her fingers in her mouth. Separate data were obtained on each of these forms of self-injury. Momentary time sampling was chosen for data collection owing to limited staff time and the high frequency of the behaviors. This observational method was carried out by having staff observe Susan for 5 seconds every 5 minutes from 8 a.m. until 6 p.m. The staff placed a check in a column for "yes" if the behavior was present and in a column for "no" if it was absent. Thus, 120 observations were made daily.

A functional analysis of the two behaviors and baseline data collection were completed. Two areas of significance were identified in the functional analysis. First, Susan engaged in self-injury only when she was not participating in an activity. Second, she would hit herself when she was asked to rise in the morning. This approach resulted in staff allowing her to stay in bed for additional time. Thus, the behavior was negatively reinforced, since Susan was permitted to avoid getting out of bed when engaging in the target behavior(s). Therefore, additional activities were provided in Susan's schedule, and she was required to arise immediately regardless of her behavior. Baseline data, which were collected for 5 days prior to adding the activities, indicated a 30% reduction in self-injury over the next week. For this reason, baseline was collected for an additional week to obtain a stable rate of responding.

SELECTION OF TREATMENT

When choosing a treatment with severely and profoundly mentally retarded persons, many factors must be taken into account, some of which have been discussed previously. However, others issues deserve some consideration here. Medical concerns and ethical issues are particularly significant when treating self-injury. Legal mandates have established that the least restrictive alternatives first must be implemented. Therefore, such techniques as differential reinforcement of other behaviors (DRO) and extinction should be carried out before punishment procedures are implemented (Matson & DiLorenzo, 1984). However, while DRO has proven to be useful with self-injury (Repp & Deitz, 1974), punishment procedures have generally been found in past research efforts to be even more effective (Matson & DiLorenzo, 1984; Measel & Alfieri, 1976) than any of the less restrictive alternatives. Because self-injury can result in serious physical consequences, it may be necessary to employ punishment procedures initially. (For a more complete review of punishment procedures, see Matson & DiLorenzo, 1984, and for treatments for self-injury, see Whitman, Scibak, & Reid, 1983.)

Many different techniques and combinations of techniques have been used to treat self-injury and similar types of behavior. For Susan, a combination of DRO and overcorrection was chosen. DRO involves reinforcement delivery when a particular response is *not* emitted. It has been attempted with many behaviors, including pica, rumination, aggression, and self-injury. Overcorrection involves two components. The first is restitution. This method involves returning the person or environment back to the original state before the behavior occurred. The second component is positive practice, which involves having the individual practice the desired behavior through repetitions. The procedure has been implemented for treatment of many behaviors, including pica, rumination, coprophagy, aggression, stereotypies, and self-injury.

In Susan's case, the combination of DRO and overcorrection was chosen for several reasons. First, Susan resided in an environment where she received little reinforcement. She was likely to respond well to the DRO procedure for this reason. Second, research has shown that overcorrection can be effective in reducing the behavior. Third, the institution in which Susan was placed historically had rejected the use of other punishment procedures, but overcorrection was approved. Finally, the direct care staff agreed to use this treatment regimen.

COURSE OF TREATMENT

This section will consist of a description of the treatments utilized, staff training, and problems encountered during the treatment process (including a dialogue between the psychologist and the direct care staff).

As already noted, the two treatments used with self-injury with Susan were DRO and overcorrection. Implementation of the program occurred between 8 a.m. and 6 p.m. daily. The DRO procedure involved giving edible and social reinforcers for displaying behavior other than self-injury. Specifically, Susan was reinforced whenever she was observed doing anything with her hands other than hitting or biting herself. Examples of behaviors reinforced are playing with a toy, holding her hands still, combing her hair, and holding her fork. The momentary time-sampling method described in the assessment section was used to determine when reinforcement was delivered. Observations occurred every 5 minutes and lasted for 5 seconds. If Susan did not engage in hitting or biting (as described previously), she was reinforced. Several edible reinforcers (raisins, nuts, sugar-coated cereal, bits of cookies, and M&Ms) were chosen from a reinforcer menu completed by direct care staff. Several reinforcers were chosen to ensure the continued effectiveness of the reward. The social reinforcer utilized was a pat on the back accompanied with a positive statement about her behavior (i.e., "Good playing, Susan"). Both edible and social reinforcements were administered together.

One of two overcorrection procedures was administered whenever Susan engaged in hitting or biting. For hitting, overcorrection involved lowering Susan's arms to her sides immediately when the behavior occurred. Her arms were then raised by the direct care worker 180 degrees until they were above her head. (This procedure had previously been documented to be effective [see Foxx & Azrin, 1973].) Some lotion was then placed on Susan's fingertips, which she was required to rub on the reddened areas she had struck for 30 seconds. This entire procedure was repeated five times after each occurrence of hitting. For biting, oral hygiene overcorrection was chosen (Foxx & Martin, 1975). This treatment involved lightly brushing Susan's teeth, tongue, and gums with a toothbrush soaked in an oral antiseptic for 3 minutes using manual guidance. Both procedures were relatively easy to administer and required less than 10 minutes to complete.

Training involved teaching four direct care staff and two supervisors in the overcorrection and reinforcement procedures. Two sessions were scheduled to train staff. First, a 1-hour classroom session was used to provide a rationale for treatment, the importance of consistent implementation, and reasons for stopping self-injury. Supervisors agreed to help direct care staff when implementation was difficult owing to inadequate time and help. Second, a 2-hour session was scheduled to demonstrate the procedures and allow staff to practice and obtain feedback. In addition, throughout the entire treatment program, a half hour of monitoring by the therapist was provided Monday through Friday. This method was followed to ensure that all procedures were implemented correctly throughout treatment.

To illustrate how training of staff was conducted, excerpts of dialogue between the psychologist and the direct care workers follow:

PSYCHOLOGIST: It is important for us to stop the hitting and biting behavior.

DIRECT CARE STAFF: Why can't we just give Susan some medicine to make it stop? I don't think that there is anything that I can do to help her.

PSYCHOLOGIST: They have tried medicine in the past and it has not helped Susan. That is why your supervisor contacted me. This time we are going to try to change her behavior without medicine.

DIRECT CARE STAFF: Does this mean that I am going to have more work to do? I already have difficulty completing everything.

PSYCHOLOGIST: With the help of your supervisor and co-workers, we are going to provide more help to you so you have time to work with Susan.

DIRECT CARE STAFF: But I don't know how to help Susan. Every time I try to help she seems to get worse. I am almost afraid to do anything with her.

PSYCHOLOGIST: I will teach you how to help Susan and provide you feedback on how you are doing when you work with her. Susan needs to have the proper consequences for her behavior. This is what I am going to teach you. First we are going to reward Susan for doing the right things and then we will punish her for the wrong behavior.

DIRECT CARE SUPERVISOR: I know this sounds like a lot of work, but we have to try and help Susan because the federal people say we have to provide active treatment. In other words, it is your job to do what we ask. We are going to help you, but nevertheless you must do the job.

PSYCHOLOGIST: I know this sounds like a lot of work, but we have had Susan for many years and she has not changed her hitting and biting. In the past we were concerned with custodial care for the residents, but now we are going to try and do more. Everyone needs to do their part. If we work together we can make many improvements in these residents' lives.

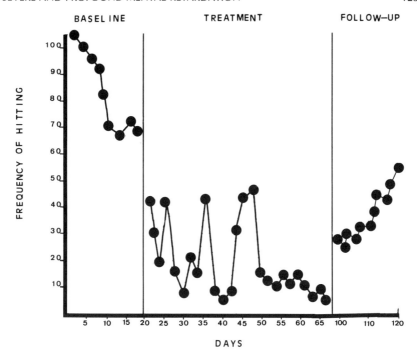

Figure 1.   The rate of hitting during baseline and during training and a 3-month follow-up. Each data point is the average of 2 days.

This dialogue illustrates the importance of "selling" the direct care staff workers on what the psychologist is planning. Without their support, it is difficult to make progress. "Selling" this idea involves training the staff in behavior therapy, providing them with answers to questions, and, most of all, doing the training with them. If they see that you are willing to help, then they become more motivated, and it enhances the likelihood that they will do a better job.

Baseline data collection began before the meeting described above. After making some changes in Susan's environment, which were described in the assessment section, a baseline for hitting of approximately 70 per day was determined. Treatment was initiated on day 20. This approach further reduced the self-injury by an additional 50%. A summary of Susan's hitting behavior is presented in Figure 1. It should be noted that problems in treatment implementation were encountered. First, the staff discovered that the amount of time required to care for Susan conflicted with caring for other residents. This problem was solved by re-

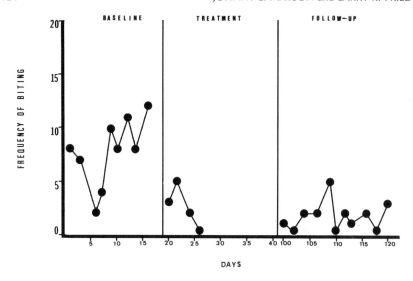

Figure 2. The rate of biting during baseline and during training and a 3-month follow-up. Each data point is the average of 2 days.

minding the supervisors of their agreement to help cover for the direct care staff when time was short. It was also pointed out that the initial stages of treatment required the greatest effort. Later, direct care staff should not be asked to implement overcorrection as frequently, thereby reducing their treatment duties. The second problem encountered was that the reinforcers used in the DRO program disappeared often and therefore were not available when needed. A cabinet was located that could be locked and kept close to Susan. The reinforcers were stored in this manner. Sufficient reinforcers for several hours were then taken from the cabinet and placed in an apron worn by the direct care staff. This overall approach solved the problems encountered early in the program.

More impressive results than those with hitting were encountered with biting. The behavior was quickly reduced when oral hygiene overcorrection was used. This procedure was implemented five times, and the behavior did not recur during the 7 weeks of treatment. A summary of the data is presented in Figure 2.

On the 5th day of treatment, yet another problem was encountered. Because of illness, no staff trained to implement treatment was available. Hitting increased on that day but was reduced the following day when the procedure was again carried out. Gradual progress was maintained until the 15th day of treatment. At that point it was discovered that staff were not following through with the five trials of overcorrection. The psychologist was monitoring the procedure for a half hour daily and the program was being carried out. However, one of the supervisors told the psychologist that the direct care person was doing the complete job only when the psychologist was present. Therefore, a 1-hour session was scheduled with all the persons involved to retrain them on the rationale for conducting the treatment and the necessity for implementing it consistently. This approach led to further decreases in the hitting behavior over the next 7 days.

Treatment was discontinued on the 23rd day for a reversal phase, which led to a rapid increase in self-injury. Treatment then was reinstituted on the 27th day, which again reduced the behavior. Low levels of responding were maintained for the next 10 days.

TERMINATION

Since the behavior was once again reduced after the program was reinstituted, a decision to fade out the reinforcers was made. This procedure was started on the 30th day of treatment and lasted for the next 18 days. Susan was reinforced frequently using the DRO procedure at this point. The social reinforcer was maintained but the edible reinforcer was administered on every other trial. Over the next 10 days the edible reinforcer was gradually faded out. Once the direct care staff actually began enjoying interacting with Susan, the social reinforcer was not reduced.

On the 35th day of treatment, the overcorrection procedure was reduced. This change led to a slight increase in the behavior, but it was not deemed significant. Susan was given social reinforcement only for not engaging in self-injury. At this time the administrative staff decided that it was no longer necessary to treat Susan's self-injury.

FOLLOW-UP

One-month follow-up data were collected. Self-injury had increased, but not to a level considered significant enough to warrant reimplementing the program.

OVERALL EVALUATION

Severely and profoundly retarded persons until recently were considered very difficult to treat. The results of this case study indicate that several behavioral techniques, as has frequently been demonstrated in the literature in the past, can help control self-injurious behavior. However, it is often difficult to work within an institutional setting. Many institutions unfortunately have followed a custodial medical model. Indeed, their staff prefer this approach since the administration of a pill to solve behavior problems takes much less effort and requires fewer skills than behavioral intervention. However, the administration of pills does not teach new behavior and in fact has led to a number of scandals and lawsuits when drugs were used to sedate clients solely for the convenience of staff. Also, drugs may have many short- and long-term side effects that are very serious. Therefore, the clinician should opt, where possible, to use behavioral methods and resort to pharmacological interventions only when all else fails. Our method is particularly recommended with problems such as self-injury, where the available research has shown behavior therapy to be the overwhelmingly better substantiated approach.

Another issue that should be mentioned is the possibility of maintaining the severely retarded person in the community. In the example of Susan, a preferred approach, and one that is beginning to receive attention, is to provide financial aid and professional support to the person in the community. Providing an aide to work in the home with Susan and her siblings would have the advantage of allowing her to stay with her family. Also, for those concerned about cost, it is highly likely that this would be less expensive for taxpayers than institutionalization. The consideration of these and other novel methods will further enhance the life of severely handicapped people. It is likely that such options will become more common in the future.

REFERENCES

Barlow, D. H., & Hersen, M. (1984). *Single case experimental designs: Strategies for studying behavior change*. New York: Pergamon Press.

Bates, P. E., & Hanson, H. (1983). Behavioral assessment. In J. L. Matson & S. E. Breuning (Eds.), *Assessing the mentally retarded* (pp. 27–63). New York: Grune and Stratton.

Berkson, G., & Landesman-Dwyer, S. (1977). Behavioral research on severe and profound mental retardation. *American Journal of Mental Deficiency, 81,* 428–454.

Cleland, C. C. (1979). *The profoundly mentally retarded*. Englewood Cliffs, NJ: Prentice-Hall.

Foxx, R. M., & Azrin, N. H. (1973). The elimination of autistic self-stimulatory behavior by overcorrection. *Journal of Applied Behavior Analysis, 6,* 1–14.

Foxx, R. M., & Martin, E. D. (1975). Treatment of scavenging behavior (coprophagy and pica) by overcorrection. *Behaviour Research and Therapy, 13,* 153–162.

Gorman-Smith, D., & Matson, J. L. (1985). A review of treatment research for self-injurious and stereotyped responding. *Journal of Mental Deficiency Research, 29,* 295–308.

Matson, J. L., & DiLorenzo, T. M. (1984). *Punishment and its alternatives*. New York: Springer.

Matson, J. L., & Mulick, J. A. (1983). *Handbook of mental retardation*. New York: Pergamon Press.

Measel, C. J., & Alfieri, P. A. (1976). Treatment of self-injurious behavior by a combination of reinforcement for incompatible behavior and overcorrection. *American Journal of Mental Deficiency, 81,* 147–153.

Mori, A. A., & Masters, L. F. (1980). *Teaching the severely mentally retarded*. Germantown, MD: Aspen.

Repp, A. C., & Deitz, S. M. (1974). Reducing aggressive and self-injurious behavior of institutionalized retarded children through reinforcement of other behaviors. *Journal of Applied Behavioral Analysis, 7,* 313–325.

Whitman, T. L., Scibak, J. W., & Reid, D. H. (1983). *Behavior modification with the severely and profoundly retarded*. New York: Grune and Stratton.

CHAPTER 11

Autism
A Case in Early Childhood

SANDRA L. HARRIS and JAN S. HANDLEMAN

DESCRIPTION OF THE DISORDER

Infantile autism is a pervasively handicapping developmental disorder that begins in the child's earliest months and often lasts a lifetime. According to the criteria of the American Psychiatric Association (1980), the essential diagnostic features for this disorder include onset before 30 months of age; a pervasive lack of response to others; gross deficits in language, with peculiar speech patterns in those youngsters who do speak; and bizarre responses to the environment, including resistance to change. These children do not exhibit the signs of thought disorder found in schizophrenia.

In spite of the severity of the symptoms of autism, the past 20 years have seen marked progress in the development of behavioral interventions, including techniques for teaching speech, social, self-help, and other desirable skills; procedures for the suppression of disruptive, maladaptive behaviors; the active use of parents as teachers; and an increasing emphasis on placing these children in the least restrictive educational setting possible (e.g., Handleman & Harris, 1986; Lovaas, 1981; Schopler & Mesibov, 1985).

The case history presented below focuses on the development of an

SANDRA L. HARRIS • Graduate School of Applied and Professional Psychology, Rutgers University, P.O. Box 819, Piscataway, New Jersey 08854.   JAN S. HANDLE-MAN • Douglass Developmental Disabilities Center, Douglass College, Gibbons Campus, New Brunswick, New Jersey 08903.

educational program to help a moderately mentally retarded, preschool autistic boy move from a highly specialized program for autistic children to a much less segregated program for children with learning disabilities.

CASE IDENTIFICATION

David Dixon was nearly 4 years old when his parents, Arnold and Ellen Dixon, brought him to the Douglass Developmental Disabilities Center (DDDC), a university-based program for the treatment of children with autism. He was the only child of this fifth-generation American family of British and Irish extraction. Mr. Dixon, age 26, dropped out of high school in the 11th grade and was employed as a plumber; Mrs. Dixon, age 25, likewise left school in the 11th grade and was at home full time as a mother and homemaker. The Dixons had a modest but adequate income, living in their own home on a quiet suburban street. They had planned to have another baby, but David's developmental problems left them fearing that the next child might exhibit similar problems.

Mr. and Mrs. Dixon had learned about David's diagnosis shortly before they came to the center to inquire about a school placement, and they were still struggling to understand both emotionally and intellectually what it meant that David was an autistic child.

PRESENTING COMPLAINTS

The Dixons had sought help for David because they were concerned about his seeming indifference to them, his lack of speech and language, his resistance to changes in routine, and his stereotyped behavior. David had perhaps 15 words in his repertoire, most of them focusing on basic needs such as *juice, soda, car,* and *ice cream.* He spent long periods rocking back and forth, appearing oblivious to the world around him. He also enjoyed clapping his hands and waving his fingers in front of his face and would continue these self-stimulatory behaviors for hours unless interrupted by his parents.

According to the Dixons, David rarely sought their company, seeming most content when he was left alone, preferring to sit in his room and rock, sift sand through his fingers, or tear paper into tiny bits.

The Dixons, while less concerned about his self-help skills than his language and interpersonal behavior, did note that David was not yet toilet-trained, although he could stay dry for several hours at a time. He did not undress or dress himself but would passively cooperate with these activities.

HISTORY

David was the product of a full-term, uneventful pregnancy. He was born by a vaginal delivery after a long 30-hour labor that left his mother exhausted. At birth he weighed 8 pounds, 7 ounces and, according to his parents, seemed quite healthy, having no problems with sucking, eating, or sleeping in his early months. It is interesting to note that Mr. and Mrs. Dixon regarded their infant son as an easy, undemanding baby who required relatively little care to remain content. In fact, David's parents felt no concern about the boy's development until beyond his second birthday, when they realized that although he remained an undemanding child, his development was unusual and some of his behavior patterns appeared increasingly rigid.

According to the Dixons, David sat alone at 11 months, stood at 12 months, and was walking by 13 months. His first word emerged sometime between 15 and 16 months, and by his second birthday he used a few simple phrases and single words such as "want juice." Sometime before 30 months David's speech began to decline and his self-stimulatory rocking, which had been present since infancy, increased. Although it is difficult for the Dixons to identify the precise date of this change, they recall that sometime between 26 and 30 months of age there was a gradual, but definite, change for the worse in their son.

David's medical history was unremarkable. There were no indications of prolonged high fever, serious accidents, seizure activity, or unconsciousness. An EEG done when he was 3 years old was within normal limits. The neurologist concluded that David, although appearing essentially normal on a general physical examination, exhibited a global developmental delay and autistic behaviors. A hearing evaluation suggested that David had normal hearing.

The Dixon family history was of some interest in that Mrs. Dixon's aunt had two mentally retarded children and Mr. Dixon had a younger sister with a learning disability. There was, however, no known family history of infantile autism.

ASSESSMENT

David's initial assessment was divided into two phases. The first evaluation focused on determining whether he was appropriate for admission to the center, and the second evaluation was done after admission to develop his individual educational plan (IEP). The IEP provided a systematic overview of our educational goals for David, as well as complying with state and federal regulations concerning the education of handicapped children.

Admission to the Center

Prior to his acceptance, David was observed in a classroom at the center. The purpose of this assessment session was to ensure that he was autistic and that his general functioning was comparable to that of the other children with whom he would be placed. In order to provide the data for those decisions, David was exposed to a range of materials from the center's curriculum.

During that session it was noted that he exhibited a number of autistic behaviors, including sterotyped rocking and active avoidance of eye contact. He did, however, sit appropriately for a one-to-one work session and made some fleeting eye contact when his name was called.

When asked to copy simple nonverbal imitations, such as standing up or touching head, David complied only with the command to clap his hands. His verbal imitative skills were likewise confined to the imitation of the single sound "bah." Indications that David had greater potential than might be suggested by his failure to follow simple commands were seen in his appropriate play with a stacking ring and shape-sorting box.

Although his fine motor skills were well below age level, David's gross motor abilities were relatively mature. It was also noted that in spite of his failure to comply with many commands, David showed a fundamental interest in the environment around him, and this, coupled with his response to food and praise as potential reinforcers, suggested that he might be quite responsive to the educational setting. Overall, David's behavior was consistent with the information provided by his parents during a detailed interview and, thus, supported the diagnosis of infantile autism and indicated that he would be a good match for his three young classmates.

Educational Planning

The development of David's IEP was done by his classroom teacher following the format provided by Romanczyk and Lockshin (1982) in the *I. G. S.*

Curriculum. This curriculum, developed for use with autistic children and accessed via one of the center's computers, allows the teacher to select from a broad menu of educational options those items that best meet the needs of the individual child.

Romanczyk and Lockshin (1982) have divided the curriculum into 16 broad areas, including maladaptive behaviors, attentive skills, speech, motor skills, and self-help skills. David's teacher chose from this menu the specific items that met David's initial needs. For example, within the domain of maladaptive behaviors, she focused on decreasing tantrums, decreasing throwing of objects, and decreasing out-of-seat behavior. Under attentional skills, she elected to increase sitting, establish eye contact, and increase visual focus on intructional materials. A complete listing of the primary objectives on David's IEP during the first year is provided in Table 1. Each of these broad goals was accompanied by a description of the specific steps involved, instructional techniques to be used, criteria for completion of the program, frequency of implementation of the program, and other related instructional guidelines selected from the menu provided by the *I.G.S. Curriculum* (Romanczyk & Lockshin, 1982).

SELECTION OF TREATMENT

One of the major attractions the center held for the Dixons was the behavioral orientation, which they viewed as consistent with their own belief that these techniques were critical to David's progress. Mr. and Mrs. Dixon were united in their opinion that the structure provided by behavioral programming was most consistent with their son's needs.

There were other components of the center's program that the Dixons regarded as vital to David's education. The center provided a full-day, year-round program to promote maintenance and prevent regression of behavior change, and the curriculum emphasized communication, cognitive, and social development. Furthermore, the availability of one-to-one teaching was viewed as very important to David's rapid mastery of basic skills. In addition, the university affiliation of the center made it accessible to current research and teaching advances.

The Dixons were also aware that the center's comprehensive family involvement program would help them begin to face the broader issues of raising a developmentally disabled child. Training seminars and evening meetings would provide them with programming assistance, and regularly scheduled home visits would support active home programming. Most important, the Dixons felt that the emotional support of the teachers and other parents would help to promote family unity and functioning.

Table 1
David's IEP Goals

  I. Reduction of madaladaptive behaviors
     A. Disruptive behavior (e.g., tantrums, throwing)
     B. Noncompliance
     C. Eating problems
 II. Attentive skills
     A. Prespeech attentive skills (e.g., remains in chair)
     B. Eye contact (e.g., on command, in response to name)
     C. Independent attentive skills (e.g., assembles puzzles)
III. Speech
     A. Nonverbal imitation
     B. Vocal imitation
     C. Verbal imitation
 IV. Receptive language
     A. Nonverbal compliance with requests (e.g., touch body parts on request)
  V. Expressive language
     A. Labeling
     B. Responds to questions
     C. Conversational skills (e.g., simple social questions)
     D. Visual discrimination (e.g., sort by color)
 VI. Motor skills
     A. Gross motor (e.g., balance, climbing stairs)
     B. Specific gross motor activities (e.g., throw ball)
     C. Fine motor (e.g., string beads)
VII. Self-help skills
     A. Self-feeding (e.g., use spoon with liquids)
     B. Self-toileting (e.g., walk to bathroom)
     C. Self-dressing (e.g., remove hat, remove mittens)
     D. Personal hygiene (e.g., wash hands)
VIII. Social skills
     A. Verbal interaction (e.g., greet people)
     B. Play skills (e.g., initiate own play)
 IX. Reading
     A. Readiness skills (e.g., discriminate same–different)
  X. Cultural skills
     A. Arts and crafts (e.g., put paste on paper)
     B. Art activities integrated into the general curriculum (e.g., manipulate clay as visual-motor activity)
     C. Music and dance (e.g., clap to music)
 XI. General information
     A. Basic awareness of environment (e.g., states name)
XII. School-related skills
     A. Appropriate classroom behavior (e.g., self-control)
XIII. Life-relevant skills
     A. Prevocational skills (e.g., sorts by color)

COURSE OF TREATMENT

David was initially placed in one of the DDDC's primary classrooms. He was one of four children in a class staffed by a professional supervisor and four undergraduate tutors. David received daily one-to-one instruction for his first year in the program.

The primary curriculum emphasized instructional control training. Initial attention was placed on teaching David to sit quietly, to establish eye contact, and to focus on environmental objects and events. Efforts were also made to improve his compliance with basic instructions and to decrease many of his self-stimulatory behaviors. Instructional activities later included teaching David the rudiments of speech and more complex communication skills.

David's progress was enhanced by his parents' participation in the center's family involvement program. In September of David's first year, Mr. and Mrs. Dixon attended a series of seminars devoted to behavior management and skill building. Upon completion of the parent training course, the Dixons demonstrated an understanding of various behavioral techniques and successfully implemented a number of programs with David at home. The Dixons also attended parent meetings at the school approximately every 6 weeks and met with David's teacher monthly in their home. These meetings focused on home programming and progress evaluation. Along with these formal encounters, there was a frequent exchange of data sheets, notes, and phone calls between school and home.

David made a smooth adjustment to the DDDC. From the very beginning, he readily boarded the small van that picked him up at home, and he entered the school without assistance. His mastery of basic instructional control tasks was fairly rapid, with the exception of some initial difficulty generalizing newly learned responses across instructors. His eye contact on request increased from a glance in September to 5 seconds of sustained attending by the beginning of October. Much of the rocking that had been observed during the early fall decreased markedly within 2 months. By November, David's improved sitting, attending, and general responsiveness prompted a decision to initiate the teaching of more complex cognitive and communication skills.

Language training first focused on increasing the consistency with which David imitated those words his parents reported hearing at home. By December, his imitative vocabulary had grown substantially and he was beginning to imitate some two-word phrases. David was also labeling some simple common objects and actions. Programming during the remainder of the school year continued to focus on promoting David's functional use of language.

David's social skills also improved during his first year at the DDDC. He was initiating more nonverbal and verbal contacts with adults, and some limited interactions with other children were reported. He would more frequently observe another child playing and on occasion would roll a ball in the direction of a nearby child. By April, David was beginning to work in a small group of two children, was participating much more in the morning group activities, and was toilet-trained.

On the basis of David's response to the primary curriculum, the staff decided to promote him to one of the center's intermediate classrooms for the next school year. During the annual review of David's educational program with his parents and professionals from the school district, interest was also expressed in moving David to a less structured educational setting in the near future. Great delight was expressed by all regarding the fine progress David had made his first year at the center.

The primary goal of the intermediate class placement was to wean David from the intensive structure of the primary program. For example, small-group programming replaced one-to-one instruction, and food was no longer used as a regular reward. Also, the curriculum was broadened to include academic readiness and life skills training. The intermediate level curriculum attempted to approximate a more traditional special educational environment and to promote more normalized experiences than were appropriate in the primary class.

David's communication and social skills continued to improve in the intermediate class. His language became more complex and he made more spontaneous requests. By December of his second year, David was consistently using three- and four-word sentences, and his conceptual understanding of language had grown. For example, David had learned to respond to yes/no questions, and he was using prepositional phrases more appropriately. David's social interactions had also increased. He frequently approached another child to make a request or to initiate limited conversation.

While David continued to develop the ability to communicate, some areas of learning remained problematic. Tasks that required a visual motor component such as writing were particularly difficult for him. He also had difficulty with activities involving visual memory or the recall of facts and details. As a result of these continuing deficits, David's educational programming remained highly systematic and structured.

The Dixons continued to support the school's efforts and to work closely with David at home. Home programming included the practice of mastered skills in the natural environment and taking David on outings to malls and restaurants to improve his ability to function in a complex environment. As a result, his tolerance of these situations was improving and his interests were becoming more varied. To provide David with some opportunity to play with less handicapped children, the Dixons enrolled David in their local recreation program.

David's success prompted the center's staff to investigate the possibility of a transition to a new school setting for the following September. During a staffing in late December, it was agreed that David could begin to benefit from less structure and more normalized programming. Together with the Dixons and child study personnel from his school district, the staff of the center began the search for a new program.

David's teacher first surveyed the public schools for possible placements. After visiting classes in David's home district and a neighboring town, she decided that the available public programs did not provide the structure that would best support David's development. Her search of local private schools identified a program for neurologically impaired and communication-handicapped children. A visit by the Dixons confirmed her choice, and an intake evaluation resulted in a recommendation for placement at the Point School.

TERMINATION

The staff of the DDDC organized a systematic transition process for David and his family. Beginning in January of his second year, the DDDC staff visited the Point School and the Point School staff visited the center several times to provide opportunities for observation and consultation regarding educational programming. These meetings helped to finalize preparations for David's transition and to firm up plans for his visits to Point School.

In February, David and another classmate, who was also in transition, spent 3 mornings a week in classes at Point School. During their visits, they participated in all classroom and school activities. Close coordination between David's teacher, the center's head teacher, and the Point School staff helped to facilitate David's initial adjustment and to promote continuity of programming. By the beginning of March, David was attending the morning session at Point School on a daily basis.

David's progress at Point School was noted in many areas. He quickly adjusted to the individualized instruction that was provided and very early in the transition was participating in group activities. He also become friendly with one of his classmates. Periodic visits by the center's administrators and the Dixons confirmed David's fine progress.

Afternoon programming at the DDDC focused on communication and social development, in addition to teaching David those school life skills he would need for success at Point School. For example, he was taught to independently use the school lavatory instead of the one in the classroom, and he was provided with furniture and workbooks that approximated those used at Point School. Classroom activities were closely coordinated between the two schools and monitored throughout the remainder of the school year and during the summer. In September, David began attending Point School on a full-time basis.

FOLLOW-UP

The cooperation between the DDDC and Point School continued following David's change in placement. During his first year at Point School there were numerous phone contacts, and David's teacher from the DDDC visited him three times. The Dixons also remained in close contact with the DDDC while actively supporting their son's new program. This spirit of cooperation was a contributing factor to the continued success of the transition process.

During her first visit in October, David's teacher from the DDDC noted some slight regression in David's overall responsiveness. This was consistent with past performance following the short summer break, and a follow-up call 2 weeks later indicated that David was back on track both socially and academically. Visits in December and March confirmed David's comfortable adjustment to Point School and his sustained growth.

Contact with the Dixons indicated their continued pleasure with the program at Point School and with David's progress. At one point Mrs. Dixon expressed the feeling that she missed the close contact with the DDDC staff and the support she received from other parents. The Dixons supported all of Point School's efforts and remained committed to increasing David's social development through community participation.

OVERALL EVALUATION

David Dixon, like most autistic children, required a highly intensive program to meet his specialized needs. The Douglass Developmental Disabilities Center provided David with behaviorally based programming designed to promote social, communication, and cognitive development. One-to-one instruction and parent training were a few of the key features of the program that supported David's progress.

The transition of autistic children to less structured and more normalized instructional settings has become a priority of many programs

(Handleman & Harris, 1986). The hierarchical nature of the DDDC's curriculum and commitment to systematic transition greatly contributed to David's success in the Point School program. The cooperative effort between the DDDC and the Point School was responsible for David's ultimate adjustment and continued growth.

The education of the child with autism must extend beyond to child to include the entire family (Handleman & Harris, 1986). The family involvement program of the DDDC provided the Dixons with the support and guidance that was initially necessary to help them adjust to David's problems. Their parental roles of teacher and advocate helped to maximize educational efforts and ensure their son's placement in the most appropriate and least restrictive program.

REFERENCES

American Psychiatric Association. (1980). *Diagnostic and statistical manual of mental disorders* (3rd ed.). Washington, DC: Author.

Handleman, J. S., & Harris, S. L. (1986). *Educating the developmentally disabled. Meeting the needs of children and families.* San Diego, CA: College Hill Press.

Lovaas, O. I. (1981). *Teaching developmentally disabled children. The me book.* Baltimore: University Park Press.

Romanczyk, R. G., & Lockshin, S. (1982). *The I.G.S. Curriculum (Individualized goal selection).* Vestal, NY: C.B.T.A.

Schopler, E., & Mesibov, G. B. (Eds.). (1985). *Communication problems in autism.* New York: Plenum Press.

CHAPTER 12

Autism
A Case in Preadolescence

LAURA SCHREIBMAN, BERTRAM O. PLOOG, and
N. JENNIFER OKE

DESCRIPTION OF THE DISORDER

Early infantile autism is a severe form of psychopathology in children originally described by Leo Kanner (1943). The disorder is relatively rare, affecting one child in approximately 2,500 births. The ratio of boys to girls is 3 or 4 to 1. Although the incidence of autism is not frequent, its occurrence has a major impact on the child, family, schools, and the community as a whole. This is primarily the case since the disorder involves so many areas of the child's functioning.

The syndrome is characterized by most, but not necessarily all, of the following characteristics. First, there are pervasive and profound deficits in social behavior and attachment. This is truly a hallmark feature of the disorder and is typically evidenced by lack of eye-to-eye contact, resistance or only passive acceptance of affection, preference for solitary activities, and lack of interest in peers. Parents of these children often report that the child does not "need" them, does not spontaneously seek affection or comfort, and seems most content when alone.

Second, there is a substantial delay or failure in the acquisition of language. Approximately half of untreated autistic children remain nonverbal, acquiring no expressive language and perhaps only very rudi-

LAURA SCHREIBMAN, BERTRAM O. PLOOG, and N. JENNIFER OKE • Department of Psychology, C-009, University of California-San Diego, La Jolla, California 92093.

mentary receptive language (e.g., respond to simple commands). Others may display abnormal, noncommunicative speech. A common form of this speech is echolalia, wherein the child repeats the speech of others, usually with minimal or no comprehension. For example, if asked, "What's your name?" the child may respond, "What's your name?" (immediate echolalia) or repeat speech he/she has heard sometime in the past, such as television commercials (delayed echolalia). Other common speech characteristics include pronominal reversals, metaphoric language, neologisms, and dysprosody.

Third, the children often have a compulsive desire for what Kanner called the "preservation of sameness." Basically, this refers to their high sensitivity to changes in their physical environment (e.g., furniture arrangements, placement of objects), routes of travel, or daily routine. Alterations of these aspects of the child's environment may lead to tantrums and, where possible, attempts to correct the changes.

Fourth, autistic children typically show unusual responsivity to the sensory environment such that most of them have histories of suspected, but unconfirmed, deafness or blindness. They may fail to respond to their name being called, to loud noises, or to salient changes in their visual environment such as the comings and goings of people. Conversely, they may be hypersensitive to stimuli and react quite strongly to a barely noticeable stimulus such as the turn of a book page.

Fifth, self-stimulatory behavior is often present. This is typically repetitive, stereotypic behavior that serves no apparent function other than to provide the child with sensory input. Examples include body rocking, arm or hand flapping, head bobbing, finger manipulations, spinning objects, repetitive vocalizations, and gazing at lights.

Sixth, some of the children exhibit self-injurious behaviors, such as head banging, self-biting, and self-hitting. The severity of these behaviors varies from relatively mild face slapping or body hitting, resulting in redness and minor bruises, to very severe self-injury that may be life-threatening. Some forms of severe self-injury may result in skull fractures, detached retinas, broken noses, loss of significant amounts of flesh, or infection.

Seventh, autistic children may show isolated, sometimes exceptional, areas of skill in the areas of memory, mechanical abilities, or music. While exceptional abilities are not as common in autistic children as once believed, one typically finds that the children's abilities exhibit a variable pattern such that deficits in language and abstract concepts are more severe than deficits in visuospatial and mechanical skills.

In addition to the above characteristics, the onset of the disorder must be prior to the age of 30 months. While autism and mental retardation are distinct disorders, they often coexist in the same child such that approximately 60% of autistic children have measured IQs below 50. However, unlike children with a primary diagnosis of retardation, autistic children typically show normal physical development and none of the physical stigmata commonly associated with retardation. While the specific etiology of autism is as yet undetermined, current research is focusing on various aspects of organic functioning, such as specific abnormal brain anatomical features and disorders in neurotransmitter functioning. This emphasis on the organic basis of autism differs markedly from the unsupported psychogenic etiology hypothesis that was advanced many years ago.

CASE IDENTIFICATION

Robert's initial intake evaluation revealed an attractive, slender 12-year-old boy with curly brown hair and brown eyes. His behavior indicated that he was a high-functioning autistic preadolescent who displayed some of the characteristic features of autism yet did not display some of the most severe and difficult-to-treat features. Thus, he showed some appropriate social behavior (to family members), no self-injury, minimal self-stimulation, and minimal unusual responsiveness to the sensory environment. He did, however, display high rates of bizarre, inappropriate speech and compulsive behaviors, and his eye contact was minimal.

Robert was the second child born to a middle-class family in California. The parents' first child, a son, died of pneumonia at the age of 2. The couple's third child, a daughter, was 8 years old and functioning normally. Both parents had college degrees and were currently employed, the father full time in sales and the mother part time for a local magazine. Both parents enjoyed good health and neither had a family history of mental retardation or other significant mental disorder. The family presented as a warm, close-knit unit where feelings were openly expressed. It was readily apparent that Robert's parents were very open about their concerns for their son and about their eagerness to learn how to help him. The nature of Robert's disorder was known to them, accepted as a lifespan handicap, and seen as something that could improve with training.

PRESENTING COMPLAINTS

At the time of his entry into our program, Robert was diagnosed autistic both by an independent agency and by our clinic. He displayed several presenting problems. Foremost of his parents' concerns was his lack of appropriate language. Specifically, he engaged in incessant repetition of television phrases, talked too loudly, had an unusual intonation pattern in his speech, did not initiate conversations, and engaged in compulsive repeating and question asking. He was compulsive about time and would ask time-related questions often and repetitively. His learning to tell time and the acquisition of a watch merely formalized the compulsions. His parents were extremely frustrated at not being able to have anything even approximating a "normal conversation" with him. When they or others attempted to engage him in conversation or ask him questions, he would often seek to avoid the interaction by saying, "That's enough," "Stop it," or "Go away."

Related to other aspects of language was Robert's lack of comprehension of reading material. While he had learned to read in school and was quite good at reading aloud, his comprehension of what he had read was minimal. Similarly, he could count and use numbers in a limited way but had no real mathematical concepts. As with reading, he had mastered the superficial only to completely miss the substantial.

Another parental concern was that his eye contact was still extremely poor and it was "almost impossible to get him to look at you." When he did look, it was for a split second. Often, he would avoid looking at others by turning in another direction. He was noted to actively avoid not only eye contact but also physical proximity. Thus, when he was required to be in the same room as others, he typically sat or stood as far away from them as possible and faced in the opposite direction.

These characteristics and presenting complaints provided initial direction in the choice of treatment targets. However, more systematically derived targets would be identified by our assessment battery, which was designed to evaluate a range of functioning areas relevant to the treatment of autistic children.

HISTORY

Robert was the product of a full-term normal pregnancy and delivery. His physical development was normally paced and uneventful. He was described as a difficult baby who was very fussy and cried a good deal of the time. He also was a poor sleeper and, in fact, did not sleep through the night until 1 year of age.

In contrast, by the time he was 2 years old, his parents began to suspect that something was wrong because Robert was just "too good." They expected the usual inquisitive "trouble" into which toddlers get.

Yet he would be content to occupy himself for hours watching television or playing repetitively with puzzles. His parents reported that they managed to paint the entire exterior of their house while Robert was alone, completely content, in the house. Robert's parents were also concerned that he seemed to ignore other people, particularly other young children who came to his home. Rather, he simply did not care about people other than immediate family members. His involvement with family members sometimes included initiations of social contact, such as sitting in a parent's lap, but the frequency of this was markedly lower than one might expect of a normal child. Another feature of Robert's behavior that concerned his parents was his ritualistic activities with toys. Instead of engaging in creative play, he had set routinized patterns of playing with puzzles or toy cars and would become upset if anyone attempted to interfere.

Despite the reassurances of Robert's pediatrician, his parents sought input that might determine whether there was indeed something wrong with their son. The accurate nature of their suspicions became apparent when they enrolled him in a normal preschool at age 3. The director of the preschool, who had had many years of experience with preschool children, told Robert's parents that he was the "most different child she had ever seen" and recommended that the family contact the local developmental disabilities office for evaluation and appropriate treatment.

Robert said his first word, *mama*, at the age of 7 months and *bye-bye* at 15 months. While he continued to use single words, it became apparent that the pattern of his speech development was abnormal. When he was about $2\frac{1}{2}$ years old his uncle noted that he did not ask for things he wanted but instead he just pointed and grunted. He told Robert's parents, "You don't make him talk to you." Soon thereafter, Robert put together his first phrase, and a pattern of aberrant speech, often seen in autistic children, was established. His first phrase was "At the sign of the cat," a phrase from a television commercial for Lincoln Mercury cars. He then added to this bizarre vocabulary with "You've got it, Toyota," "Century City Ford," and other television commercial phrases. He also repeated phrases from game shows (e.g., "You've just won $7,000!") and from "Sesame Street." By the age of $3\frac{1}{2}$ he would engage in this delayed echolalia frequently and would spend extensive amounts of time "talking to himself" in this manner. The intent of the speech was clearly noncommunicative, yet his desperate parents soon learned that it was the only way to communicate with their son. Thus, if they wanted to get him to talk to them they would have to initiate a phrase from a television commercial, a game show, or "Sesame Street." He would respond with another such phrase. His teachers similarly noted this echolalia and that he would sometimes ramble incessantly, mixing television speech with other contextually inappropriate speech, such as "two plus two equals four, four plus four equals eight. . . ." It was not until Robert was approximately 9 years old that he began to use language in a communicative manner. While this language was communicative, it retained the pronominal reversals and inaccurate syntax characteristic of echolalic speech. Such functional language was very limited and occurred only after years of very intensive efforts by teachers, speech therapists, and his parents.

As Robert matured from infancy to childhood, several other features of the autistic syndrome emerged. His social behavior remained localized to his parents and younger sister, and he continued to ignore other children. Generally, he preferred to be alone. He did not join group activities and, in fact, became extremely upset in crowds. He resisted eye contact and did not show even minimal eye contact until he was 7 years old.

Robert displayed many of the compulsive and ritualistic behaviors so characteristic of autism. His parents reported that "everything had its place," and Robert made sure that things were put away where they belong. He would line up his toy cars and become quite upset if anyone disturbed them. For approximately 1 year, his mainstay meal was Braunschweiger and crackers. While he had always refused to wear anything on his head, one Christmas he received a blue-and-white billed cap on which was printed "Ford Mustang." He became compulsive about wearing the hat, and this lasted for 2 years. One of Robert's most consistent compulsions was time. If things were not on time he became very upset. He knew what was on television at any specific time and on which channel. He repeated the times of day when specific events would occur (e.g., "You go to school at seven o'clock"). He would repeat these statements until someone would confirm it (e.g., "Yes, you go to school at seven o'clock"). Reassurance was short-lived, and he might begin the same process, with the same statement, a few minutes later.

His parents also reported that sometimes it was impossible to direct his attention to something in the environment. For example, his mother remembered driving in the car with him when a fire engine went by with its flashing lights and blaring siren. She said, "Look at the fire engine, Robert!" yet he just stared straight ahead, in his own world.

Robert's self-stimulatory behaviors included rocking on hobby horses or swinging chairs. He would rock on one of these objects for hours, and, in fact, his mother has a baby book entry describing when he rode a spring rocking horse for a total of 4 hours in one day. It was also noted by teachers that even though he would engage in this kind of activity for long periods, oblivious to anything else, he did not seem to have a look of enjoyment on his face. He also would flip through the pages of telephone books with lightening speed for lengthy periods. The majority of the physical self-stimulatory behaviors gradually disappeared by the time he was 10 years old. Another behavior that consumed much of his time was watching television. He particularly liked game shows and "Sesame Street" and would watch them whenever possible. As noted above, his television viewing provided the basis of much of his language, and this behavior was evident up to the time he entered the present treatment program.

Robert's isolated skill areas centered on letters, numbers, and his immediate memorization of specific verbal input. He memorized the alphabet and numbers at a very early age and could count in both English and Spanish, all acquired from watching "Sesame Street." He readily memorized and used numbers in his speech (however, his comprehension of the abstract conceptual properties of mathematics was very limited). Most striking, however, was his phenomenal memory for songs and verbal information from records, tapes, and television. His mother reported that he had memorized literally hours and hours of this information, including TV show theme songs, "Sesame Street" songs and dialogue, and the ubiquitous television commercials.

Robert's performance on intellectual assessments was typical for an autistic child in that there was a sharp discrepancy between his abilities on nonverbal and verbal tests. A few years prior to his participation in the present treatment program, an intellectual evaluation yielded a Leiter International Performance Scale IQ of 80. However, looking at the verbal and performance scales of the Wechsler Intelligence Scale for Children (Revised), the contrast in his abilities was apparent. While he earned an 81 IQ on the performance scale, his score on the verbal scale was 45. This places his nonverbal abilities within the low average range and his verbal abilities within the moderate retardation range. His strengths were in visual-motor perceptual organization, spatial abilities, and nonverbal concept formation. His major weaknesses were in the areas of abstract concepts and expressive language. However, his verbal abilities were difficult to assess using standardized tests. Examiners noted that he tended to echo questions rather than to supply answers and would often repeat the questions several times over the course of the test.

As is the case with many autistic children, Robert has been given a number of diagnoses over the years, including autism, pervasive developmental disorder, aphasia, atypical development, and retardation. Sometimes the diagnosis was changed to provide access to appropriate school programs. After his first unsuccessful attendance at a normal preschool, Robert entered a private school for retarded children when he was 4 years old. A year later he attended a class for severely handicapped children in a public school. Since he was not as severely impaired as the children in this class, he was transferred to another school and entered a program for aphasic children. At this time, his family moved into the local area and he entered a summer program for autistic children. The next school year he entered a public school aphasia class, where he was with children who also had language disabilities but were socially normal. He remained in this program for 4 years until his entry into a public school program for the severely learning handicapped.

ASSESSMENT

Identifying Problem Behaviors

In order to design an effective treatment program, we first attempted to identify excessive and deficient behaviors in Robert's behavioral repertoire. "Excessive" refers to behaviors that were undesirable, and which therefore were to be either decreased or eliminated. "Deficient" refers to behaviors that were in principle desirable, but which were either not sufficiently developed in Robert's repertoire, or which existed only in some deviant form. We also considered Robert's strengths and abilities as a basis to build new, and maintain already existing, behaviors.

In addition to information obtained from medical, psychological, and school records, his mother provided valuable information in the initial intake interview for our clinic. And, of course, during the following 2 years of treatment, the parents and schoolteachers continued to exchange important information with us.

More formally, Robert was assessed in our clinic at the beginning of his treatment (pretreatment), and from then on approximately once every 6 months. These formal assessments consisted of (a) videotaping (and evaluating) Robert in a structured laboratory setting, (b) administering standardized tests, and (c) administering a test curriculum.

Videotaped Assessment. These observations were conducted to evaluate Robert in a room separated from, and not associated with, treatment. The room resembled a typical waiting room, with toys to which Robert had free access. During the first segment of each of these videotaped probes, an adult present in the room with Robert sat quietly in the room and watched Robert play without making any attempt to initiate an interaction with him. After 10 minutes she or he left the room in order to allow us to assess Robert's dependence or attachment to the other person in the room. The next segment in these observations involved 10 minutes in which the adult tried to engage Robert in conversation, cooperative and compliant behavior, and toy play. At the end of this segment, the adult again left the room and we assessed Robert's reactions. Finally, in the last segment of these observations, the person interacting with Robert attempted to evoke affection from him and to elicit laughter.

Different adults were present for each of these sessions. The first probe was conducted with Robert interacting with his mother, and also with a person ("stranger") he had not met before. (The "stranger" was included to assess for generalization.) From then on, every 6 months the probe was repeated with a parent, a stranger, and a therapist. This was done to assess his behavior in the presence of a variety of different individuals.

During these sessions, multiple response measures were obtained using an interval scoring procedure to measure percent occurrence of various appropriate and inappropriate behaviors. The following were scored as appropriate behaviors: (1) playing with toys in a way that suited their purpose (e.g., stacking blocks or putting a puzzle together, rather than just holding the objects or mouthing them), (2) nonpsychotic, functional, in-context speech (e.g., answering a question or tacting objects correctly rather than echolalic verbalizations or "word salad"), and (3) social nonverbal behaviors such as compliance, cooperation, affection, or initiating play with the other person (e.g., following requests, sharing a toy with the adult, or inviting the adult to play a game). At the pretreatment assessment, the obtained percent occurrence of those behaviors were 47%, 58%, and 27%, respectively.

Scored as inappropriate behaviors were (1) tantrums (i.e., fussing, crying, yelling, or physical agitation), (2) self-stimulation (including repetitive inappropriate sounds), (3) psychotic speech such as "word salad," echolalia, or meaningless, out-of-context speech, and (4) noncompliance (e.g., refusing to follow reasonable requests by the adult, such as "Come over here, and let me see the truck!"). The obtained percent occurrence for those four behavioral categories were 0%, 7%, 78%, and 3%, respectively.

Standardized Measures. We conducted two standardized tests to evaluate Robert's language and social development. The tests used were the Assessment of Children's Language Comprehension (ACLC) and the Vineland Social Maturity Scale.

The ACLC provided an analysis of Robert's level of language development with respect to population norms. Specifically, it measured his vocabulary and his ability to attend to one or several relevant information cues that would enable him to select the correct picture out of a series of alternatives. For example, Robert was asked to point to the "dog" (vocabulary test), to the "chicken in the basket" (three critical elements), or to the "dog sleeping behind the chair" (four critical elements). The scores obtained for Robert at pretreatment level were 94%, 100%, 80%, and 80%, for vocabulary, two, three, and four critical elements, respectively, indicating some weakness in vocabulary and difficulties with attending to more than two relevant verbal cues.

The Vineland Social Maturity Scale yielded both a social quotient and a level of social maturity in years with reference to population norms. The items in this questionnaire were answered by his mother, but they strictly pertained to Robert's behaviors or social functioning level. For example, typical questions included whether Robert knew how to tell "time to the quarter hour" or whether he was able to make "minor purchases" by himself. Deficiencies in Robert's social development were mainly evident in a lack of age-appropriate independence.

Test Curriculum. This instrument was previously developed in our clinic to assess children's behaviors and performance in the areas of learning readiness, fine and gross motor skills, expressive and receptive language skills, conceptual abilities, socialization, and self-help skills. Testing was conducted by asking Robert to perform or imitate these behaviors upon request, using body parts, games, picture books, picture cards, and other objects, such as plastic animals and food items, dollhouse furniture, and geometric shapes. Performance was tested on behaviors such as holding eye contact, drawing geometric shapes, writing, self-help skills, simple arithmetic, verbal imitation, money concepts, identifying emotions, delayed recall of remote past, and causal relationships. In the course of testing, each of these behaviors was then scored in respect to the frequency of the response (e.g., often, sometimes, or never).

Defining the Problem Behaviors

The next step was to examine the data obtained from the various observations, tests, and the curriculum, in order to specify precisely the treatment goals by defining operationally what exactly Robert was to learn in our clinic and at home. As pointed out earlier, Robert is a relatively high-functioning autistic child. Thus, unlike many other autistic persons, he did not exhibit problem behaviors that centered on self-stimulatory, tantrumous, or self-injurious activities. Instead, it became clear that his main problems were associated with many different aspects of speech and compulsive behaviors. For example, from our videotaped observations it became evident that self-stimulatory and tantrumous behaviors were low (7% and 0%, respectively), but psychotic speech occurred at an unacceptably high level of 78% of the time intervals scored. This was consistent with reports we had obtained about his earlier history.

Behavioral excesses relating to speech included delayed echolalia ("TV talk," repeating TV commercials, game shows, or whole episodes from "Sesame Street") and compulsive repetitive speech (i.e., asking his mother 20 times within half an hour if they would go to Hawaii in the summer, even after he had already received an answer). In fact, it was common for Robert to have the last word in any verbal interaction in the clinic and at home, and this resembled some of the compulsive behaviors often seen in other autistic individuals.

Other problem behaviors were yelling (answering in an inappropriately loud voice) and verbal statements indicating avoidance, such as "Cut it out, guy!" "That's enough!" and "Be quiet now!" He engaged in these behaviors when approached or when demands were placed on him.

Often his functionally appropriate speech sounded bizarre, because of various language deficits. The main deficits of concern at the time of the pretreatment assessment were pronoun reversals, failure to answer yes/no consistent with his actual desire, and failure to relate past events. In addition, Robert's reading comprehension was poor, and he needed to learn certain self-help skills such as going to the store and making small purchases.

SELECTION OF TREATMENT

A behavioral approach to treatment was selected because it has been empirically proven to be effective and is used extensively for the treatment of behavioral excesses and deficits displayed by autistic children. It was necessary to decrease Robert's behavioral excesses that interfered with learning of appropriate behaviors. Thus, clinic treatment was designed to decrease these behaviors and to address his deficits in language skills and other areas.

Parent training was selected as an equally important aspect of the treatment. Lovaas, Koegel, Simmons, and Long (1973) demonstrated the importance of parent training in a follow-up study of a behavior modification program for autistic children. The results showed that 1 to 4 years after termination of treatment, those children whose parents were trained in behavior modification principles in addition to receiving clinic treatment continued to improve. On the other hand, children whose parents did not receive training lost gains previously acquired in a clinic setting. There are several advantages to training parents. First, Robert's parents would learn to teach him new skills and thus provide a round-the-clock treatment environment. Second, they would learn to deal effectively with present behavior problems and new problems as they arose. Finally, it would help ensure that treatment gains would generalize and be maintained in the home and other extratherapy environments.

COURSE OF TREATMENT

Clinic Treatment

Throughout the course of treatment Robert was seen in the clinic once a week for 90 minutes. (Under normal circumstances we would see a family two or three times a week, but because Robert's family lived a long distance from the clinic and because of both parents' work schedules, once a week was determined to be feasible. In addition, given his level of functioning, we determined he could make substantial gains even given our limited contact.) The training in each clinic session consisted of presentation of consecutive learning trials in a discrete trial format (see Koegel & Schreibman, 1982).

During the first month of treatment a token economy was established. Robert received pennies contingent upon correct responses. Pennies could buy backup reinforcers such as food or access to an activity (e.g., seeing and hearing himself live on a video monitor or listening to music). The use of a token economy was established for three reasons: (1) It was easily administered and would not interrupt his responding, (2) it was appropriate given Robert's level of functioning and his chronological age, and (3) it would allow us to use a response-cost procedure to reduce behavioral excesses and other inappropriate behaviors.

Behavioral Excesses. When Robert first began treatment, he displayed a high rate of verbal avoidance behaviors. By eliminating these avoidance behaviors we could make longer verbal exchanges with therapists, family, and others more likely, thus allowing him to learn more appropriate speech through interaction with others. A response-cost procedure (losing one penny for each occurrence of the behavior) was implemented and effectively decreased the avoidance behaviors.

One of Robert's verbal compulsions was "repeating." He would repeat a phrase or sentence several times (up to 50) during a half-hour period. An effective consequence for this behavior was implemented in which Robert was asked "rapid-fire" questions for 1 minute. This procedure was chosen because, although Robert liked to talk on his own terms, he disliked this type of intensive demand. In short, repeating was followed by an aversive stimulus (a punishment procedure). An example of an instance of "repeating" and the consequence is as follows: The therapist would tell Robert to put his hands down. He would comply with the request and then say, "I did put my hands down." The therapist would acknowledge his statement, "Thank you, Robert." Robert would then repeat the statement, "I did put my hands down." After this second occurrence of the behavior, the therapist would rapidly ask questions about his statement for 1 minute (e.g., "What did you do?" or "Why did you put your hands down?").

When "repeating" was eliminated, the topography of this compulsive behavior changed and Robert began "commenting" on other people's statements. This behavior, while less obviously bizarre, also retained the compulsive nature of his autistic speech and still made him appear abnormal. For example, when told, "Robert, read this," he would immediately reply, "Yes, I will read this." Initially he was just told, "No commenting," to label the behavior, to which he would inevitably respond, "Okay, I won't comment." Because a verbal reprimand was ineffective in reducing the occurrence of the behavior, a response-cost program was implemented. However, losing only one penny was ineffective. Typically he would "comment" four or five times in immediate succession before engaging in the behavior became "too expensive" and he would stop. Therefore, the procedure was changed. Robert lost all his pennies for one occurrence of the behavior. A second occurrence of "commenting" resulted in the loss of half of the food item he was earning pennies to buy (e.g., half of a bag of chips would be taken away).

As soon as the above program was implemented, the topography of his compulsive behavior changed again and Robert began whispering (presumably commenting under his breath). When the program was extended to include whispering, this behavior was also eliminated. Whispering was replaced by a subtle, but still inappropriate, behavior: head nodding. A verbal reprimand was sufficient to eliminate this behavior.

Behavioral Deficits. Our main emphasis in the treatment of Robert's behavioral deficits was to improve his language skills. Both our assessment and parental information indicated that one important goal was to work on conversational skills. Thus, treatment focused on teaching Robert to respond appropriately to a variety of questions. For instance, he displayed pronomial reversals characteristic of echolalic speech. Initially, the language program focused on teaching the receptive and expressive skills for the correct use of pronouns. Robert was taught to correctly respond to questions such as "Who has on blue pants?" using the pronouns *I*, *you*, *he*, and *she*.

A second target behavior of the language program was to teach Robert to answer questions appropriately with the response "yes" or "no." Robert was taught to respond correctly to questions such as "Is my sweater red?" After he mastered this task, these types of questions were interspersed with the questions above requiring the correct use of pronouns. For example, while playing a matching game, the therapist might ask both "Is this a frog?" and "Who has the frog?"

A third deficit in language skills was Robert's failure to answer questions about past events such as "What did you do at school today?" and "What did you eat for lunch?" In order to begin to address this problem, he was first taught to recall a very recent event. After the therapist modeled or had Robert perform a sequence of two and later three actions, he learned to recall the events in the correct order. For example, the therapist would stand up, knock on the door, and touch the table and then ask him, "What did I just do?" Although he learned to recall the order correctly, he had difficulty with sentence structure, pronouns, and verb tense in his responses. Therefore, we shifted the emphasis of the task to teaching him grammatically correct responses. It was necessary at first to limit the task to one event and a few simple verbs that were quickly learned, allowing us to gradually add more and work toward generalization to all verbs.

The assessment also revealed that Robert had difficulty answering "why," "when," and "where" questions. Initially, we began with only "why" questions and structured the task to make the questions concrete. For example, the therapist performed an action (e.g., putting her keys on the table) and then asked him about the causal relationship (e.g., "Why are the keys on the table?"). Again, it was necessary to limit the task to a few verbs and teach him correct grammar. Once he mastered the limited task, more verbs were added as before. Next, the questions shifted to more abstract questions, such as "Why do you go to school?" and similar "when" and "where" questions (e.g., "When do you eat breakfast?" or "Where do you sleep?") were added.

One major function of communication is to get information from others (e.g., ask questions). We felt this was another important conversational skill to teach Robert, particularly because he never showed interest in other people by asking questions. This skill would enable him to acquire information relevant to him (e.g., "Mom, what are we having for dinner?") and serve to initiate social interchanges. Thus, during each clinic session Robert was required to ask five questions of various people in the clinic. He also had to remember the answer when he was asked after a short delay (3 minutes). It was necessary to require him to remember the answer to increase his motivation to listen (otherwise he would ask the question but not wait for the reply). Initially, a token system was necessary to increase his motivation to ask questions and listen to the answer. We subsequently began bringing this skill into contact with naturally occurring reinforcers such that asking questions could be maintained without artificially programmed reinforcement. That is, he could ask, "Where are the potato chips?" to obtain that reinforcer.

It was also important to address reading comprehension. Robert's oral reading skills were quite good but he showed little comprehension of what he read. Both his parents and his teacher emphasized this as an important behavior to focus upon because he was having considerable difficulty with the reading program at school. Our assessment of his comprehension skills indicated that, while he had a good vocabulary, he had difficulty comprehending a sentence. Thus, we began by teaching him to follow written commands, beginning with one-step commands and increasing the difficulty to two-step and then three-step commands. When written commands were mastered, we began teaching him to answer questions based on the content of two-sentence stories. An effort was made to make these stories age-appropriate and interesting.

Finally, we have also taught Robert functional, independent living skills, such as purchasing items at a store. These skills were identified by his classroom teacher for intervention. He has received training and practice both in the clinic and at school. Initially, he learned coin labels receptively and expressively. He then learned money values up to $5. He has also learned how much change he should receive for a small purchase (i.e., up to $.50). Since early in his treatment he has practiced going to a small store on campus during each clinic session. At first, his performance was aided by learning to recite the steps involved in shopping and by role-playing in the clinic with a therapist. He has learned to independently go to the store and buy an item. In general, we have attempted to teach him various smaller skills incorporated into a larger context relevant to his environment outside the clinic setting (Koegel & Schreibman, 1982).

Parent Training

Both of Robert's parents have participated in the parent training aspect of his treatment. For the first 7 months of treatment, Robert's father brought him to the clinic, and contact with his mother was limited to telephone conversations. For the remainder of his treatment, his mother has brought him to the clinic. Throughout treatment both parents have been extremely active and effective in carrying out programs in the home.

In this research program, parent training utilizes a wide variety of training materials. First, Robert's parents read a manual on behavioral management techniques (Baker, Brightman, Heifetz, & Murphy, 1976) and a manual on the use of behavior modification procedures with autistic children (Koegel & Schreibman, 1982). Parent training sessions included discussion of the reading material and viewing a parent training videotape showing correct and incorrect use of the procedures. His parents also learned to identify, define, and assess target behaviors. With the help of the parent trainer, they began to develop and implement programs in the home to deal with these behaviors. For example, initially, the parents learned to successfully use extinction to reduce inappropriate behaviors, such as asking repetitive questions (e.g., "What time does the bus come for Robert?") and making compulsive statements about dates, times, and activities (e.g., "Robert goes to school at 8:15" or "We are going to the beach on Saturday, right?"). They also observed Robert's clinic treatment sessions and began working with him in the clinic, with the therapist providing feedback.

A token economy was established at home for the same reasons given for adopting it in the clinic: (1) It was easily implemented since the parents could readily administer programs in public as well as at home, (2) it was more age-appropriate; that is, it was more similar to earning an allowance like other children his age, and (3) it would allow the parents to use response-cost programs for inappropriate behaviors as well. As is sometimes the case, the parents were resistant to the idea of a token economy when it was first introduced. They were concerned that rewarding him with pennies for appropriate behavior was a "bribe" and worried that he would expect to be paid for everything he did. However, once the effectiveness of the token economy was established, their reservations were dispelled. Not only did it provide a specified structure for contingency management, it also reduced aversive interactions and yielded immediately effective results. It did not lead to Robert's expecting to be "paid" for every behavior. Importantly, the parents saw how the token economy would evolve with changes in Robert's behavior.

Behavioral Excesses. "Repeating" was a problem at home as well as in the clinic setting. At first, Robert's parents implemented the same program that was in effect during clinic sessions—specifically, asking him "rapid-fire" questions about his statement for 1 minute. In the home setting this consequence did not decrease the behavior to an acceptable rate. The parents implemented another program to decrease repeating at home. Differential reinforcement of other behaviors (DRO) was put into effect. That is, Robert could earn pennies for each half hour he did not repeat (i.e., reinforcement was given for behaviors other than repeating). This program was effective in decreasing the behavior to a rate acceptable to the parents (i.e., once or twice a day). As in the clinic setting, "commenting" replaced "repeating." A response-cost procedure was implemented to decrease this behavior as well. In addition to losing a penny for commenting, Robert also earned pennies for appropriate responses (i.e., just saying, "Yes," rather than "Yes, Mom, I do want ice cream").

Robert's mother noted that she sometimes lost objective perspective as to the appropriateness of his behavior because she saw him on a day-to-day basis. To compensate, she has used other people's reactions to Robert's behavior as a gauge to determine appropriate and inappropriate behaviors. For instance, she would let him walk ahead of her and watch to see if people looked at him when he talked too loud, talked to himself, or walked inappropriately (e.g., skipping). One behavior that reliably elicited stares was his loud talking. As a result, a program was implemented for loud talking; pennies were lost for talking in a loud voice and earned for talking in a normal speaking voice. In public, a DRO procedure was implemented in which Robert could earn mints for not speaking in a loud voice for increasingly longer periods of time.

Both parents have become skilled at identifying target behaviors and incorporating these behaviors into the token economy program. Robert has earned pennies for appropriate behaviors including age-appropriate play, appropriate speech, compliance, and performance of household tasks. He has lost pennies for inappropriate behaviors such as hiding his face, avoidance behaviors, TV talk, and running in the house.

Behavioral Deficits. One emphasis throughout parent training has been to increase age-appropriate activities. His parents designed and implemented a program to decrease the amount of time Robert spent watching television programs and to increase time spent in more age-appropriate play. They limited the hours during which he could watch television and also limited his choice of shows to only age-appropriate programs. In addition, they encouraged and reinforced age-appropriate play. At age 14, Robert now does not watch shows like "Sesame Street" and spends some of his time shooting baskets, biking, or swimming. They also make an effort to get Robert active in family activities such as board games and bowling.

The family is also working on interacting with Robert in an age-appropriate manner. Understandably, because he is not functioning at his age level, they tended to use childlike language with him and engage him in inappropriate play. For example, his father would demonstrate affection in public by tickling as one would a young child. This type of interaction in public tended to stigmatize Robert. They have also worked on behaviors such as teaching Robert to say, "Mom," rather than "Mommy," and asking him, "Do you want dessert?" rather than "Does Robert want dessert?"

Both parents have been involved in working with Robert during clinic sessions on behaviors such as shoe tying and telling time (using the concept appropriately as opposed to compulsively). For shoe tying, the parents decided upon the steps and taught the behavior using forward chaining. They have also worked extensively on language skills. His mother designed and implemented a program to teach Robert to answer "who," "what," "where," "why," and "when" questions using pictures as prompts. In a typical trial, she would show him a picture of winter, ask him, "Why is it cold?" and reinforce any appropriate response such as "because it is snowing." The program also involved requiring him to formulate the same type of questions to ask her.

Both parents have learned the principles of behavior modification and how to apply these principles to increasing and decreasing behaviors at home. They have been consistently motivated, cooperative, hardworking, and dedicated. The substantial gains in Robert's behavior are due primarily to the efforts of these parents.

FOLLOW-UP

Since autism is a life-span disability, Robert will probably remain in some therapeutic environment for many years or perhaps throughout his life. Thus, for autism, as with other disabilities such as mental retardation, it is perhaps inappropriate to speak of termination of treatment. Rather, treatment programs and environments should be evaluated and alterations be made as the client's behavior changes.

Robert's improvement is somewhat apparent in the data obtained from the formal assessments. When we compared Robert's score on the ACLC obtained at the beginning of the treatment (pretreatment) and after 24 months, we observed only a slight improvement (average of 88.5% correct increased to an average of 91.5% correct). The main improvement occurred in the test category involving three critical elements: Robert improved from 80% to 100%. Test scores at the 24-month level, however, involving four critical elements dropped by 10% to 70% correct.

Similarly, the Vineland Social Maturity Scale scores revealed only

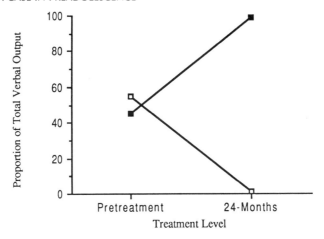

Figure 1.   Proportion of total verbal output at pretreatment and 24-month level. The open squares indicate inappropriate speech (such as echolalia and inappropriate noises), whereas the solid squares indicate appropriate speech (such as asking questions, answering appropriately, and initiating verbal communication). The data are expressed as proportions from the total number of time intervals when Robert spoke.

a slight increase in social maturity (from 11.1 years to 11.6 years). When Robert's social maturity was expressed in terms of the social quotient, however, a drop was observed (from SQ = 92.5 to SQ = 81.3), since Robert was 2 years older at that point, but his social maturity improved by only half a year.

The results from these standardized measures are not surprising and should not be considered as discouraging. Robert's overall functioning level (including social maturity and language development) is, and was, fairly high when compared with other autistic children or teenagers. With only 2 years of treatment these measures might not reflect changes in the relative complex behaviors we addressed in Robert's treatment. That is, his problem behaviors targeted for therapy were mostly very subtle when compared with the rather global behaviors measured by the two standardized tests.

One of the most striking behavioral changes in this child is apparent from our measures of appropriate versus inappropriate speech, as can be seen in Figure 1. (Other behaviors assessed during the videotaped observations are not reported, since their pretreatment and 24-month levels were quite low. The majority of Robert's inappropriate behaviors were related to speech.) There has been a substantial increase in appropriate speech. During the pretreatment assessment, Robert engaged in inappropriate speech during 55% of the intervals during which he spoke. Only 45% of his speech was appropriate. Assessment on this measure, obtained 2 years after treatment began, indicated a substantial increase in the proportion of appropriate speech (i.e., 99%). This change has been accompanied by other improvements in his language, as indicated by his increased use of correct grammar and verb tenses, expanded vocabulary, more proficient command of conversational skills, and understanding of more abstract concepts. Especially encouraging is his increased use of spontaneous speech since we did not explicitly train this skill. Robert uses phrases like "Whoops, wrong answer" when he makes a mistake, or corrects himself by saying "—er—I mean, . . ." It is becoming apparent that Robert can now generalize his language skills and, importantly, learn the appropriate speech forms as modeled by others.

Robert's increased spontaneity was noted in nonverbal as well as verbal behavior. One day, for example, his parents returned home unexpectedly while he was watching "Sesame Street" (which he is not allowed to watch anymore). Just before his parents entered the room where he was watching, he changed the channel to a different program, looking "guilty," and now pretending that he had not watched the children's program. In addition, his mother reported that he shows more and more interest in associating with peers. When his sister brings friends over to their home, Robert now often wants to participate in the activities with the others.

OVERALL EVALUATION

Looking back over the previous 2 years in our treatment program, we can be very pleased with the progress Robert has made. Of course, much of the success is to be attributed to his family's participation in parent training and their admirable dedication to Robert's therapy as described above. In addition, the contribution to Robert's improvement by his school program must be considered.

Robert's steady improvement, as indicated by the data of our assessments, is consistent with a more general impression obtained from less formal observations. Robert appears much more like other young teenagers now. According to his mother, he seems to enjoy his accomplishments when working on the various tasks at home and at school. In the clinic, this is also apparent by the drastically reduced amount of avoidance behavior, and by an increase of positive affect, such as smiling, eye contact, and spontaneity. These impressions were recently further validated when his mother reported that Robert's improvement pleasantly surprised several visiting relatives who had not seen Robert for a few years.

As a result of Robert's general improvement toward normalization, the rest of his family also enjoys a more normal family life. It has become easier for Robert to participate in family activities without becoming a burden or an embarrassment for the rest of the family. Robert's mother told us about an outing the entire family recently took together to a local aquatic park. Of particular interest was Robert's reaction when he was told he could not go on one of his favorite rides because it was for younger children only. Rather than becoming agitated, as he would have in earlier years (when his routines were disturbed or when he did not get what he wanted), he accepted the fact in a calm and controlled manner. Also of note, he imitated many of his sister's behaviors at the park, such as feeding dolphins and picking up starfish (which he would have never done in earlier years). Reporting on this recent outing, his mother enthusiastically announced that he "was a normal child!"

Despite the most favorable treatment success in Robert's case, cautions are warranted to guard from exaggerated expectations for comparable success with other autistic children. First, it has to be kept in mind that tremendous treatment efforts from his family, teachers, and therapists were (and continue to be) implemented. Robert was in treatment for virtually all his waking hours. In school he received intense training (including socialization training). At home his parents and sister took over direct treatment with admirable dedication by consistently applying the skills they had learned in our clinic. In addition, Robert received direct treatment in our clinic. Second, Robert is a fairly high-functioning autistic child. This fact obviously indicates a relatively positive prognosis in general. Lower-functioning autistic children might not achieve his level with the same treatment effort.

Keeping in mind that the syndrome of autism is best considered a life-span disability, we are confronted with still another series of problems in Robert's treatment. As yet autism cannot be "cured"; thus, continued treatment will always be necessary. A complicating factor is that many of Robert's behavior problems have become increasingly more subtle and therefore more difficult to operationalize. With Robert growing up and looking more and more like an adult (Robert is now 14 and 6 feet 2 inches tall), even these subtle behavioral abnormalities become a concern, since they may be more stigmatizing in an adult than in a prepubescent child.

For example, Robert still occasionally engages in bizarre vocalizations when his parents or therapists are not around. (His mother noticed from a distance that passers-by at a public beach looked at Robert in a strange way, which indicated that he probably was engaging in inappropriate behavior.) We started taping his speech with a tape recorder when he was sitting by himself in a public area or when he was in a public restroom. In the course of the treatment we planted in those locations people he had never met before ("strangers") to apply unexpectedly an aversive consequence for inappropriate speech, such as telling him sternly, "Stop whispering, it really bothers me!" This form of treatment proved effective in virtually eliminating his inappropriate vocalizations in those areas. (We made use of "strangers" because Robert had learned to suppress bizarre vocalizations in the presence of the therapists and his parents but still showed an unacceptably high rate of psychotic speech when he was by himself or with people who had not been associated with applying consequences.) Some audio recordings indicate that he still whispers in locations where the treatment has not been implemented yet. Our treatment plan to increase generalization of the treatment effects entails applying the consequences for inappropriate vocalizations in additional novel settings, such as on the beach, in a student lounge, in a cafeteria, and in different public restrooms.

Another problem behavior is his gait, walking pace, and posture. When he walks Robert often holds his arms in an unusual position and walks in a loping manner two steps behind the person with whom he is walking. We plan to modify his behavior by giving him cues or corrective instructions (i.e., "Put your hands down and keep up with Jennifer while you are walking") while he practices normal walking, using a wireless radio transmitter with an earphone.

In general, we are confronted with still another set of problems if we want to be most effective in further normalizing Robert. We will have to continually reassess what activities are age-appropriate, and which activities may be feasible for Robert. For example, in what kind of group sport can he participate, what goals should we aim for in terms of making him more and more independent of supervision, how can we help Robert to learn to relate to peers including the opposite sex, how can we teach him to comply with authority without becoming too compliant and thus becoming an easy victim?

We will continue to work with Robert, and the focus of treatment will change to new directions addressing the more subtle behaviors. Thus, therapy with Robert will also become more challenging. In the months and years to come we will have to adapt our treatment methods to Robert's becoming older and his behavior more differentiated. Since Robert is relatively high-functioning, does not have any of the severe behavior problems usually associated with autism, and has responded extremely favorably to the treatment programs so far, we feel that his prognosis for making maximal improvements is generally very good.

ACKNOWLEDGMENTS

   Preparation of this chapter and the clinical research reported herein
were supported by U. S. P. H. S. Research Grants No. 39434 and No.
28210 from the National Institute of Mental Health, and by University of
California, San Diego, Academic Senate Grant No. RJ 138-G. The authors
wish to express gratitude to David Corina and Wendy Tada for helpful
comments on an earlier draft of this manuscript, and to "Robert's" parents, who have contributed substantially to the treatment of their son and
to the preparation of this chapter.

REFERENCES

Baker, B. L., Brightman, A. J., Heifetz, L. J., & Murphy, D. M. (1976). *Behavior Problems.*
    Chicago: Research Press.
Kanner, L. (1943). Autistic disturbances of affective contact. *Nervous Child, 2*, 217–250.
Koegel, R. L., & Schreibman, L. (1982). *How to teach autistic and other severely handi-
    capped children.* Lawrence, KS: H & H Enterprises.
Lovaas, O. I., Koegel, R. L., Simmons, J. Q., & Long, J. S. (1973). Some generalization
    and follow-up measures on autistic children in behavior therapy. *Journal of Applied
    Behavior Analysis, 6*, 131–166.

CHAPTER 13

Stuttering

GORDON W. BLOOD

DESCRIPTION OF THE DISORDER

Descriptions and definitions of stuttering vary with the observer's perception and with the agreement the individual finds with other observers' perceptions at a specific time. Most definitions of stuttering include primary characteristics and some accessory features. For the purposes of this chapter, stuttering is the involuntary prolongation and repetition of sounds and syllables, often accompanied by tension, struggle, and concomitant physical movements. Some researchers and therapists believe that preschool children, school-age children, and adult stutterers share similar symptoms but should be treated as having different disorders. I agree that preschool child stutterers are not adult stutterers in size-4 toddler clothing. In a sense, stuttering is a disorder of children. It has a gradual onset between the age of 3 and 5 years and tends to be a problem that many children manifest and fortunately recover from before the onset of puberty. Studies indicate that between 50 and 80% of children who stutter recover from their stuttering. There are approximately three to four male stutterers for every one female stutterer. There also exists an increased likelihood of stuttering in families where there are other stutterers. Variability, within individual stutterers and among other stutterers, is a major descriptor. The variable and cyclical nature of stuttering in the preschool child stutterer presents a dilemma in treatment for the therapist. One of the frustrating problems therapists must confront is whether ther-

GORDON W. BLOOD • Department of Communication Disorders, Pennsylvania State University, 105 Moore Building, University Park, Pennsylvania 16802.

apy is intervention or interference. Most nonstuttering children go through a period of "normal nonfluency" as part of their development. This period coincides with the onset of stuttering and shows similar symptoms of repetitions and prolongations of sounds and syllables. However, these repetitions and prolongations are usually effortless nonfluencies, which vary in topography and type from stuttering, with not a great deal of awareness or concern by the child. In contrast, the young stuttering child may display sound and syllable repetitions and prolongations in greater quantity, may manifest concern, tension, and struggle behavior, and may develop compensatory actions to alleviate the problem. A number of authors have suggested that duration of the problem, awareness of the disorder by the child as demonstrated by avoidance of speaking, quantity and type of nonfluent behaviors, parental concern, observable tension, effortful vocal and articulatory attempts at speaking, and concomitant facial and body movements associated with disfluent speech serve as indicators of a chronic stuttering problem. The fact remains that no objective diagnostic tool can predict which four out of five children will outgrow their stuttering. Therapists must decide how to treat a child's normal nonfluency to prevent it from becoming a chronic problem and a child's stuttering from becoming a more severe disorder.

Once the decision to treat a child has been made, the therapist is presented with three options: direct therapy for the child, indirect therapy for the child through parental therapy, or a combination of the first two options. Like many therapists, I prefer an eclectic combination approach of treating both the child and the significant others in the environment.

CASE IDENTIFICATION

This client's stuttering was identified from audiotape recordings of the child's speech provided by the parents, audiotape and videotape recordings of the child's speech with the therapist, and fluency questionnaires filled out by the parents at home and during a direct interview. The client is a firstborn male, aged 4 years 7 months. The child presents strong evidence for some type of immediate therapeutic intervention. There appeared to be a familial history of stuttering, increasing the likelihood of a chronic problem. The onset or identification of the stuttering problem was 22 months prior to contacting the clinic, suggesting a persistent problem. Analysis of the disfluencies showed multiple syllable and sound repetitions, with an average of 4 repetitions per stutter and a range of 2 to 13 repetitions per stuttering moment. Prolongations were present in the child's speech, with an average of 7 seconds for the three longest prolongations. Observable tension in the lips, long silent pauses, and a rapid rate of speaking (201 syllables per minute) were also noted. The parents manifested a heightened concern, coupled with self-reported attempts at controlling the stuttering. These indicators served to identify the child's problem as stuttering not associated with normal fluency development.

PRESENTING COMPLAINTS

The parents' complaints are summarized in the history section. These briefly included a desire to help the child by increasing fluent speech and decreasing his stuttering. The stuttering was reported to occur at home, preschool, restaurants, and church with parents, relatives, teachers, child care attendants, and strangers. The parents were concerned that the child would grow into a stutterer, and the paternal grandmother had described this as a "terrible, lifelong struggle that hampers a man's success." The mother indicated that although the problem started with just repeating and prolonging words, now the child was pursing his lips, closing his eyes, and locking his breathing. The increase in the severity of stuttering symptoms and the client's entrance into the public school system within the year prompted the mother to contact the clinic.

The child's complaints were less dramatic. After about 5 minutes of play, the child confided that he had trouble with his talking. He explained that his words got stuck in his mouth and that he talked too fast. He said that if he slowed down he could talk better. He indicated that a peer made jokes about his speaking and that he did not like that boy anymore. He said that his talking did not bother him all the time. When asked if he would like some help with his talking, he sat up attentively and answered with an emphatic affirmative.

HISTORY

The mother of this client telephoned and set up an interview to discuss her child's stuttering problem. The parents were college graduates, living in close proximity to both sets of grandparents, with one younger son. When asked to describe the problem, the mother indicated that the child repeated words, parts of words, and prolonged endings of his words for at least 5 seconds. The parents indicated that they first noticed the problem when he began combining two and three words during a holiday season at 2 years 6 months of age. It was labeled stuttering at that time by the parental grandmother. Her sensitivity may have been heightened by the fact that her father (the child's great-grandfather) and her brother (the child's great-uncle) both stuttered. The grandmother also disclosed to the child's mother for the first time that the child's father and his sister manifested a stuttering problem from childhood until adolescence. The mother also reported that the child was unintelligible at times, and his entrance into a preschool had made his preschool teacher request suggestions for dealing with the stuttering problem. The mother indicated that she had read that ignoring the problem was the right thing to do and told the teacher not to draw attention to the stuttering. The mother also did not know if the problem was worse at school. The child's peers at school and play were imitating his disfluent speech pattern. The mother stated that the stuttering became a problem at 3 years of age, when other people started asking the child to repeat what he said or simply looked at her for an interpretation. It was around this time that the child also began asking why he was talking so funny. A frequent question was "Why can't I talk?" The mother recalled a drive to the supermarket, approximately 2 minutes from their residence, during which the child repeated the same interrogative "Where" until she turned the car off and unbuckled his seat belt, at which time he finished the question "are we going?" It was at this time she decided to abandon her "leave it alone and it will disappear" philosophy. Instead, the parents began telling the child to stop and think of what he wanted to say and slow down. They also began filling in his words and completing phrases to save him from embarrassment and frustration. Around this time the second child was born, and the mother believed that the client's stuttering became worse for a short period of time. The mother stated that the child went through periods of remission where he might not stutter for an entire week. On numerous occasions he identified the behavior as stuttering and himself as a stutterer, according to the mother. She also noticed that he tended to shy away from most social and verbal interactions, but she indicated that both parents are shy in nature. The client was known to avoid certain words (especially words starting with p and g).

ASSESSMENT

When a parent makes telephone contact, I send out a case history questionnaire for speech, language, and fluency development and also request that the parent make a 10-minute audiotape recording representative of the child's speech. My assessment is a combination and modification of Costello and Ingham's (1984) and Ryan's (1974) assessment techniques, which provide a detailed behavioral analysis of the child's speech in a number of situations and contexts. The Riley Stuttering Severity Instrument (1981) is used to evaluate the frequency, duration, and physical concomitants of the child's stuttering and to derive a stuttering severity rating. Finally, a series of attitudinal questionnaires (Cooper, 1985) are administered to the parents about their perceptions of the stuttering disorder.

Child's Evaluation

Initially, the child's hearing is screened and receptive language skills are evaluated. These tests do not require the child to respond in a verbal manner and help to establish a rapport. Later during the evaluation an articulation or phonology test, expressive language tests, and an oral peripheral examination are completed. The child is requested to play with some toys (He-Man, Go-Bots, cars) that elicit dialogue with the parent. At this point, the therapist begins interacting with the child, sharing pictures of his own children, showing how he plays with the toys, and asking the child to share some stories about the toys. All these interactions are videotaped and audiotaped for later detailed analysis. Assessment of the stuttering is accomplished by asking the child to recite the alphabet, answer information questions (e.g., "How old are you? Where do you live? What is your best friend's name?"), respond in an echoic fashion, recite a nursery rhyme, and ask the therapist five questions. These tasks help to (a) determine if stuttering occurs as a result of the type of linguistic demands placed on the child, (b) examine changes in the stuttering, and (c) evaluate the child's attempts to regain fluency. The specific analyses include examination of speech quality (prosody and tension), rate of speech (measured in syllables and words per minute), and the stuttering moments (measured in percent of stuttered syllables and words and the average duration of the three longest stutters). The articulatory rate (total number of nonstuttered syllables/total amount of talking time), types of stuttering behaviors (whole-word or part-word repetitions, prolongations, presence of "ah" hesitations), and concomitant posturing, respiratory, facial, syntactic, and vocal behaviors are also measured.

The child's summary sheet revealed that his speech was characterized by sound and syllable repetitions and prolongations, abnormal pitch and intensity levels during stuttering moments, unusual prosodic patterns, obvious physical tension and struggle behaviors, an average duration of the three longest stutters of 7 seconds, insertion of "ah" during stuttering moments, mild extraneous hand and head movements, an average of 8.9%

stuttered syllables, and a speaking rate of 201.6 syllables per minute during conversation with parents in and out of the clinic. A stuttering severity score of 18 was obtained on the Stuttering Severity Instrument, which suggests a moderate stuttering problem.

Stuttering behavior was also evaluated through a series of probes. Costello and Ingham (1984) call these Talking Logs. They are simply probes examining changes in stuttering using a simple ABAB design. The interruption probe evaluates the changes in stuttering while the client is being interrupted. It is possible that the listener plays a significant role in this child's stuttering disorder. After a baseline of approximately 1 minute of client talking time free from interruption, the therapist begins to interrupt by looking away, playing with a toy, pushing papers around, and whistling to himself for 1 minute. This is followed by intense interest and attention for the next 1 minute, and, finally, the interruption is administered during the final minute. The next probe asks the child to speak as "best he can, without any bumpy speech" for 1 minute using the same paradigm. This is used to determine what strategies the child may be using to enhance his fluency. The third probe consists of having the child speak to the therapist and then to a puppet. Children often become fluent when the listener is perceived as nonrejecting and nonthreatening. The fourth probe consists of having the child speak to the beat of a metronome. This helps to determine if there are certain rhythmic fluency enhancers. The fifth probe consists of having the child slow down his talking after a model from the therapist. One-word, three-word, and then five-word utterances are recorded using picture stimuli. The sixth probe is also a modeled probe using slow, prolonged, and continued speech. The child is instructed to bump his words together while responding to picture stimuli. These two probes help to determine if specific fluency shaping measures should be attempted during therapy. The last probe is a distractor probe, where the child is asked to talk and draw a picture at the same time. This helps to determine if stuttering changes when the child focuses on something other than his speech.

Fluency was enhanced during the slowdown, "bump your words together," puppet, distractor, and metronome probes. Fluency decreased during the interruption and perform as "best you can" probes.

Parents' Evaluation

A number of questionnaires are administered to the parents to determine their knowledge and perceptions of the disorder. These include the Stuttering Chronicity Prediction Checklist, the Parent's Attitudes toward Stuttering Checklist, and the Situation Avoidance Behavior Checklist (Cooper, 1985). The parents were very aware of the disorder. There appeared to be a familial problem of stuttering. The father was certain that his family history was responsible for the problem. Neither parent thought the child would outgrow his stuttering. They reported doing a number of activities to decrease the stuttering and indicated that they were embarrassed in public when they heard their child stuttering.

Each parent's speech was also analyzed for rate, linguistic complexity, and the number of questions during the samples obtained in the clinic and at home. A change in the parents' speaking pattern may provide a more permanent and rapid change in the child's fluency pattern. Results of the speaking analyses revealed that the father spoke at a rapid rate (253 syllables per minute) and the mother averaged (home and clinic) 221 syllables per minute. It was also noted that 75% of the father's and 45% of the mother's interactions were questions or statements that demanded a response. Both parents interrupted their child, filled in words for him, and told him to take his time when he began to stutter.

SELECTION OF TREATMENT

The treatment selected for this child was a combination and modification of the Gradual Increase in Length and Complexity of Utterance (GILCU; Ryan, 1974) and the Home Intervention Program (Johnson, 1984), based on the child's response to the probes, parental concern, and rate of speaking. GILCU is a fluency-shaping applied behavioral analysis technique, which is easy to conduct, does not require the child to speak in an abnormal speech pattern, and tends to produce good transfer and generalization. The GILCU program gradually increases the length and complexity of the child's utterances (e.g., one word, two words, three words, . . . up to 5 minutes of fluent speech). The consequences for the program include "good" plus tokens for a fluent response and "oops, that was bumpy speech" and no token for stuttered responses. The tokens are used throughout the establishment phase of the program. Modifications of the programs included reducing the child's and each parent's rate of speaking to a rate between 140 and 180 syllables per minute during short phases. The criterion level for this child was set at 95% fluent speech and recovery within three stimulus presentations. This helped to reinforce the concept that fluent speech is desirable, but recovering from disfluent speech is also an acceptable goal. The parent program consisted of modeling the slow speech patterns, teaching the parent(s) to attend to their child's fluency, instructing them to insert pauses in their speech, and training each parent in a number of conversational and pragmatic activities.

COURSE OF TREATMENT

The therapy program for this child is summarized in Table 1. The treatment consisted of three sessions a week and began with instructing the child about the token system and the reinforcers that would be administered. After baseline measures for one- through six-word utterances, small sentences, and 30-second through 10-minute monologues were obtained, therapy was initiated. Probes were administered after successful completion of each of the 36 steps to determine if certain stages of therapy could be eliminated owing to generalization. The first step of treatment was simply having the child look at 100 pictures of one-word objects (e.g., ball, rope, hat, cat), with the instructions to produce slow and fluent speech. The child reached the 95% criterion with no errors. The child was then asked to produce two words fluently. These were word combinations that had semantic meaning (e.g., red ball, blue hill, nice lady, good man, happy dog). The child reached criterion on the first set of 100 two-word utterances. The third through sixth steps of the therapy con-

Table 1
Therapy Intervention Protocol

Child	Parent

Steps 1–6
  Child produces 1 to 6 words fluently
  using at least 100 picture stimuli with
  95% accuracy
	Parents are provided information about
	  stuttering, discuss their feelings, and
	  observe the child in therapy sessions

Steps 7–10
  Child produces 1 to 4 sentences fluently
  using the same criteria as above
	Parents are trained in conversational skills
	  and reduction of stress in the
	  environment

Steps 11–18
  Child speaks from 30 sec to 10 min
  fluently using same criteria and/or
  recovery from stuttering
	Parents report on progress in home
	  environment and changes in child's
	  fluency

Child taught to reduce rate	Branching step: Parents taught to reduce rate

Child recycled through steps 1–18 during
  conversation
	Report on home activities and changes in
	  fluency

Transfer activities in and out of clinic	Transfer activities at home Interview/telephone follow-up

sisted of having the child look at pictures of three-, four-, five-, six-word utterances and tell what they were. The stimuli consisted of three to six pictures placed in front of the child on a table. The child was required to produce the utterance fluently. Again, these were word combinations that had semantic meaning (e.g., little red barn, a small blue ball, a big dog and cat, the mean man with a stick). The client was able to reach criterion level for three-word utterances with one set of 100 stimuli. The 95% criterion was not reached until 200 stimuli were employed for the four-, five-, and six-word utterances. Steps 7 through 10 consisted of having the child produce one, two, three, and, finally, four sentences from the pictures. A token and verbal reinforcer was given only if the child responded fluently. The client completed the three sentence levels with slow, fluent speech. Steps 11 through 18 consisted of having the child look at picture stimuli and generate monologues for 30 seconds, 1 minute, $1\frac{1}{2}$ minutes, 2 minutes, 3 minutes, 5 minutes, and 10 minutes. At this stage of the program, a branching step was necessary. The child's rate of speaking was so rapid (201 syllables per minute) that he was unable to produce the fluent pattern. At this step, the child was taught to produce slower, easy, continuous speech. The following is the excerpt of the therapy between the child and the therapist.

CLIENT: I-I-I-I-I just c-c-c-an't get the wah-ah-ah-ah-ah ords right.

THERAPIST: What I want you to do is pretend you are moving very, very slow. Watch me (demonstrates by getting up and moving slowly around the room). See my hands are moving slow. Now my feet are moving slow. Now I am walking slow and even talking slow. You try it with me.

CLIENT: N-ah-ah-ah-o. It looks silly.

THERAPIST: Come on. If you can do this you can earn some chips (tokens).

CLIENT: M-m-m-m-y body is going so slow and so are my feet. . . .

THERAPIST: Let your talking slow down too.

CLIENT: Like (pause) a (pause) robot?

THERAPIST: Not that slow, how about like a fish who swims up and down on the waves. In fact, I've got a clock we can watch to see how slow you and I can talk.

CLIENT: F-f-fish don't swim u-u-u-u-p a-ah-ah-ah-nd down on waves, th-th-they stay i-(prolongs for 4 sec)n the water.

THERAPIST: These fish (gesturing to child and therapist) do. Come on, move your hands and use easy, slower speech.

CLIENT: Now (pause) I (pause) am (pause) a (pause) slow (pause) fish.

THERAPIST: That's great. The clock says you are slower, but can you bump your words together like this, so you don't sound like a robot fish? (Child laughs and therapist demonstrates easy, slower, continuous phonation with normal stress and prosody.)

CLIENT: You (pause) mean (pause) this (pause) kinda (pause)?

THERAPIST: I am going to put chalk on the board and whenever you talk like a robot fish, like this—my (pause) name (pause) is (pause), I'll lift the chalk off the chalkboard. Whenever you use fish, nice, easy, slower talking like this—my (prolonging into) name (prolonging into) is (prolonging into), I'll keep the chalk on the board.

CLIENT: (tries and it doesn't work)

THERAPIST: (tries the same script with his finger on the child's arm) When I lift my finger off, you'll know it's a robot fish. Okay? You talk and see if you can make my finger stay on your arm for the whole five seconds like a fish swimming nice and easy, up and down on the waves.

CLIENT: The (prolonging into) little (prolonging into) barn (prolonging into) had (prolonging into) one (prolonging into) lamb.

THERAPIST: Terrific, I knew you could do it. Great let's do another.

Again, a 95% criterion and a recovery of fluency within three words were employed. Once the child was at the 2-minute level of therapy, his speaking rate began to increase. He was allowed to maintain an increased rate as long as he was fluent.

It was also at this time that the parents' involvement in the therapy was increased. The parents were informed that the child was unable to progress through a 30-second monologue without stuttering. The branching step was explained, and then the results of their baseline speech sample and the possibility that the child might be trying to model their rapid rate was reintroduced. This was initially suggested earlier at the end of the assessment. Prior to this session, the parents' involvement consisted of sharing a number of their feelings about the problem and observation through video camera monitors. The parents had been given factual information about stuttering and pamphlets to read. It was explained that they would have to make some temporary adjustments in their life-style to enhance their son's fluency. It was pointed out that the therapist spoke at a rapid rate but slowed his rate upon entrance into the therapy room. They were asked to observe the slow, easy, and continuous speech that was used while interacting with their son. The next part of the session was devoted to changing the parents' rate of speaking. The father and mother were audiotaped for 10 minutes of talking with the therapist. At the end of the 10 minutes, the audiotape was reviewed and the parents' rate of speaking was calculated. The therapist then made suggestions, such as pausing after every third word, setting a stopwatch, and allowing a specific number of words per minute. After the parents achieved 30 seconds of slower, easier speech, they practiced for 1 minute with the therapist. The first assignment was to practice only at dinnertime, using the slower, easier rate of speaking. The mother reported that she and her husband noticed a change in the child's fluency. The father was unable to attend the next 10 sessions, but the mother and the therapist reviewed the reduced rate of speaking and increased it to 5 minutes with the therapist. The mother also practiced her reduced rate with the therapist and the child in the therapy room. The slower, easier talking was extended to other times during the day and different situations. On the father's return to observe at the clinic, he indicated that "the kid is doing great, but we all act and sound like we're comatose." At this time the parents had already begun to increase their rates of speaking but were now practicing other skills. The parents were also trained in basic pragmatic skills, including turn-taking in conversation, interrupting each other, allowing the child to complete his utterance, being a good listener, and avoiding verbal performances from their child.

The client completed the remainder of the first 18 steps with 95% accuracy or recovery from stuttering within three syllables, words, or phrases. He was then recycled through all 18 steps during conversation with the therapist. The client successfully completed the second 18 steps of program. Transfer activities included speaking with the therapist outside of the therapy room, down the hall, walking around the building, and walking in other buildings. Additional activities including speaking fluently with one additional person in the room, with two additional persons in the room, with the parents and the therapist, and with the parents and no therapist. Reports by the mother of interactions with peers, preschool teacher, and relatives were also recorded.

TERMINATION

Therapy sessions were reduced from three times a week during the establishment phase to twice a week during the transfer stage. When fluency rates stabilized at above 95% for 10 minutes in four transfer activities, the mother was instructed to bring the client once weekly for sessions and report on his fluent behavior. The parents had already increased their speaking rates to slightly slower than their original rates and indicated they were still incorporating the pragmatic activities in their daily routines. The client's speaking rate was also rapid, but fluent. The client was dismissed after 63 therapy sessions and considered a fluent speaker. He was told to come to the clinic for speech checkups (just like a dental checkup) as soon as there were any problems with his talking, or every 6 months, whichever came first. The parents were told that small setbacks at certain times (e.g., holidays, overtiredness, stressful days at school, initiation of new learning activities) might occur and not to become overly concerned.

FOLLOW-UP

During the first and second 6-month checkup spontaneous speech samples of the child were elicited with the parent and the therapist. Ten-minute speech samples in the clinic and outside clinic settings were also obtained from the mother. Fluency was above criterion in all situations, and the mother reported two incidents of relapse. She indicated that the child had been stuttering for approximately 1 day each time and recovered the next day. She also indicated that she reduced her own rate of speaking, attempted to listen better, and tried to determine what had changed in the child's routine. The parent telephoned for her third checkup to indicate that she saw no further reason for evaluating her son's stuttering. She reported that no stuttering had been observed. A telephone follow-up 3 years later indicated that the child had had a relapse at a family holiday celebration that lasted "about a week." During that time, both parents reduced their rate of speaking, practiced the conversational activities, and allowed the child to talk about what was happening to his speech They reassured him that it would dissipate and that he should not be overly concerned. The client has been relapse-free for 2 years.

OVERALL EVALUATION

There are a number of uncontrolled variables that confound this client's success. The client's positive response to a combination of fluency-shaping behavior therapy and parent intervention suggests that an appropriate therapy technique was selected. A number of therapists and researchers have recommended that each child be examined carefully to determine the most effective therapy or combination of therapies to be conducted. Although selection of a technique is based on a number of observable and measurable behaviors, there are also some "X" factors present in this and most cases that should be addressed. First, the possibility exists that this child could have outgrown his stuttering without intervention. The predictors employed suggest that such would not have been the case, but it was possible. Second, the parents in this case were cooperative participants in the therapy. This is not always the case. The father's initial resistance was quickly resolved, and the mother's concern may have been diminished by merely seeking and obtaining any type of therapy. The effect of being treated may have eased the parental tension that spilled over into the child's world. This specific approach gave everyone involved something constructive to do. This appeared to be critical and helped the parents and child feel responsible for the therapy's success. I think the results of the therapy were successful; however, some researchers indicate that at least a 5-year follow-up is necessary to determine therapeutic effectiveness. Another researcher/therapist may have dealt with this child in an entirely different manner, but ideally concluded in a similar manner. In view of the fact that no two stutterers are identical, one can safely assume that no two therapy programs would be identical. Often in therapy, the differences among stutterers eclipse the similarities.

REFERENCES

Cooper, E. B. (1985). *Personalized fluency control therapy* (2nd ed.). Austin, TX: Learning Concepts.

Costello, J., & Ingham, R. J. (1984). Assessment strategies for stuttering. In R. Curlee & W. H. Perkins (Eds.), *Nature and treatment of stuttering: New directions* (pp. 303–334). San Diego: College Hill Press.

Johnson, L. (1984). Facilitating parental involvement in therapy of the preschool disfluent child. In W. H. Perkins (Ed.), *Stuttering disorders* (pp. 29–40). New York: Thieme-Stratton.

Ryan, B. P. (1974). *Programmed therapy for stuttering in children and adults.* Springfield, IL: Charles C Thomas.

Riley, G. (1984). *Stuttering severity instrument.* Tigard, OR: C. C. Publications.

CHAPTER 14

Oppositional Disorder

ALAN M. GROSS

DESCRIPTION OF THE DISORDER

Disobedient, negativistic, and provocative opposition to authority is the essential feature of Oppositional Disorder (APA, 1980). The oppositional attitude is directed toward family members and teachers. Parents are the most frequent target of the child's maladaptive responses.

The persistence of the oppositional style is striking. Oppositional children will exhibit this type of behavior even when it is destructive to their well-being and self-interests. For example, rules are routinely broken, requests refused, and suggestions opposed. If asked to refrain from engaging in an activity, the child appears compelled to perform it. This negative pattern of responding often leads to a decrease in productive activity and pleasurable relationships. It is the persistent nature of the oppositional attitude that differentiates oppositional children from youngsters who occasionally engage in noncompliant responding.

Oppositional children should also be distinguished from conduct-disordered youngsters (Gross, 1985). In conduct disorder, the child displays responses that violate the basic rights of others or major age-appropriate rules. The behavior of the oppositional child is not so severe as to include persistent lying, theft, aggression, or vandalism.

The occurrence of oppositional behavior between the ages of 18 and 36 months is considered to be a normal part of development. As such, the diagnosis of oppositional disorder is used only when severe opposi-

ALAN M. GROSS • Department of Psychology, University of Mississippi, University, Mississippi 38677.

tional behavior continues beyond this period of time. While the age of onset can be as early as 3 years, it occurs more commonly in late childhood or adolescence. The disorder usually lasts for several years and can interfere with social relationships. Oppositional behavior in school also frequently results in academic problems, and school failure is a common complication.

CASE IDENTIFICATION AND PRESENTING COMPLAINTS

Zack was a 6-year-old boy who lived with his mother and father in a large southeastern city. His parents reported that in the past 8 months Zack had become impossible to manage. His mother (Mrs. D.) stated that he had a very negative attitude. She indicated that he was noncompliant to almost all requests from her and her husband, and that he exhibited severe temper tantrums when he did not get his way.

His negative attitude was also becoming a source of concern at school. Mr. D. stated that Zack's teacher had recently complained that it was difficult to prompt Zack to do his schoolwork. It was reported that he frequently refused to do his assignments. He was also noted as being defiant and noncompliant to her requests. In particular, his refusal to remain in his seat and not talk out in class was disruptive to the entire class.

HISTORY

Mrs. D. recalled no problems during her pregnancy or the birth of her son. She stated that, as an infant, Zack had a wonderful temperament. Getting along with him had become difficult only within the past year. It was reported that Zack had reached all the developmental milestones within normal limits.

Zack's parents had been married 2 years when he was born. Mr. D. owned a very successful advertising agency. Because of the financial security his business success provided, Mrs. D. chose to stay home with her son rather than work. Prior to his birth she had worked as a flight attendant.

At the time of their first clinic visit Mr. D. was no longer required to do much business-related travel. However, approximately 1 year earlier he was out of town an average of 2 nights a week every other week. Mr. D.'s business activity had not required him to travel prior to this period. This schedule lasted approximately 6 months and was the result of a decision to expand his business into another city.

Mrs. D. indicated that Zack reacted poorly to his father's absences. He and his father spent considerable time together, and Zack appeared to miss very much the daily time with his father. Moreover, during the period that Mr. D. was frequently away from home, Mrs. D. was pregnant with their second son, Jack. They hired a live-in housekeeper to help Mrs. D. during this period. Mrs. D. also suggested that as a result of the physical exhaustion the pregnancy produced, she was unable to be as attentive as Zack required during this time.

Initially, when his father was away Zack demanded a tremendous amount of attention. He constantly wanted his mother to act as a play-mate. He would whine and cry if she refused. It was also at this time that he began to exhibit tantrums when he did not get his way. He began to display problems at bedtime. She reported that the only way to get him to go to sleep was to allow him to sleep in her bed. This was still a problem.

The birth of Jack coincided with an increase in Zack's behavior problems. Mr. and Mrs. D. emphasized, however, that these difficulties were evident prior to Jack's birth. His parents reported that since the arrival of their second son they had made a concerted effort to give individual attention to Zack. This did not seem to have any effect on his behavior. Zack was reported as getting along very well with his baby brother.

Despite their efforts, Zack's behavior had progressively deteriorated at home. It was stated that Zack appeared to go out of his way to break household rules. He had become extremely argumentative. Tantrums occurred when he did not get his way, and almost any request evoked an automatic "no" response. Mr. and Mrs. D. felt as if they were starting to plan their lives in a manner to minimize their interactions with Zack.

ASSESSMENT

The assessment process was implemented at the initial interview. The therapist met first with Mr. and Mrs. D. During this meeting an attempt was made to obtain a general description of the presenting problem and relevant historical information. The therapist asked Zack's parents to describe in detail an example of a recent problem interaction with Zack. This was done in order to identify antecedent and consequence stimuli that might have been contributing to their difficulties. A portion of the initial interview follows:

THERAPIST: Please describe in detail a recent incident you had with Zack.

MRS. D.:   This happened three days ago. We were pretty upset about it and it is really what prompted us to call. Zack has a little battery-operated riding toy. He really loves those kind of toys. My husband had just come home and we were in the backyard. Well, Zack jumped on his car and started riding on the cement patio next to the pool. I asked him to come ride over next to us and he ignored me.

THERAPIST: What did you do then?

MR. D.:   I asked him if he had heard what his mother had said. He just looked at me and kept doing what he had been asked not to do.

THERAPIST: What happened next?

MRS. D.:   We had been having a pretty good day and I didn't want to spoil it with a fight so I told him he could continue to ride by the pool as long as he kept outside the blue tile line. That seemed to prompt him to ride inside the line.

THERAPIST: Then what did you do?

MRS. D.:   I tried to explain to him that I wanted him to ride elsewhere because I was afraid he might fall in the pool. Upon hearing that he turned the car and rode directly into the pool.

MR. D.:   After we pulled him out of the pool and saw that he was all right, I really started yelling at him. He really could have been hurt. He just acted like he hadn't done anything wrong.

THERAPIST: Did you punish him?

MR. D.:   I told him he could not use any of his riding toys for a week.

THERAPIST: Did you follow through with this plan?

MR. D.:   For a day or so.

After the therapist finished talking with Zack's parents he met alone with Zack. During this interview he attempted to measure the youngster's understanding of why he and his family had come to the clinic. He also tried to determine potential reinforcing and punishing stimuli for use in treatment planning. Zack felt that things at home were all right, even though his parents sometimes did yell at him for being bad. It was explained to Zack that his parents didn't like it when they yelled, and that the reason the family came to the clinic was to learn how to get along at home without hollering. This was done in order to stress to the child that he was not the sole focus of the problem.

The first interview was concluded with the therapist's presentation of a brief summary of his assessment observations. As a homework assignment, Mr. and Mrs. D. were asked to record in detail two examples of family arguments that occurred during the week prior to the next session. This was done in order to gather further data concerning possible antecedents and consequences of the family's problem interactions. This procedure was conducted throughout the course of treatment. These weekly reports helped the therapist monitor treatment progress, as well as providing useful data upon which adjustments in treatment could be made. Permission to call Zack's teacher on the telephone to discuss his behavior in school was also obtained during the first interview.

Zack's teacher indicated that Zack was a bright boy. However, it was rare that he displayed these abilities in his schoolwork. Zack's teacher noted that he had a "terrible attitude" and was "rebellious." He failed to follow her instructions whether they concerned academic tasks or classroom rules. She reported that he was not aggressive. His resistance most commonly involved ignoring requests. Displays of disobedience and passive resistance to authority figures characterized his interactions with other school personnel. She also suggested that he seemed to be well liked by his peers and that he did not have any difficulties socially.

An analysis of the data that Mr. and Mrs. D. brought back on their next clinic visit revealed a specific pattern in their interactions with Zack. Zack's noncompliant behavior resulted in a great deal of one-to-one attention. Following an oppositional response, Mr. and Mrs. D. usually explained to Zack the reasons that it was important to follow their instructions. When this failed, they usually threatened him with punishment or tried to persuade him to comply. More important, if their efforts failed to prompt the desired behavior from Zack, they would frequently become frustrated and perform the task themselves. For example, after an argument concerning keeping his toys out of the living room failed to produce the desired effect, Mrs. D. usually put the toys away for him. This sequence of events resulted in his parents' inadvertently reinforcing noncompliant behavior. A similar pattern of experiencing no immediate aversive consequences for inappropriate behavior characterized many of the problem interactions with his teacher.

Data also indicated that Zack's parents were very inconsistent in their attempts to use punishment procedures. While they would frequently impose a punishment for some transgression, they rarely followed through with the application of the contingency. For example, in the dialogue presented from the first interview it can be seen that his parents told Zack that because of his disobedience he would not be able to use any of his riding toys for 1 week. However, he was allowed to use them after a day or so.

SELECTION OF TREATMENT

Results of the assessment indicated that Zack's parents were inadvertently encouraging his inappropriate behavior. Their attempts to discipline him using punishment procedures were failing. This was due to the inconsistency with which they imposed their contingencies. Therapy, therefore, consisted of training Mr. and Mrs. D. in child management skills. This consisted of teaching them to observe and monitor Zack's responding as well as their own parenting behaviors. They were then taught to develop specific behavioral contingencies. Emphasis was placed on the importance of clearly defining target behaviors and associated consequences. The child management techniques taught included reinforcement, punishment, extinction, and negotiation skills. It was expected that teaching Mr. and Mrs. D. to reward Zack's appropriate responses and punish his inappropriate responses would result in an improvement in his behavior. It was also expected that helping Mr. and Mrs. D. develop a consistent parenting style, in which rewards were frequently delivered for good behavior, would help Zack learn to obtain attention from his parents via more socially acceptable methods. Last, it was predicted that improved parenting skills and the decrease in parental yelling it produced would lead to an improvement in the nature of the relationship that existed between Zack and his parents.

COURSE OF TREATMENT

The first session of treatment (session 2) began with the therapist's explaining to Zack's parents the relationship between their son's inappropriate responding and their own behavior. This was carried out in order to begin to educate them concerning the relationship between behavior and the consequences it produces. The basics of using reinforcement were also introduced in this session. A segment of the interview follows:

THERAPIST: Let me give you an example of what I mean about behavior being a function of its consequences. In particular, I want to start by discussing the concept of reinforcing a respone. One of the situations you reported this week involved an argument about keeping his bicycle out of the driveway. You asked him to move it and he didn't. Then you lectured him and hollered at him. Finally, you put the bicycle away.

MRS. D.:   Sometimes it is easier to do it myself than fight with him.

THERAPIST: In the short run that is correct. However, looking at it from the response– consequence analysis, we see that in this situation the consequence for disobedience is one-to-one parental attention. I know that this kind of attention seems aversive to you and me. However, it is attention. Frequently, when a child is good, parents don't comment on the act and as such he gets very little attention for it. A second consequence for his noncompliance is that he avoids having to perform an undesirable task. His experience has taught him that when you finish yelling at him you will do his work for him. From this point of view, it appears that noncompliance is inadvertently reinforced with attention and avoidance of an unpleasant task.

Following the above discussion, the therapist began instructing Mr. and Mrs. D. in specific parenting skills. An attempt was made to teach them to issue clear and direct commands, specify response–consequence relationships, and to deliver rewards for the display of target behaviors. Furthermore, the importance of consistently using these procedures was emphasized. A segment of the discussion concerning this topic follows:

THERAPIST: We have been talking about how important it is in your interactions with Zack to clearly convey what behaviors you expect performed and what consequences he will receive when he displays them. There is a thought I would like to suggest in order to help you train yourself to communicate this way. I call it the if–then statement. That is, when I want a child to do something I try and verbalize it in an if–then statement. For example, getting back to the bicycle incident. Rather than simply ordering him to put his bicycle away it would be better to say, "I want you to put your bicycle away during the next TV commercial. *If* you put it away, *then* you can continue to watch TV. *If* you don't put it away, *then* I am going to turn the TV off until you do what I ask."

MRS. D.:   That doesn't sound too hard to remember.

THERAPIST: In fact, you probably use this procedure from time to time already. Most parents use some variant of it at the dinner table; eat your vegetables before you can have dessert. In essence, what you are doing is making the occurrence of a highly desirable event contingent or dependent on the occurrence of a low-probability behavior.

The second session was concluded with a homework assignment. Mr. and Mrs. D. discussed two problematic situations that they were experiencing on an almost daily basis and generated a number of possible contingencies that they could impose. They were asked to attempt to use this new procedure when the situation was appropriate, but in particular when the two target situations occurred. They were also asked to record in detail what happened in these targeted situations on two occasions. This information would be discussed at the next session.

The results of Zack's parents' attempts to use contingency statements was the focus of the third session. They indicated that in instances where they used this technique it proved fairly successful. However, thinking of a reward was at times problematic. It was also reported that they could be doing much better at attending to Zack's good behavior. Suggestions were made concerning ways to notice and praise Zack's appropriate responding.

In order to assist Zack's parents in developing their management skills, a portion of the third session was spent enacting role-plays. Various problematic situations were discussed and examples of potential contingency strategies were developed. The role-play procedure also allowed the therapist to provide Zack's parents with feedback regarding use of the procedures. At the conclusion of the session the therapist instructed Mr. and Mrs. D. to use these procedures throughout the following week and record an instance when the procedure was successful and an occasion when it failed.

At the fourth session it was reported that things were going much better at home. Mr. and Mrs. D. were becoming very comfortable with using contingency statements when making requests of Zack. They also noted that this had resulted in an improvement in their son's behavior and a remarkable decrease in yelling and arguing. The increase in pleasant interactions also seemed to facilitate their ability to attend to his appropriate responding.

After providing Zack's parents with feedback concerning their application of the contingency procedures, the therapist prompted them to discuss how they were allotting their time between Zack and his younger brother. While there was no doubt that Mr. and Mrs. D. were attempting to spend a great deal of time with their children, it was apparent that Zack was not receiving nearly as much individual time with his parents as he had before his brother was born. It was explained that while Zack had to experience a decrease in one-to-one time with his parents as a result of having a sibling, it was still very important that he receive some parental attention that did not include his brother. In addition to their regular assignment (using contingency statements, praising good behavior, recording a successful and unsuccessful attempt to discipline), Mr. and Mrs. D. were each asked to spend a small amount of individual time with Zack before the next session. Suggestions of possible strategies for achieving this goal were discussed.

As did the previous sessions, the fifth meeting began with a review of the week's events. It was reported that things were continuing to improve at home. Along with a further decrease in disobedient behavior, there was a noticeable increase in pleasant family interactions. Mr. and Mrs. D. also reported experiencing successful individual outings with Zack. The parents were praised for their outstanding efforts and were urged to continue using these skills. Spending further individual time with Zack was also suggested.

Since Zack's parents had demonstrated good general skills regarding applying contingency management procedures at home, the therapist shifted the focus of the treatment session to Zack's school difficulties. His parents indicated that in a discussion the previous week with his teacher they had learned that Zack was still disrupting his class. It was suggested that his academic problems could also be attacked using a contingency management approach. Moreover, allowing Zack to participate in the development of school contingencies would be useful. This type of involvement frequently increases the likelihood of treatment success. Mr. and Mrs. D. were asked to speak with Zack's teacher and determine specifically what behaviors needed to be altered. They were also instructed to have Zack accompany them to the next session.

The therapist began the following session by meeting alone briefly with Zack's parents. The information Mr. and Mrs. D. obtained from Zack's teacher was discussed. Appropriate target behaviors and potential rewards were also generated. The therapist then met alone with Zack. They discussed Zack's perceptions about what had been going on at home. Zack reported that he was pleased with his situation at home. He was told that his parents shared this feeling, and that they were proud of how hard he was working on improving his behavior. However, they were still concerned about how he was doing in school. Conferences with his teacher indicated that he had trouble staying in his seat, talking out of turn, and following instructions. Zack was told that the reason he asked to come to this meeting was to assist him and his parents in developing a plan that would help him do better at school and help his parents learn not to yell at him about his schoolwork. Following his meeting with Zack, the therapist asked Mr. and Mrs. D. to join Zack and him. A portion of the remainder of the session follows:

THERAPIST: Mrs. D., why don't you tell us what you want from Zack concerning his schoolwork.

MRS. D.: I know that he can do better in school then he has been. His teacher says that when he tries he does really well. She says he needs to learn to follow her instructions. In particular, she wants him to stay in his seat and not talk out of turn.

THERAPIST: School can be hard work, right, Zack? Sometimes there are other things you would rather be doing. Such as talking to your friends or going to the pencil sharpener. However, its important that you try your best in school. Its also true that when people work hard they get rewarded. Do you think that it would be easier to remember to work hard all day, and not just part of the day, if you were going to get rewarded that day for doing well?

ZACK: I guess so.

MR. D.: We would be willing to reward you for working harder and doing better in school.

THERAPIST: In order for your folks to know how hard you worked in school the teacher has to send them a note about your behavior. Your parents tell me that your teacher gives out Happy Faces and Frowny Faces for some of the work you do in class.

ZACK: Yeah.

THERAPIST: Starting Monday, at the end of each school day your teacher is going to give you a sheet of paper to take home to show to your parents. If you worked hard all day and followed instructions she will put a Happy Face on the paper. If you haven't had such a good day, then she will put a Frowny Face on the sheet. Mr. and Mrs. D., you said that if he did well he would earn rewards. What do you suggest?

MR. D.:   How about an extra half hour of TV?

MRS. D.:   We could play a game for 30 minutes each day he gets a Happy Face.

ZACK: How about both?

THERAPIST: What about a compromise. On days that you bring home a Happy Face you can choose either extra TV or to play a game with your parents.

MRS. D.:   That sounds fine.

THERAPIST: Is that alright with you Zack?

ZACK: Yeah.

At the completion of the session Zack's parents were instructed to implement the school contingency the following Monday. They were also urged to continue with the other aspects of the program.

The focus of the next couple of sessions was to help Zack's parents perfect their newly acquired behavior management skills. When Zack demonstrated an improvement in his academic behavior, adjustments in the contingencies were discussed. More important, a portion of each of these latter sessions was devoted to instructing Mr. and Mrs. D. in how to apply contingency management methods in novel situations. This was accomplished by having the therapist suggest potential problem situations and asking Mr. and Mrs. D. to role-play solutions.

TERMINATION

The termination phase of treatment was conducted over two sessions. The aim of treatment was to teach Mr. and Mrs. D. a set of child management skills for general use. As such, the focus of the final phase of treatment was on emphasizing the importance for them to continue to use these methods. The therapist pointed out that at the onset of therapy Zack was receiving attention for inappropriate behavior and his good behavior was going unnoticed. A crucial factor in the successful treatment of Mr. and Mrs. D.'s difficulties was learning to attend consistently to appropriate behavior and to punish or extinguish inappropriate behavior. They were told that many parents revert to their old habits when problems are eradicated. Their experience with treatment demonstrated that Zack's behavior changed as a function of changes in their behavior. If they reverted to the previous manner in which they interacted, it is most likely that his behavior would also revert to what it once was. In order to help them remember to continue to employ their new parenting skills, it was proposed that they monitor each other's interactions with Zack and deliver praise when good parenting skills were displayed.

In addition to reminding Zack's parents of the importance of continuing to be systematic in their discipline, a large portion of the session was devoted to explaining formal procedures for promoting maintenance of behavior change. The school contingency provided the focus for this discussion. The therapist explained that when attempting to shape a new behavior it was extremely important to make the relationship between the response and its consequences very salient. That was why treatment emphasized the use of immediate reinforcement. However, the majority of behavior is supported by intermittent or delayed rewards. In order to teach Zack to display appropriate responding in the absence of immediate reinforcement, and learn to delay gratification, it was considered useful to slowly fade the more formal aspects of the school contingency. An example of this portion of the session follows:

THERAPIST: One possible way to modify the school contingency would be to reduce the frequency with which the teacher sends home notes. For example, you might ask her to send them home on Wednesdays and Fridays, or just on Fridays.

MRS. D.:   I assume that when we do this he gets his special privileges until we get a bad report.

THERAPIST: That's correct. You would tell him that he has been doing great and as such you don't see the need for daily checks. As long as he keeps bringing home good reports he has earned his rewards.

MR. D.:   What do we do if he brings home a bad report?

THERAPIST: He should be told at the time that you reduce the frequency of reports that a bad report means the loss of privileges until he brings home a good report. It might also be a good idea to ask the teacher to send hom a report the next day so that he doesn't have to go a week without privileges while he is being good at school.

Zack's parents were also told that continuing to praise his efforts was important and that delivering unexpected rewards for good behavior would help him learn to delay gratification. Zack's parents were instructed to implement these changes and return in 2 weeks with Zack.

In the final session, the therapist first met alone with Zack's parents. They reviewed the week's treatment progress. Mrs. D. indicated that things were continuing to go very well at home and that Zack had brought home a good school report in each of the previous weeks. When asked about their success at continuing to attend to unprompted good behavior from Zack, they reported that they were doing above average. Mr. D. stated that having his wife comment on his performance was a very useful reminder. Once again they were reminded of the importance of consistently using their new skills and were praised for their efforts.

Following the brief interview with Zack's parents the therapist met alone with Zack. During this meeting the therapist praised Zack for the dramatic improvement he had displayed in his behavior. He was also asked about his feelings concerning home life. Zack was enthusiastic about the changes that had occurred at home. He said that he felt as if his parents didn't get mad at him as frequently as they did before they started coming to therapy. He also liked the individual attention he was receiving. The therapist praised Zack for his hard work and explained that since things were going so well as home, he and his parents were not going to return for quite a while.

The session was concluded with a meeting with the entire family. Once again, all of them were praised for their hard work. They were encouraged to continue with what they had been doing. The therapist explained that since they were doing so well it was not necessary to see them again for 1 month. However, if problems arose, or if they had questions about how to handle a particular situation, they should feel free to call him.

FOLLOW-UP

Three days prior to their follow-up meeting Mrs. D. called the therapist to cancel the appointment. At this time she indicated that because things were going so well at home she did not see a need for the family to return. Upon further questioning it was revealed that Zack was doing very well in school and that his teacher suggested that there was no longer a need for her to continue to send home weekly reports. While there were occasional arguments at home, Mrs. D. felt that they were nothing unusual. Zack had become a pleasure to deal with and the level of family interaction had dramatically increased. She also felt that she and her husband had been successfully working together to maintain a high level of consistency in their application of their new parenting skills. The therapist praised their efforts and told her to feel free to call if he could be of any assistance in the future.

OVERALL EVALUATION

This case represents a fairly straightforward example of treating an oppositional child using contingency management procedures. A young boy was brought to the clinic by his parents because of behavior problems at home and in school. The assessment procedures involved interviewing the youngster's parents. This procedure revealed a number of target behaviors and their associated maintaining stimuli. Treatment consisted of training the child's parents in child management skills. In particular, they were instructed to issue commands clearly, specify response contingencies, and praise appropriate behavior. A home-based reward program was also implemented to improve his behavior in school. Data collected by the parents throughout treatment indicated a large increase in appropriate behavior and a corresponding decrease in inappropriate responding. These changes were maintained at follow-up. Overall, the child and his family responded very positively to treatment.

REFERENCES

American Psychiatric Association. (1980). *Diagnostic and statistical manual of mental disorders* (3rd ed.). Washington, DC: Author.

Gross, A. M. (1985). Oppositional behavior. In M. Hersen & C. G. Last (Eds.), *Behavior therapy casebook* (pp 304–317). New York: Springer.

CHAPTER 15

Learning Disabilities

NIRBHAY N. SINGH, IVAN L. BEALE, and
DEBORAH L. SNELL

DESCRIPTION OF THE DISORDER

The National Joint Committee for Learning Disabilities has defined *learning disabilities* (LD) as a generic term that refers to a heterogeneous group of disorders manifested by significant difficulties in the acquisition and use of listening, speaking, reading, writing, reasoning, or mathematical abilities. These disorders are intrinsic to the individual and presumed to be due to central nervous system dysfunction. Even though a learning disability may occur concomitantly with other handicapping conditions (e.g., sensory impairment, mental retardation, social and emotional disturbance) or environmental influences (e.g., cultural differences, insufficient/inappropriate instruction), it is not the direct result of those conditions or influences (Hammill, Leigh, McNutt, & Larson, 1981). The usual criterion for a diagnosis of LD, consistent with this definition, is a substantial discrepancy between level of ability in one or more academic skill areas and the level of general ability as indicated by an intelligence test.

Although various classifications of LD have been attempted based on the type of psychological process thought to underly the academic deficit, such classifications are widely regarded as unreliable and invalid. In addition, they are probably irrelevant to treatment decisions and treat-

NIRBHAY N. SINGH • Educational Research and Services Center, Inc. 425 E. Fisk Avenue, De Kalb, Illinois 60115.   IVAN L. BEALE • Department of Psychology, University of Auckland, Auckland, New Zealand.   DEBORAH L. SNELL • Department of Psychology, University of Canterbury, Christchurch, New Zealand.

ment outcome. A better case can be made for classification based on the type of academic skills showing deficits.

Specific reading disability is the most common of the academic disabilities, arguably because of the complexity of the reading process. Subclassifications of reading disabilities vary considerably, but there is some agreement on the usefulness of a distinction between individuals unable to identify words on the basis of the sounds of the component phonemes and individuals who cannot identify words or letters on the basis of what they look like. The first type seems much more common than the second. There is also evidence of individuals with both types of problems, often severely affected. Attempts to characterize these types in terms of presumed underlying perceptual or cognitive abnormalities are still controversial and of dubious relevance to treatment decisions. Prevalence of reading disabilities is around 3% of the school population, with a male/female ratio of about 3 to 1.

Specific arithmetic disability can occur with or without accompanying reading disability. Where the two occur together care must be taken to note whether the arithmetic deficit is not wholly due to using an arithmetic test that must be read. There is evidence of two major types of arithmetic disability. One is associated with difficulty on visuospatial tasks, such as some performance subtests of the WISC-R, and is not accompanied by reading or spelling problems. The second type is associated with reading disability and poor performance on verbal subtests of the WISC-R. Prevalence of arithmetic disability is lower than in reading disability and may be higher in females than in males.

Specific writing and spelling disabilities may occur together with, or separate from, reading disability. Two types of disability have been described that seem to parallel the two major types of reading disability. One common type of spelling disability is characterized by phonetic confusions and often occurs with reading disability. A second type is often phonetically correct but shows poor visual discrimination skills. It is more often associated with arithmetic disability than with reading problems, and the spelling problem is usually less severe than in the first group. A third type of disability is not associated with either reading or mathematical disability but is confined to severe problems with written expression.

CASE IDENTIFICATION

Nigel is a right-handed boy of 13 years 4 months. He is in grade 5, having been held back for 2 years in this grade because of slow academic progress. He is the third of five children in a family of seven. Nigel has been repeatedly assessed from an early age by various professionals, and at present participates in special class activities (although he is not mentally retarded) 1 day a week at his school. He is having a series of cranial manipulations by his chiropractor and has been on a strict no-sugar diet for 2 years. His homework is closely supervised by his parents and he participates in a special remedial class.

PRESENTING COMPLAINTS

Nigel was referred for psychological assessment and treatment for academic problems in school. According to his teachers, his major problems were in reading, both oral reading and comprehension, and in spelling. In addition, he performed poorly in mathematics. His parents and teachers requested assistance with his reading and spelling in the first instance and suggested that remediation for mathematics be provided once his proficiency in the other two areas had increased.

HISTORY

Nigel's developmental history was clinically insignificant. His mother had a normal pregnancy but had an early induced birth. Motor and speech development was reported as being slightly delayed. Nigel received speech therapy from the age of 3 and began school with his age-peers. He performed well academically until he reached grade 3, when difficulties with reading and spelling were noticed by both his teacher and his parents. He was also observed to have extremely poor memory and concentration. Nigel has been described as being a shy and slightly anxious child, and not considered a conduct problem either at home or at school. A review of family history indicated that both parents and their siblings had significant learning problems in school. In addition, four of Nigel's five siblings (including his twin sister) have learning problems.

ASSESSMENT

There is no consensus on a standard battery of tests that can be used to assess learning disabilities. However, regardless of the test(s) used, one of the basic requirements is that the assessment show a discrepancy between intellectual functioning and academic performance to meet the criteria for most definitions of learning disability. For this purpose, a psychometric assessment is necessary but not sufficient by itself since it does not lead to treatment options. Thus, we used psychometric assessment to establish the diagnostic status of the child and behavioral assessment for consequent remediation.

Psychometric Assessment

The WISC-R and McCarthy Scale of Children's Abilities are two scales that have excellent psychometric characteristics and are recommended for this purpose. While we believe that children's performance on these tests provides us with essential information necessary for making a diagnostic classification of learning disabilities, we have some problems with the notion that the pattern of performance on certain subtests reliably characterizes learning-disabled children. For example, some investigators maintain that learning-disabled children with reading disorders perform especially poorly on arithmetic, coding, information, and digit-span subtests (ACID pattern) of the WISC-R. However, there are no data to show that the ACID pattern reliably characterizes learning-disabled children or is useful in prescribing appropriate interventions.

As shown in Table 1, Nigel was of average intelligence, with an extreme performance IQ–verbal IQ discrepancy. He had greatest difficulty with verbal subtests, especially vocabulary. On these subtests, he tended to give up more easily on more difficult items. On performance subtests, in particular block design and object assembly, Nigel scored extremely high, having the effect of elevating his overall performance IQ score. On these items, Nigel was systematic, fast, and accurate; however, he indicated that he had had a lot of practice on these types of tasks.

Behavioral Assessment

Since academic behaviors are of interest with learning-disabled children, it is best to focus on them during assessment. In line with other investigators (e.g., Treiber & Lahey, 1985) we think that functional or molar units of academic performance (e.g., oral reading of stories, writing words) rather than molecular units (e.g., phonic discriminations) should be assessed in the first instance for the purpose of remediation. Achievement tests that include tasks approximating those the child might encounter in class are appropriate for this purpose. Good examples of such tests include the Wide Range Achievement Test-Revised (WRAT-R), the

Table 1
Test Results for Nigel on WISC-R, WRAT-R, and ARI

WISC-R

Full scale IQ	96
Verbal IQ	78
Performance IQ	120

Subtest	Scaled score
Information	7
Similarities	7
Arithmetic	7
Vocabulary	5
Comprehension	6
Digit span	5
Picture completion	11
Picture arrangement	11
Block design	16
Object assembly	19
Coding	7

WRAT-R

Subtest	Grade	%
Reading	<3	.1
Spelling	<3	1.0
Arithmetic	<3	.06

Analytic Reading Inventory

Level	Grade
Estimated reading level	
Independent	Primer
Instructional	2–3
Frustration	—
Listening	—
At frustration level	
Word recognition	Prefirst
Comprehension	Prefirst
Listening level	2–3

Spache Diagnostic Reading Scales, and the Analytic Reading Inventory. In addition, fully inclusive samples of the student's written work and direct behavioral observations of ongoing classroom activities should be included in any behavioral assessment.

Nigel was tested on the Analytic Reading Inventory (ARI) and the WRAT-R. The ARI is an informal reading inventory that can be used by teachers to observe, record, and analyze a student's reading performance. It can be used to identify students' reading levels and their strengths and weaknesses in word recognition and comprehension. This information can be used to formulate a remedial reading program for individual children. The student's oral reading ability is graded on the following basis: Independent (99% word accuracy and at least 90% accuracy on comprehension), Instructional (95% word accuracy, at least 75% on comprehension), Frustration (less than 90% word accuracy, comprehension below 50%; level beyond which reading has little meaning), Listening (i.e., hearing comprehension level, 75% of passage read by examiner or teacher is comprehended by the student).

Word Recognition. On the ARI, Nigel's oral reading was slow and broken, with frequent pauses. He displayed poor word-recognition skills, tending to look at the first letter of words and guessing the rest. He was unable to make use of context and had difficulty monitoring the meaning of passages, although, from the pattern of his self-corrections, it was evident that he attempted to do so. It was clear that Nigel had difficulty with both word recognition and comprehension at the Primer reading level (see Table 1), and it was at this level that the Frustration level was set. His word-recognition skills were so poor as to render the passage meaningless.

Comprehension. Retelling of stories was generally poor, with Nigel failing to comprehend most of the material read. Although he was able to state broadly the main idea of the passage, he was rather vague about the main idea and was unable to elaborate on the theme even when he was prompted. When responding to comprehension questions, he performed better on those involving factual rather than inferential material. He scored at an instructional level of 2–3 on listening capacity. Although this is higher than his scores for word recognition and comprehension, it is still below that expected for his age and IQ level. Nigel's story-retelling ability fell in the poor to moderate range when tested on listening levels 1–3; however, his responses to comprehension questions were much better when compared with his oral reading performance. That is, Nigel could comprehend slightly more challenging material when not confronted with the task of recognizing the words in context as well. Finally, he failed to reach an independent reading level and was performing at an instructional level only on listening tasks.

Behavioral Observations

Classroom observations indicated that Nigel was quiet and shy in class. He appeared to be popular with his peers and well liked by teachers. During observation, Nigel was able to work independently on projects and tended to ask peers rather than the teacher for assistance. Overall, his classroom productivity and accuracy appeared to be around 60–70%, although this was rather difficult to assess, particularly in relation to his classmates, since he was in a special remedial class with other children having various learning, social, and/or emotional difficulties. In addition, tasks were structured for him so that he could complete them with few errors.

Summary of Assessment

Nigel is of average intelligence, with an extreme performance–verbal IQ discrepancy. He had greatest difficulty with verbal subtests, especially vocabulary. On the performance subtests, Nigel scored extremely highly on block design and object assembly tasks, thereby elevating his performance IQ score. On these two tasks, Nigel responded quickly, systematically, and with accuracy; however, when questioned on his performance, he indicated that he had had some practice on similar tasks in the past.

Analysis of achievement test scores indicate greatest difficulty with word recognition and written spelling. When his performance on the reading subtest of the WRAT-R is compared with that on the ARI, it is clear that he is performing at or below first-grade level for word recognition on both tests. Consistent difficulties involved frequent letter substitutions, omissions, and wild guesses at difficult words. On the ARI, his poor word-recognition skills had the effect of rendering passages meaningless, thereby resulting in low scores on comprehension during oral reading. There is every indication, however, that Nigel can comprehend some challenging material when he is not confronted with the task of recognizing words in context; i.e., he has good listening comprehension.

His performance on the written spelling subtest of the WRAT-R indicates that Nigel' spelling errors are not phonetically correct. He was able to recognize and spell correctly simple monosyllabic words but had difficulty when faced with words of more than one syllable. His performance on the arithmetic subtest of the WRAT-R was compounded by difficulty in recognizing mathematical symbols and words (e.g., multiply). He was slightly better on the oral arithmetic items on the WISC-R, where word-recognition skills are not important.

These tests suggest that Nigel has a reading disability characterized by dysphonetic reading and spelling errors, and related difficulties with arithmetic. The history of mild developmental language delay, and lower verbal IQ when compared with performance IQ, is consistent with this pattern of findings.

SELECTION OF TREATMENT

After discussions with Nigel, his teacher and his parents, it was decided that the initial focus of treatment should be on his reading and spelling. An analysis of his oral reading showed that Nigel is a dysphonetic reader. That is, he has a very limited sight vocabulary and is not able to decode unknown words through word analysis. He guesses from the first letter and length of the word.

The treatment of choice for a dysphonetic reader like Nigel is to improve his sight vocabulary through increased word-recognition skills. Initially, new words should be taught using a whole-word approach, and when he has a sizable sight vocabulary, he should be taught word-analysis skills so that he can become an independent reader. Since reading is a contextual exercise, word-recognition skills should be assessed and remediated within the context of a meaningful sentence or story. Thus, remediation of errors during oral reading was chosen as the mode of treatment, using a number of error correction procedures for enhancing word recognition.

Procedures that have been found to be effective in remediating oral reading errors require the teacher or reading tutor to make changes in the antecedent and consequent conditions that control the accuracy of a child's reading. Previewing the target text with the teacher, delayed attention to oral reading errors, and overcorrection of error words have been used for this purpose (see Singh & Beale, in press) and found to increase both word-recognition skills and comprehension. These procedures were chosen for use with Nigel, with the provision that once his sight vocabulary increased substantially, he could be given training in word analysis (i.e., phonics, structural analysis, syllabication, and blending).

To improve his comprehension, Nigel was provided with a series of question prompts (Wong, 1980) during oral reading. Research has shown that learning-disabled children do not appear to make inferences about what is read as actively as a peer who is a good reader. Thus, using questions/prompts "activates" the learning-disabled reader into generating needed processing strategies to answer inferential questions.

As for spelling, a whole-word spelling approach was taken, with the provision that once Nigel began word analysis training during oral reading, he could be provided additional training that would make him a phonetic speller. It was decided that Nigel be taught new words at his instructional level of achievement through overcorrection (Ollendick, Matson, Esveldt-Dawson, & Shapiro, 1980). Spelling remediation was linked to his reading, with the words being taken from books that he had successfully read. To ensure that the words learned were functional for him and not learned just in isolation, his spelling of these words was tested periodically in written composition during both assessment and intervention.

COURSE OF TREATMENT

Reading

Storybooks chosen for Nigel were at his reading level and were from a series graded in terms of reading age and written to appeal to adolescents. His reading level was determined by having him read 100-word passages of increasing difficulty and counting his oral reading errors. An oral reading error was defined as a mismatch between a word in the text and the reader's oral response to the word. An error rate between 8 and 20 words per passage indicated the appropriate instructional level. During baseline, Nigel was required to read a new 100-word passage from a long story in each session. Stability on the number of oral reading errors was achieved in five sessions.

Remediation began on the sixth session. Each daily remediation session lasted 15 minutes and was carried out in a 1:1 format with a reading teacher. Before instructing Nigel to read the 100-word text chosen for the session, the teacher previewed the story with him. She provided a background to the story, talked with him about the story by using the title as a cue, and explained new words in the title. During preview, the teacher introduced new words, phrases, and expressions orally but did not identify them visually in the text. In addition, the teacher discussed the meanings of new words in the text and answered all of Nigel's questions about the target story. Following this, he was required to read the target text. If Nigel made an error, a delayed-attention procedure was used. That is, the teacher was required to delay her attention to his errors until the end of the sentence in which the error occurred or, if he paused after making an error, delayed attention was provided between 10 and 15 seconds later. This allowed Nigel to self-correct his error through contextual information without being preempted by the teacher. If Nigel did not self-correct in this time, an overcorrection procedure was used. The teacher pointed to the error word and said the correct word. Then Nigel was required to point to the word and say the same word five times. Following this, he was required to repeat the sentence in which the error word occurred. In addition to the above three procedures, all correct first attempts at self-correction of errors were followed by descriptive praise. No edibles were used.

To aid comprehension, Wong's (1980) question/prompts procedure was used. That is, while Nigel read the text he was questioned and prompted by his teacher (i.e., "What do you think happens after [the stated event] in the sentence? and "Tell me more"). Ten comprehension questions, prepared in advance for each reading passage, were presented to Nigel at the end of each session.

Results of Reading Remediation

Nigel's oral reading errors during baseline ranged from 10 to 20, with a mean of 16. During remediation, this decreased on average to about 13 errors per session by the end of the first 4 weeks, decreased further to 9 per session by the end of 10 weeks, and fluctuated between 4 and 7 over the next 16 weeks. His self-corrections increased from 2 per 100 words in baseline to 8 during the last 4 weeks of remediation. Nigel's comprehension scores showed that he averaged 1 correct answer per passage during baseline. This was usually a question that required him to recall factual material. During remediation, his scores increased to an average of 3 correct answers by the end of the first 4 weeks, increased to about 5 by the end of another 4 weeks, and ranged between 7 and 10 during the last 4 weeks of intervention.

Spelling

Target spelling words were taken from Nigel's reading books that were not currently being used for reading remediation. Stimulus words were selected on the basis of two paper-and-pencil tests, and only words that were mispelled twice were selected for training. Nigel was asked to write down each word that the teacher asked him to spell, and an error was recorded when a target word was spelled incorrectly. A misspelled word was not recorded as an error if the subject spontaneously self-corrected the word within 20 seconds of being asked to spell that word. An initial pool of 50 words was established and further words were added as new reading material became available.

Each daily assessment and instruction session, which lasted about 15 minutes, was taken by Nigel's teacher in a 1:1 format. During baseline, a set of 10 randomly chosen words from the pool of 50 was chosen for assessment and intervention. The teacher instructed Nigel: "I will ask you to spell some words. Write down each word as I ask you to spell it. Try your very best." She then read the words from the spelling list, and Nigel was given 20 seconds to respond to each word. Feedback on accuracy was provided after each attempt. Only three baseline sessions were necessary to establish that Nigel could not spell any of the words correctly.

Overcorrection for errors was introduced in the fourth session. The teacher pronounced the word and Nigel was required to write the word. If the word was spelled correctly, the teacher provided descriptive praise. If the word was spelled incorrectly, the following sequence was used: The teacher pronounced the word, Nigel pronounced the word, the teacher said aloud each letter of the word, and Nigel said aloud each letter of the word as he wrote the word correctly. This sequence was repeated five times and then the teacher moved on to the next word on the list. Following training in each session, Nigel was tested on his current list of 10 words under baseline conditions. The posttest provided data on his learning of new words. Words that were spelled correctly in three consecutive sessions were replaced by unknown words from his word pool. All correctly spelled words were tested under baseline conditions every 4 weeks to assess maintenance.

In addition to spelling instruction on isolate word lists, Nigel was also required to write a short sentence in which at least one target spelling word was used. This requirement, which was in operation on every third or fourth day during both baseline and intervention, enabled us to assess whether Nigel could spell these words when used in context. The sentence was provided by the teacher, who made sure that all but the target words were in Nigel's spelling repertoire. These sentences were written under test conditions, feedback on accuracy of the target words was provided immediately after the session, but overcorrection was not instituted for errors.

Results of Spelling Remediation

While Nigel had no correct responses during baseline, his spelling improved dramatically once overcorrection was introduced. He learned an average of three to four words in each session over a period of 30 weeks and had 90 to 95% accuracy on tests for maintenance. His spelling performance in context matched his performance on isolate words.

TERMINATION

Formal intervention was terminated after 30 weeks when Nigel had reached a level of performance that showed increasing gains in oral reading skills, comprehension, and spelling. The teacher felt that she could maintain and enhance Nigel's academic gains within the classroom setting and gradually began fading out her 1:1 teaching format. In addition, at this stage Nigel's parents and teacher felt that it was appropriate for the parents to take a more active role at home in terms of assisting Nigel with his reading and spelling homework. We concurred with their decision and trained the parents in the remediation procedures we had used with Nigel at school. The question of Nigel's poor mathematics performance was raised, and consensual agreement was that it should be referred for assessment and intervention in the following year.

FOLLOW-UP

A 6-month follow-up was scheduled during the first month of school the following year, and it was found that Nigel was still having some problems in reading when compared with an average age-peer. However, his new teacher was pleased with the substantial gains he had made in both academic areas and showed an interest in learning the remedial procedures. Observations and assessments indicated that Nigel was now only about 6 months behind his age-peers in his reading and spelling, and was progressing at a rate that would enable him to match his peers in the near future. His parents expressed their appreciation of what had been achieved.

As a consequence of participating in Nigel's remedial instruction program, his teacher is now using similar procedures with other academically delayed children, and his parents are doing the same with Nigel's twin sister. In addition, Nigel has now been referred for remedial instruction in mathematics. In terms of his school behavior, Nigel now appears to be better socialized, has more self-confidence, and is increasingly motivated to undertake academic tasks.

OVERALL EVALUATION

The clear advantages of the behavioral assessment used in this case are that it was treatment-oriented and had an interactive character that was sensitive to the ongoing effectiveness of treatment. The behavioral assessment placed emphasis on obtaining a full description of what Nigel could and could not do when reading and spelling. The monitoring of targeted skills on a session-by-session basis provided the teacher with a clear indication of the effects of treatment and any variability in Nigel's response to it.

A traditional assessment approach might have placed emphasis not on what Nigel could and could not do but on what this implied regarding deficits in the underlying neuropsychological process. The dysphonetic character of Nigel's reading and spelling errors, together with his low scores on verbal subtests of the WISC-R, might have typed him as having a dysphonetic reading and spelling disorder. According to one developmental-lag theory of this disorder, Nigel would be unable to progress in reading before neurological functions matured sufficiently to permit the development of phonological coding skills. According to another theory, the missing phonological coding skills would need to be directly taught. Neither theory seems consistent with treatment outcome in this case. In the event, adequate progress was made without the need to address the phonological deficit. The targeting of molar units of performance would seem to be endorsed by the effects of treatment so far. Whether a program to teach phonetic word-analysis skills would now be needed to facilitate further progress is a matter for conjecture.

REFERENCES

Hammill, D. D., Leigh, J. E., McNutt, G., & Larson, S. C. (1981). A new definition of learning disabilities. *Learning Disability Quarterly, 4*, 336–342.

Ollendick, T. H., Matson, J. L., Esveldt-Dawson, K., & Shapiro, E. S. (1980). Increasing spelling achievement: An analysis of treatment procedures utilizing an alternating treatments design. *Journal of Applied Behavior Analysis, 13*, 645–654.

Singh, N. N., & Beale, I. L. (in press). Learning disabilities: Psychological therapies. In J. L. Matson (Ed.), *Handbook of treatment approaches in child psychopathology*. New York: Plenum Press.

Treiber, F. A., & Lahey, B. B. (1985). A behavioral model of academic remediation with learning disabled children. In P. H. Bornstein, & A. E. Kazdin (Eds.), *Handbook of clinical behavior therapy with children* (pp. 742–771). Homewood, IL: Dorsey Press.
Wong, B.Y.I. (1980). Activating the inactive learner: Use of questions/prompts to enhance comprehension and retention of implied information in learning disabled children. *Learning Disability Quarterly, 3,* 29–37.

CHAPTER 16

Attention Deficit Disorder with Hyperactivity

MARK D. RAPPORT

DESCRIPTION OF THE DISORDER

Attention deficit disorder with hyperactivity (ADDH) is a serious and pervasive psychopathological disorder of childhood characterized by inattention, impulsivity, and excessive gross motor activity (American Psychiatric Association, 1980). Associated features of the disorder frequently include poor peer relationships, learning disabilities, academic failure, conduct disturbance, and aggression.

A first step in the clarification of the diagnosis of ADDH is to note the distinctions among inattention, impulsivity, and overactivity as symptoms (i.e., discrete behaviors), as a syndrome, and as a nosologic disorder. Being inattentive, impulsive, or overactive is a subjective state experienced by most children at various points in their lives, and by itself it is not necessarily pathological. Most of us can recount times in our lives when we have been "hyper" or unable to pay attention as the situation demands it. In contrast, ADDH as a syndrome implies more than an isolated incidence of these behaviors and occurs in combination with other symptoms such as those described above to form a symptom-complex or syndrome. When this clinical syndrome is characterized by a particular symptom picture with a specifiable course, duration, outcome, response

MARK D. RAPPORT • Department of Psychiatry and Behavioral Science, Putnam Hall, South Campus, State University of New York, Stony Brook, New York 11794-8790.

to treatment, and potential familial, psychological, and biological correlates, then it is referred to as a discrete nosological entity or disorder.

The controversy in the literature surrounding the classification of ADDH in childhood has been concerned primarily with the description and definition of the characteristic clinical symptomatology constituting the disorder of ADDH in children, rather than inattention and/or hyperactivity as an isolated event or symptom. In reviewing the literature thus far, it appears that ADDH meets most of the requirements of a clinical disorder. There are several behaviors common to children with ADDH, although children with ADDH do not exhibit all of these behaviors to the same degree. The disorder begins early in life and runs a fairly consistent developmental course. Impairment ranges from mild to severe, and most symptoms continue to be displayed throughout adolescence and into adulthood. Response to rigorous and continuous treatment is fairly predictable, although it may be inconsistent with some children. There is a fairly robust relationship between ADDH and various psychological, genetic, and familial markers in the families of these children

CASE IDENTIFICATION

For purposes of illustration, a case study that is characteristic of children with ADDH is presented herein. It is important to note, however, that no two cases are identical, and many children undergoing a diagnostic evaluation will present with both qualitative and quantitative differences in presenting history and symptomatology.

Al was an 8-year-old Caucasian male of average intelligence whose physical stature and features were largely unremarkable for his stated age. Al lived at home with his two parents, an older brother, and a younger sister. Their house was located in a suburban, mostly middle-socioeconomic-class township several miles from the nearest city in the northeast section of the United States. Al was attending the third grade at a public elementary school within walking distance from his house. He had qualified for, and subsequently received, special educational assistance 6 hours per week from a learning disabilities specialist during the past year in the areas of reading and auditory sequential memory/processing skills.

A detailed family history revealed that Al's father had experienced considerable difficulty in school, beginning around the second or third grade and lasting throughout high school. He denied being "hyperactive" and described most of his problems as involving difficulty paying attention, a general lack of interest in most subjects, acting up in class, and frequently getting into trouble for misconduct with school officials. He later attended junior college and obtained an associate of arts degree. His ability to pay attention and his scholastic grades were noticeably improved in subject matters that interested him and that were immediately relevant to real-life situations. The father had been married once previously for 6 months, denied being an alcoholic but admitted to frequent and chronic drinking, and was currently employed as an on-site supervisor for a construction company. His usual extracurricular activities involved outdoor activities and going out with the boys. The father denied having excessive difficulty in controlling Al's behavior at home and felt that his son was a "typical boy" with a lot of energy who would eventually outgrow his problems.

Al's mother described her early educational history as largely unremarkable. She had relatively few problems in school, obtained a B.A. degree in business management, and was currently employed part time as a sales representative for a local firm. She enjoyed reading and decorating but admitted to having little or no time for these activities owing to child-rearing demands. Al's mother was responsible for initiating the diagnostic appointment, was the primary care-provider for the children, and experienced chronic difficulty controlling her son's behavior.

The extended family history was remarkable for hypertension, mild diabetes, alcoholism, and hyperthyroidism. A history of other psychological/psychiatric disorders in extended family members was denied.

PRESENTING COMPLAINTS

Al's mother initiated the referral for evaluation because of her son's chronic difficulties in school and behavior at home. Despite her being told that her son would eventually "outgrow" his immaturity, his problems in school appeared to be worsening. He was described by his past and current classroom teachers as immature, fidgety (frequently out of his seat or shifting seat positions), lacking motivation, inattentive, into everyone else's business, and easily distractable. His current teacher felt that Al could indeed function at or slightly below grade level if he simply applied himself. His lack of motivation and poor self-control were believed to underlie most of his problems in school. He completed academic assignments on an erratic basis and frequently missed easy problems owing to his rushing through them or beginning the assignment before understanding the instructions. Al's handwriting was illegible at times, and he handed in most of his assignments with little regard for neatness.

Aside from his academic difficulties, Al experienced considerable difficulty initiating and maintaining peer relationships at school. He enjoyed playing with other children but tended to overwhelm them with his robustness and, at times, bossiness. Most children in the classroom disliked him for these reasons and because he wasn't good at taking turns during games, was somewhat uncoordinated at sports, and tended to get them in trouble during classroom activities.

Al's mother stated that she experienced considerable difficulty managing his behavior at home on a day-to-day basis. Al required constant supervision, frequently irritated his siblings, and was easily bored. Despite being provided with frequent reminders, Al appeared to experience considerable difficulty remembering what he was supposed to do from one moment to the next, and everything seemed to "go in one ear and out the other." Conversely, Al was reportedly able to play solitary games such as Lego, dismantle old household appliances, watch highly stimulating video movies (e.g., *Star Wars*), and play games on his Commodore computer for extended periods of time without distraction or diminution of interest. Punishments ranged from spankings and restriction of activities to brief time outs in his room—nothing seemed to work, however, and the mother had begun to ignore much of his misbehavior in an effort to "maintain her sanity."

HISTORY

Al's parents reported a normal pre-, peri-, and post-natal history. No alcohol or nicotine was ingested during the full-term pregnancy. The mother did ingest two to three cups of caffeine daily in addition to caffeine-laden substances (e.g., colas). Al was delivered within 1 week of his expected due date and received an Apgar score of 8 and 9 (immediately and shortly after the delivery, respectively). Total amount of time spent in labor was estimated to be 14 hours, with a spinal block administered after 8 hours of labor without complications. The delivery itself was without complications, and the use of forceps was unnecessary owing to the correct positioning of the head and appropriate dilation of the cervix. Birth weight and length were 7 pounds 8 ounces and 20 inches, respectively.

Developmental milestones were accomplished according to age-appropriate norms. Phonemes were emitted around 3 to 4 months, morphemes around 10 months, short sentences by age 2 years. Al took his first steps by 11 months of age and proceeded to walk and then run almost immediately. He incurred several accidental falls owing to his "getting into everything" and crawling up on high objects within the house. A negative history of traumatic head injuries or periods of unconsciousness was reported. The parents "child-proofed" the house almost immediately after Al became mobile. No allergies or untoward reactions to specific foods were reported, although Al had an early history of projectile vomiting that necessitated a change in formula.

Although Al's early history within the familial environment necessitated continuous parental supervision, the parents did not feel that he was "hyperactive." In kindergarten, Al was described as being a very sociable but somewhat immature child who required frequent redirection and reminders to stay on task. It was recommended at the end of the academic year that he be retained because of his immaturity. After consultation with school personnel, it was decided that Al be promoted to the first grade but placed in a transition classroom (i.e., consisting of kindergarten and first-grade children and emphasizing basic academic skills).

The parents became increasingly concerned after Al entered the first grade. His ability to sustain attention and to inhibit his behavior appropriately in accordance with situational demands, as well as his disruptive behavior in the classroom, appeared to worsen as correspondingly greater demands for self-control and task completion were required of him. The course of Al's problems showed a gradual worsening and exacerbation in the second and third grade despite his receiving special education remedial services and being placed on a home-based management program by the school psychologist.

ASSESSMENT

Both of Al's parents were present at the initial diagnostic appointment. After a detailed developmental, medical, social, educational, and family history was obtained, Al's parents were questioned regarding the occurrence of (1) unusual behaviors (to rule out psychotic disturbance, pervasive developmental disorder, obsessive–compulsive disorder); (2) behaviors characteristic of anxiety in children (e.g., sleep disturbance, frequent and recurring nightmares and/or terror, somnambulism, nervous habits, bruxism, overconcern regarding competence, school refusal, simple phobias, motor tension, anxiety when separated from parents, unexplained physiological symptoms such as dyspnea, paresthesias, and physical discomfort); (3) behaviors characteristic of an affective disorder (e.g., insomnia or hypersomnia, suicidal ideation, flat or constricted affect, dysphoric mood [persistently sad facial expression], irritability, difficulty concentrating, withdrawal from normally attended social activities, changes in appetite with or without corresponding weight gain or loss, psychomotor retardation or agitation, sulkiness, and poor self-esteem);

(4) past and recent psychosocial stressors or changes in the environment (to rule out adjustment reactions); (5) child or sexual abuse; (6) periods of staring or incomprehension (to rule out absence seizures); (7) conduct, oppositional, and antisocial behavior; and (8) recurrent, involuntary, repetitive motor movements (tics), and other behaviors consistent with Tourette's disorder (e.g., tongue protrusion, throat clearing, vocal tics, copralalia, sniffing).

Other than occasional occurrences of moderate oppositional behavior, aggression with peers, a general dislike for school, low self-esteem, and nightmares after viewing frightening movies, the parents reported a negative history of the above behaviors and an unremarkable medical history. The parents were each requested to complete several questionnaires and rating scales to provide additional information regarding Al's behavior. These included the Werry-Weiss-Peters Activity Rating Scale (WWPAS; primarily a measure of gross motor activity), the Barkley Home Situations Questionnaire (HSQ; indicates occurrence and severity of problems at home), the Conners Parent Rating Scale (CPRS; the most widely used measure to assess parental perceptions of hyperactivity), the SNAP Rating Scale (covers DSM-III diagnostic criteria for ADDH), and the Personality Inventory for Children (PIC; provides a comprehensive personality profile). The parents were also requested to complete several side effects rating scales to assess the presence of physical and somatic symptomatology in the absence of medication.

Results of these rating scales indicated that Al experienced severe difficulty (i.e., greater than 2 standard deviations above the mean according to developmental norms) in the areas of inattention, impulsivity, and excessive gross motor activity. He was also found to be moderately oppositional to authority figures and deficient in social skills and peer relationships (see Rapport, 1987, for a description of these instruments). It was interesting to note that there were some rather remarkable differences in the ratings obtained from Al's parents. Al's father tended to deny significant problems at home but did agree that his son experienced difficulty at school, which he blamed primarily on the school system. Conversely, the ratings obtained from Al's mother were more consistent with the classroom teacher's report (see above and below) and clinical examination (see below) regarding severity and breadth of behavioral difficulties.

The classroom teacher was requested to complete the Abbreviated Conners Teacher Ratings Scale (ACTRS; the most widely used measure to assess teacher perceptions of hyperactivity), the ADDH Comprehensive Teacher Rating Scale (ACTeRS; a relatively new measure of ADDH across four dimensions—inattention, activity level, oppositional behavior, and peer relationships), the Humphrey Teacher's Self-Control Rating Scale (TSCRS; to assess the child's ability to exhibit self-control and perceived competency), the SNAP Rating Scale, and Achenbach's revised Child Behavior Checklist (CBC; assesses a broad band of behavior problems in children). Results obtained from the ratings and checklists were consistent with the core characteristics exhibited by children with ADDH (i.e., an inability to sustain attention and inhibit impulsive responding and activity level with respect to the child's age; poor peer relationships, and academic difficulties).

In examining the aforementioned rating scales, questionnaires, and information obtained from parent/teacher reports as they relate to a diagnosis of ADDH, we were essentially looking for a consistent, pervasive (i.e., across settings) pattern of behavior that varied from day to day but was consistent across months and years, and that showed a gradual worsening of expressed symptomatology as a function of increasing demands on attention and inhibition of behavior and activity level.

Al was seen separately from his parents for a clinical interview as well as being administered a comprehensive diagnostic test battery. During the interview, the child was questioned regarding his school performance (in a nonthreatening manner), peer relationships, difficulties at home, sibling relationships, greatest worries/fears, frequency of nightmares, best and worst skills, general likes and dislikes, mood/affect, and occurrence of unusual behaviors, thoughts, and intrusive stimuli. He was moderately concerned with his poor school performance but admitted to being concerned only because of his parents' desires for him to succeed academically. His mood was euthymic, affect was broad, speech was spontaneous, relevant to questioning, articulate, and without pressure. Al showed no evidence of thought disorder or signs of anxiety or affective disturbance. He did admit to having difficulty maintaining friendships.

A brief neurological screening examination was administered and showed evidence of mild spillover effect (during finger tapping, foot tapping, and finger roll), mild difficulty with balance and gross motor coordination (tandem walking front- and backwards, hopping on each foot, hand-to-nose movements), adequate muscle tone and strength, and appropriate discrimination of fingers touched and left–right body parts (with eyes closed).

A test battery was administered subsequently and consisted of the following instruments: Continuous Performance Test (CPT; a frequently used measure of sustained attention); Paired Associates Learning (PAL; a measure of a child's ability to learn new associations and short-term memory); Delay Test (DT) and Matching Familiar Figures (MFFT) Test (provides information regarding a child's ability to inhibit impulsive responding and the type of search strategy used to solve matching-to-sample problems, respectively); Peabody Picture Vocabulary Test-Revised (PPVT; to provide a brief assessment of verbal intelligence given that a full-scale battery was recently completed and available); the Southern California Motor Accuracy Test (to provide an assessment of the child's hand–eye motor accuracy as it relates to using a writing instrument); and Porteous Mazes (to assess planning and foresight with regard to ability to withhold responding under appropriate circumstances).

The results of testing, when compared with the previous information elicited from the parents and classroom teacher, were consistent with a diagnosis of ADDH. Al's ability to sustain attention and inhibit impulsive responding were both within the "abnormal" range according to developmental norms. His verbal intelligence was within the "average" range and consistent with the results obtained on a previously administered WISC-R. He experienced considerable difficulty in concentrating and learning paired-associate relationships, and his level of motoric activity showed a clear increase as the testing session progressed. Eye–hand fine motor coordination was 1½ years below expected performance criteria, but it was not possible to discern whether this was due to an actual deficit in this area or secondary to the child's impulsivity. Al's performance on the Porteous Maze Test revealed poor planning and foresight and a lack of fine-motor inhibition.

SELECTION OF TREATMENT

Approximately 1½ hours were allotted for debriefing Al's parents on the various test results and synthesizing the information obtained from school, interview, history, questionnaire, and rating scale instruments. Prior to a discussion of treatment options, the diagnosis of ADDH was explained at length. Al's parents asked several questions regarding the "cause" of ADDH, and previously held notions related to causal factors (e.g., poor/inadequate parenting, dietary factors, immaturity, brain damage) were examined. Selected articles and books were recommended for additional reading.

A trial of stimulant medication (methylphenidate and specifically Ritalin), with behavioral treatment (response-cost during academic periods in school) added if necessary, was recommended to the parents for several reasons. Our clinical experience with over 120 children with ADDH has shown us that a carefully controlled and individually titrated dose of psychostimulant medication can produce significant treatment gains in a relatively brief period of time. Moreover, clinical improvement is usually found throughout the day as well as across settings (i.e., home and school). Conversely, various forms of behavior therapy have been shown to be equally effective, and at times more effective (depending on the specific measure used), with some children, but they necessitate the continuous cooperation and consistency of school personnel within each day, across days, and over a period of several years. Thus, from a cost-effective and practical point of view, we typically recommend a trial dose of methylphenidate (MPH) as the first treatment of choice.

The word *trial* is always emphasized in our recommendations to parents. We have never encountered parents who were particularly fond of the idea of treating their child with any type of medication, much less a psychostimulant. Inherent in the word *trial,* however, is that the willingness to try the medication is always within the parents' control. Moreover, MPH is a very fast acting medication whose clinical effects can be assessed 45 minutes to 1 hour after ingestion. Thus, if clinical effects are not immediately apparent or untoward effects occur, the medication can be discontinued and its effects diminished completely within hours. It is equally important to emphasize that there are favorable and adverse responders to MPH—which must be determined in a carefully controlled clinical trial. Given that a child shows a favorable response, it is still incumbent upon the clinician to determine the minimally effective dose (i.e., the lowest dose that results in the greatest amount of improvement without untoward side effects).

After providing the parents with the information above, we require them to consider the options for at least 48 hours. Our policy is never to allow them to select a particular treatment immediately without thinking about it first, discussing it with one another, and considering other available treatment options.

COURSE OF TREATMENT

Al's parents contacted the clinic 2 days following the diagnostic evaluation and had agreed upon a trial of psychostimulant medication for their son. The parents were instructed to contact their pediatrician to arrange for a complete physical examination and discuss the recommended treatment. A complete report of the results of the evaluation was forwarded to the physician prior to the appointment. Al's pediatrician concurred with the diagnosis, found no contraindications for using the medication, and prescribed the recommended dosage of MPH for the clinical trial (see below).

General Procedure

Al was subsequently scheduled for a concurrent 6-week evaluation consisting of clinical testing and school observation. He was seen once per week at the clinic for approximately 2½ hours. During the first week, Al's performance was assessed without medication to establish a baseline level for future comparison. He was also observed unobtrusively in his regular classroom placement for 3 days during the morning hours of this week by trained graduate and undergraduate students who were blind regarding his medication status (observers were introduced as student teachers who would be observing normal classroom functioning).

During each of the ensuing clinic visits, Al was administered an encapsulated single oral dose of MPH (5 mg, 10 mg, 15 mg, or 20 mg) or a placebo 45 minutes prior to testing. The order of drug administration across weeks was counterbalanced and determined by random assignment owing to the research-practitioner nature of the clinic. If Al showed no untoward emergent symptoms during the clinic testing, his parents were given a 6-day supply of the medication containing the same dose (to begin each Sunday; Saturday was used as a "washout" day between dosages) in precoded, dated envelopes. Al and his parents were purposefully kept "blind" regarding medication status throughout the evaluation. The parents were instructed to give Al one capsule each morning, approximately ½ hour prior to his leaving for school. This was to ensure that the medication was active during the morning hours in which he was to be observed (i.e., 3 of the 5 school days each week). This procedure was followed until Al had undergone clinical testing and school observations at each of the above MPH doses.

Assessment of Treatment Effects

The effects of MPH on Al's behavior and test performance were assessed in the clinic using each of the following instruments: PAL test, CPT, Southern California Motor Accuracy Test (SCMAT), and MFFT. In addition, several side effects rating scales were administered prior to and during the active medication period on each testing day. Al's weight, height, and heart rate were routinely measured over the 6-week assessment period.

Information obtained during the active life of the medication (i.e., 1 to 4 hours) from Al's classroom included (1) the percentage of time he spent attending to his academic assignments (% on task), (2) the percentage of academic assignments completed during this time, (3) the percentage of academic assignments completed correctly, and (4) teacher ratings (ACTRS, ACTeRS, TSCRS) based on morning behavior only (owing to the relatively short half-life of MPH).

Al's parents completed two rating (WWPAS, Barkley's HSQ) and two side effect scales (Barkley's Side Effects Questionnaire and the NIMH STESS) to provide information regarding perceived changes in his behavior and the presence of treatment-emergent symptoms on Sunday. We routinely ask the parents to limit their ratings to Sunday only since this is the only time in which they observe the child under active medication (i.e., the effects of MPH have long worn off by the time the child returns home after school).

Results of Medication Trial

The results of the medication trial across the 6-week evaluation period are presented separately across the three assessment settings (clinic, school, and familial environment).

Clinic Assessment. Al's performance on each of the clinic-based assessment instruments across the various MPH doses are presented in Table 1. The medication doses are arranged in hierarchical order for pre-

Table 1
Clinic Assessment Data across Dose[a]

		Dose			
	Placebo	5 mg	10 mg	15 mg	20 mg
CPT performance					
Omission errors	16	15	9	4	7
Commision errors	14	9	8	2	2
PAL Performance					
Percent correct	60	58	66	78	74
MFFT performance					
Total errors	12	13	7	3	2
Latency (in sec)	5	7	11	14	22
SO CAL total score	175	177	182	195	192

[a] CPT = Continuous Performance Test, PAL = Paired Associates Learning Test, MFFT = Matching Familiar Figures Test, SO CAL = Southern California Motor Accuracy Test—Revised. Lower scores indicate improvement on the CPT and MFFT (errors). Higher scores indicate improvement on the PAL and SO CAL.

sentation purposes—Al did not receive them in this order, as indicated earlier.

Several points are worth noting in the results obtained from the clinic assessment. Al tended to show minimal or no improvement on the various instruments until the 10-mg MPH dose was administered. His optimal performance was exhibited at the 15-mg and 20-mg doses on most of the assessment instruments, depending upon the specific domain measured. For example, CPT omission errors (ability to sustain attention and scored by not detecting the paired target stimuli) were optimally reduced at the 15-mg level yet showed a slight increase under the 20-mg dose. CPT commission errors (more indicative of impulsivity and scored by responding to other than paired target stimuli), however, showed no change from the 15-mg to the 20-mg dose. Similarly, MFFT errors (primarily a measure of impulsivity) were reduced considerably at both the 15-mg and 20-mg doses, whereas MFFT latency (mean time to the first response for the entire test) increased fairly evenly as a function of increasing dose until the 20-mg dose was administered. When the four measures obtained from the two assessment instruments are considered together, they suggest that Al was somewhat "overfocused" at the higher 20-mg dose (i.e., he began missing target stimuli on the CPT without a concomitant increase in commission errors and took much longer to respond on the MFFT without a noticeable reduction in error rate). The results obtained from the PAL test and the SCMAT were similar in that performance was enhanced up to 15 mg MPH, then showed a slight decrease (i.e., motor accuracy on the SCMAT actually remained stable, whereas latency to completion was longer under the 20-mg dose).

Observations of Al's behavior during clinical testing and side effect ratings completed by the child indicated an absence of untoward emergent symptoms except at the higher 20-mg-MPH dose. Al reported feeling somewhat tired and jittery under this dose, with mild stomach distress occurring 20 to 40 minutes postingestion. Observations of Al's behavior during the 20-mg clinical testing day indicated that he rubbed his eyes frequently, was moderately withdrawn in his social interactions with the staff, and fixated on visual stimuli during testing for a longer than necessary period of time.

School Assessment. The results obtained from the school assessment over the course of the 6-week evaluation are depicted in Figure 1. Al's initial mean weekly rate of attending to his academic assignments (on task) prior to receiving active medication (i.e., during the placebo week) was approximately 35%. He typically completed only 40% of his academic assignments without the benefits of active medication but tended to com-

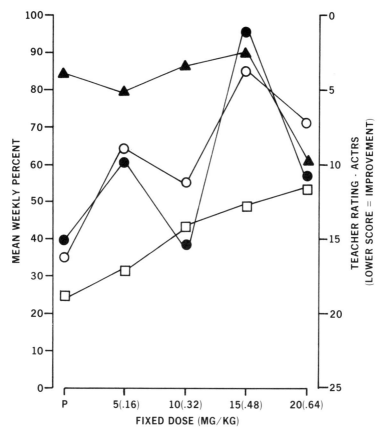

Figure 1. The dose–response curves for Al are depicted for each of the four dependent measures across dose levels (mg/kg shown in parentheses) using the left-hand ordinate for percentages of on-task behavior (open circles), academic assignments completed (closed circles), and academic assignments completed correctly (closed triangles); right-hand ordinate for ACTRS weekly teacher ratings (open squares). P = placebo.

plete most of them correctly. Teacher ratings (ACTRS) for this week indicated a score of 19, which is approximately 3 standard deviations above the mean according to normative values. Moderate improvement in Al's attention (on task) to, and completion of, academic assignments was noticeable under the 5-mg MPH dose. Teacher ratings indicated gradual but sustained improvement in social deportment as a linear function of increasing dose, with optimal improvement seen under the highest MPH dose (i.e., 20 mg). Conversely, Al's ability to attend to and complete his academic assignments was optimally enhanced under the 15-mg (0.48-

mg/kg) dose, without a corresponding loss of accuracy. Under the 20-mg (0.64-mg/kg) dose, however, his attention, completion of academic assignments, and accuracy in completing assignments showed a rather dramatic decrease compared to the lower 15-mg condition.

Parent Assessment. The two parent rating scales and treatment emergent symptoms questionnaires completed each Sunday throughout the medication trial indicated that Al's behavior at home showed the most improvement under the 10-mg and 15-mg MPH doses, respectively. His behavior was actually rated as most improved under the 20-mg dose; however, both parents felt that their son appeared socially withdrawn from ongoing activities in and around the house under this dose. A slight increase (compared to ratings obtained under baseline and placebo conditions) in the number and severity of somatic complaints was also evidenced under the higher 20-mg dose.

Child Assessment. Al was questioned regarding his perceptions of the MPH treatment each week following clinical testing, as well as being debriefed prior to termination of the case. Although Al was purposefully kept "blind" regarding medication status throughout the evaluation, he was quite perceptive regarding his improvement in school under several of the doses. For example, he was able to state quite assertively that he could better attend to his assignments in school and, consequently, was not getting into as much trouble with his teacher or classmates. Only under the 20-mg dose did he complain of physical discomfort and felt that we were giving him too much medication because it was making him tired.

TERMINATION

Al and his parents met with the director of the CLC for a complete debriefing of the obtained results and recommendations for continued treatment, prior to the forwarding of a full report to the child's pediatrician and debriefing involving school personnel. (Note: we recommend that a copy of the report *not* be placed in the child's school records owing to its sensitive and confidential nature.) In Al's case, we recommended to the parents and the pediatrician that he be placed on a maintenance dosage regimen consisting of Ritalin SR-20 mg plus a 5-mg tablet in the a.m. (equivalent to a 15-mg a.m., 10-mg afternoon dose).

Our rationale for recommending this particular dosage schedule was twofold. Ritalin SR-20 mg (a sustained release formula that contains a *total* of 20 mg, but purportedly releases an equivalent amount of drug to a 10-mg b.i.d. or twice-per-day dose) tends to have a more gradual onset and longer active period of effect (typically between 6 and 10 hours, although there is disagreement among professionals regarding this issue) compared with single oral doses using standard Ritalin tablets. By adding the 5-mg tablet in the morning, we were hoping to mimic the effect obtained under the previous 15-mg MPH dosage trial. The second, related reason for using this dosage schedule was to circumvent the need for in-school administration of medication, which can prove to be both embarrassing and unreliable in certain schools. For example, we have encountered situations in which a child has been requested over the school intercom to come down to the main office for "his pill," or situations in which the time of medication depends entirely on the availability of the school nurse on any particular day. Finally, most children tend to work on the majority of their "hard-core" academic assignments during the morning hours, thus necessitating that the most potent dose be active during these hours. Needless to say, the use of this dosage schedule as a viable substitute for a twice-a-day regimen awaits empirical investigation, and the clinician should exercise appropriate caution (e.g., additional follow-up assessment) if recommending it to the child's pediatrician.

In completing our recommendation to the parents and their son's pediatrician, we felt that Al should receive the lower Ritalin SR-20 mg alone (i.e., 10-mg b.i.d. equivalent) on weekend days throughout the remainder of the school year. This recommendation was based on Al's continuing difficulties with his parents and peer relationships. During the medication evaluation, he exhibited improved self-control in his peer relationships (e.g., he was not so intrusive with peers and was able to take turns while playing games that required cooperation both at home and at school) and was noticeably more compliant with parental requests according to his own and his parents' accounting.

Following the debriefing meeting, Al and his parents were referred back to their pediatrician with our recommendations for continued treatment and monitoring.

FOLLOW-UP

Al was placed on the recommended dosage schedule by his pediatrician and continued to receive medication throughout the school year. He showed continued progress in most areas of academic functioning, completed his daily assignments on a fairly regular basis, and was subsequently promoted into the fourth grade. He continued to receive special-education remedial intervention throughout the academic year and appeared to be making steady progress in reading comprehension and auditory processing skills.

Al's fourth-grade classroom teacher contacted his parents and the clinic on several occasions throughout the academic school year. She was concerned that Al's behavior and school performance were occasionally erratic and that he might not be receiving his prescribed dosage on a regular basis. After checking with the parents, the teacher was assured that Al was receiving his medication as prescribed and (reminded) to expect a moderate degree of fluctuation in his effort and daily performance throughout the school year. The point to keep in mind here is that children with ADDH continue to experience difficulty even under an optimal medication regimen, and that it is important for the clinician to help establish reasonable expectations on the part of parents and teachers. In Al's case, he was earning mostly B's and C's on his report card compared with C's and D's prior to treatment. His classroom teacher, however, felt that he could perform academically at an even higher level. Similarly, Al's parents agreed that his behavior was much improved at home, yet they complained that he still experienced moderate difficulty with peer relationships and frequently fought with his siblings.

Although we agreed with Al's parents and teacher that he indeed appeared to have considerable ability and might at some time perform at a higher overall level, they were gently reminded that medication does not in and of itself "teach" children new skills or adaptive behavior and that additional therapies could be applied if warranted. Both the teacher and the parents requested that Al receive additional therapeutic intervention to help him attend to and complete academic assignments in school. A recently developed Attention Training System (ATS—Gordon Systems, Inc., P.O. Box 746, DeWitt, New York 13214) was selected as the treatment of choice owing to its demonstrated success in helping children with ADDH attend to and complete academic assignments in classroom settings (Rapport, 1987; Rapport, Murphy, & Bailey, 1982). The ATS is based on a response-cost paradigm and requires the child to attend to and complete school work to gain points. A small electronic device is placed on the child's desk during periods of academic seatwork and automatically awards one point per minute that the child attends to his assignments. If the child wanders off task, the teacher, by remote control, can cause the counter on the child's apparatus to decrement by one point. On these occasions, a small light on top of the child's module lights up, signaling the child that he has been off task and has lost one of his earned points. Thus, the teacher can silently but effectively deliver immediate feedback to the inattentive child without disrupting other children or hurriedly rushing about the classroom administering tokens or checkmarks.

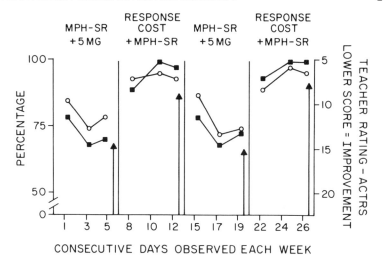

Figure 2.   The mean percentage of intervals of daily on-task behavior (open circles) and academic assignments completed correctly (closed squares) across alternating experimental conditions (MPH-SR + 5 mg = methylphenidate [Ritalin]- sustained release formula + 5 mg MPH tablet administered in a.m.; Response Cost + MPH-SR = implementation of behavioral program + administration of MPH [Ritalin]- sustained release formula in a.m.). Teacher ratings (ACTRS) are depicted as vertical arrows at the end of each week and interpreted using the right coordinate.

Accumulated daily points are traded in by the student at the end of the morning and afternoon academic periods for structured free-time activities (i.e., each point earned represents one minute of earned free time).

Because of Al's favorable response to MPH, we recommended that he be continued on the medication, with attentional training (response cost) implemented during periods of academic seat work on an alternating-week schedule. By using this schedule, we were able to evaluate whether attentional training enhanced Al's classroom performance and behavior over and above the effects of MPH alone in the context of an ABAB treatment design. The differential effects of MPH and the combined treatment regimen are depicted in Figure 2. Al's on-task behavior, academic efficiency (percent of daily academic assignments completed correctly), and teacher-rated social deportment (using the Abbreviated Conners Teacher Rating Scale—ACTRS) were clearly accentuated as a function of combining the two treatments.

Al continued to receive the combination of treatments throughout the fourth grade. Toward the end of the academic year, the ATS was gradually withdrawn and replaced with a free-time product contingency, wherein Al earned ½ hour of structured free-time activities following the morning and afternoon academic sessions if he was able to successfully complete all of his academic assignments. During the summer months, we recommended to Al's pediatrician that he be discontinued from the medication for a period of 6 weeks. A combined treatment approach consisting of medication (Ritalin-SR 20 mg a.m. dose only) and behavior therapy (free-time product completion) was initiated upon Al's entrance into the fifth grade and continued throughout the year with consistently successful results.

OVERALL EVALUATION

The case study presented herein represents a fairly typical and uncomplicated example of assessing the effects of psychostimulant treatment and a combination of psychostimulant and behavioral treatment on a child with ADDH. Despite the relative synchrony obtained among measures and across settings in assessing medication effects, several considerations should be observed.

Individualized Titration

Psychopharmacological investigations conducted over the past 10 years have clearly shown that children's response to CNS medication is not only idiosyncratic but frequently specific to the type of measure or behavior being examined. Differences in psychopharmacological response also appear to depend on a number of setting variables. Thus far, neither mg/kg nor fixed-dose guidelines appear sufficient in determining the minimal effective dose for a particular child (Rapport, DuPaul, Vyse, & Kelly, in press).

Titration Based on a Range of Doses

Because of the inherent difficulties associated with individually titrating MPH and the scope of potentially effective dosages for various behavioral domains, it would be prudent to subject children to a relatively wide dosage range during the course of a medication evaluation.

Titration Based on Learning and Academic Performance

Children with ADDH are frequently referred because of their disruptive social conduct. Nevertheless, there appears to be increasing concern for their continuing academic failure in the academic environment. During the past several years, we have systematically treated over 120 children with ADDH in the manner described above and have come to believe that dosage should be regulated according to demonstrated gains in learning and/or academic functioning—regardless of whether or not social behavior is optimized. Evaluating drug response on the basis of target symptoms only, or until untoward effects occur, may inadvertently compromise adaptive behavior. Thus, monitoring the academic performance of children undergoing stimulant treatment should be viewed as the *sine qua non* in conducting therapeutic drug trials.

Unfortunately, few practitioners have the time and/or resources to observe children in classroom settings over a period of several weeks. Past research findings, however, suggest that direct observations may not be critical in establishing therapeutic dose levels, given the relationship between observations of on-task behavior, academic performance, and teacher ratings (Rapport, DuPaul, Stoner, & Jones, 1986; Rapport, Stoner, DuPaul, Birmingham, & Tucker, 1985). The latter two variables are relatively easy to monitor on a weekly basis if teacher cooperation is solicited. Additional information gathered from drug-sensitive clinic-based instruments such as the MFFT, PAL test, CPT, and classroom analogue tests may facilitate clinical decision making, but this remains an empirical issue.

Combining Treatment Modalities

Despite the relatively wide use and pronounced clinical effects psychostimulants exert, alternative and/or combined treatments are frequently necessary to help children with ADDH function successfully in academic environments. In selecting alternative or additional treatments, the clinician must consider critical treatment parameters, specific needs of the child, and relevant exigencies with the classroom before deciding upon a particular intervention strategy (see Rapport, 1983, for a review). The most successful ones appear to include active treatment components that (a) focus the child's attention directly to ongoing task demands, (b) do not disrupt the child once he or she is successfully engaged in the task, and (c) provide rapid feedback of both a positive and a corrective nature based on the child's performance.

REFERENCES

American Psychiatric Association. (1980). *Diagnostic and statistical manual of mental disorders* (3rd ed.). Washington, DC: Author.

Rapport, M. D. (1983). Attention deficit disorder with hyperactivity: Critical treatment parameters and their application in applied outcome research. In M. Hersen, R. Eisler, & P. Miller (Eds.), *Progress in behavior modification* (Vol. 14, pp. 219–298). New York: Academic Press.

Rapport, M. D. (1987). Attention deficit disorder with hyperactivity. In M. Hersen & V. B. Van Hasselt (Eds.), *Behavior therapy with children and adolescents: A clinical approach* (pp. 325–361). New York: Wiley.

Rapport, M. D., DuPaul, G. J., Stoner, G., & Jones, J. T. (1986). Comparing classroom and clinic measures of attention deficit disorder. Differential, idiosyncratic, and dose-response effects of methylphenidate. *Journal of Consulting and Clinical Psychology, 54,* 334–341.

Rapport, M. D., DuPaul, G. J., Vyse, S. A., & Kelly, K. L. (in press). Assessing ADDH children's response to methylphenidate: Molar, intermediate, and molecular level analysis. In L. M. Bloomingdale (Ed.), *Attention deficit disorders.* New York: Spectrum.

Rapport, M. D., Murphy, H. A., & Bailey, J. S. (1982). Ritalin vs. response cost in the control of hyperactive children: A within-subject comparison. *Journal of Applied Behavior Analysis, 15,* 205–216.

Rapport, M. D., Stoner, G., DuPaul, G. J., Birmingham, B. K., & Tucker, S. (1985). Methylphenidate in hyperactive children: Differential effects of dose on academic, learning, and social behavior. *Journal of Abnormal Child Psychology, 13,* 227–244.

CHAPTER 17

Conduct Disorder

ALAN E. KAZDIN

DESCRIPTION OF THE DISORDER

Conduct disorder encompasses a broad range of antisocial behaviors in children and adolescents, including fighting, stealing, vandalism, truancy, and running away. The central feature of the disorder is the violation of major social rules. Although all children at some point are likely to get into fights or to lie, the diagnosis of conduct disorder is reserved for those who exhibit extremes of these and related behaviors. More specifically, the diagnosis is provided for children and adolescents who evince a *pattern* of antisocial behavior, who show *significant impairment in everyday functioning* at home and at school, and who are *regarded as unmanageable* by their parents and teachers. The frequency, severity, and repetitiveness of the antisocial behaviors depart from what one usually sees in children over the course of development.

Conduct disorder is a significant clinical and social problem because of the relatively high prevalence and clinical referral rates. Between 4 and 12% of children in the population show major symptoms of conduct disorder. Most of the cases are boys, with the ratio of boys to girls ranging from 3:1 to 10:1. Among children and adolescents who are seen in treatment, between 33 and 50% are referred for various antisocial behaviors.

The significance of the problem also derives from the fact that the prognosis is relatively poor. Conduct disorder in childhood portends psychiatric dysfunction and poor adjustment in adolescence and adulthood

ALAN E. KAZDIN • Department of Psychiatry, Western Psychiatric Institute and Clinic, University of Pittsburgh School of Medicine, 3811 O'Hara Street, Pittsburgh, Pennsylvania 15213.

Table 1
Symptoms That Are Included in the Diagnosis of Conduct Disorder[a]

A disturbance of conduct lasting at least 6 months, during which at least three of the following have been present:

1. Has stolen without confrontation of a victim on more than one occasion (including forgery)
2. Has run away from home overnight at least twice while living in parental or parental surrogate home (or once without returning)
3. Often lies (other than to avoid physical or sexual abuse)
4. Has deliberately engaged in firesetting
5. Is often truant from school (for older person, absent from work)
6. Has broken into someone else's house, building, or car
7. Has deliberately destroyed others' property (other than by fire-setting)
8. Has been physically cruel to animals
9. Has forced someone into sexual activity with him or her
10. Has used a weapon in more than one fight
11. Often initiates physical fights
12. Has stolen with confrontation of a victim (e.g., mugging, purse-snatching, extortion, armed robbery)
13. Has been physically cruel to people

[a] In addition to the presence of the diagnosis, criteria are also provided for severity of the disorder (mild, moderate, and severe) and for alternative subtypes (Group Type, Solitary Aggressive Type).

and predicts similar behavior in one's offspring (see Kazdin, 1987). The problem is not one in which merely the children, adolescents, and adults are miserable. The antisocial acts they may commit, ranging in degrees of severity (e.g., firesetting, homicide, theft, driving while intoxicated), have significant consequences for innocent victims in society at large.

Psychiatric Diagnosis

In the *Diagnostic and Statistical Manual of Mental Disorders* (DSM-III-R; American Psychiatric Association, 1987), the essential feature of conduct disorder is a "repetitive persistent pattern of conduct in which the basic rights of others and major age-appropriate societal norms or rules are violated". For the diagnosis to be made, one or more problematic behaviors must be evident for a period of at least 6 months. Table 1 provides the list of behaviors or symptoms that are likely to be evident in a child who receives a diagnosis of conduct disorder.

Usually, several symptoms of conduct disorder are evident and hence constitute a symptom constellation or syndrome. The precise set of symptoms that individual children will show may vary widely. However, there has been some consistency in two general types of conduct disorder (Kazdin, 1987). In the first type, *aggressive behavior* is the major symptom. Children are likely to engage in frequent fighting with others, although a variety of other symptoms, such as those listed in Table 1, are likely to be present as well. In the second type, *delinquent activity* is the central feature. In this type, the unique characteristic is that the child engages in antisocial behavior in the presence of the group or gang. Usually, stealing is the core feature, but other symptoms are likely to be evident. There remain major questions regarding how to delineate subtypes of conduct disorder. Also, various subtypes are not mutually exclusive. For example, youths who engage in gang behavior often are aggressive, and youths who do not engage in gang activities often steal.

Associated Features

Children who are diagnosed with conduct disorder often show a variety of other features that are not central to the diagnostic criteria (see Kazdin, 1987). Such youths usually show academic deficiencies at school, as evident in their grades, achievement level, and specific skill areas such as reading. They are also likely to be seen by their teachers as overactive and generally disruptive. They often show poor interpersonal relations with both peers and adults, a consequence that might be expected from their aggressive and defiant acts. A variety of other characteristics have been found, such as cognitive and attributional processes and deficits in their interpersonal skills, each of which contributes to poor interpersonal interaction.

The characteristics of conduct disorder are conveyed more concretely in the case described below. The case shows many of the characteristics of the disorder. In addition, the description includes a discussion of the assessment and treatment of the child and an evaluation up to 1 year after treatment was completed.

CASE IDENTIFICATION

Cory is a 10-year-old boy who lives at home with his mother, stepfather, two younger brothers, and a sister. He attends regular elementary school but is in a special classroom for socially and emotionally disturbed children. His placement in a special class began when he was 8 years old because his behavior could no longer be managed in the regular classroom. Cory is physically healthy and developed normally in terms of the usual milestones (e.g., walking, talking). He is somewhat small for his age (55th percentile in height, 45th percentile in weight). Psychological testing has shown that his intelligence is within the normal range (Full Scale IQ = 102 on the Wechsler Intelligence Scale for Children-Revised).

PRESENTING COMPLAINTS

Cory was referred to treatment by a school counselor who was in close contact with the family because of his protracted history of disruptive behavior. At home, Cory constantly fights with his siblings. He steals personal possessions of all family members, swears, disobeys family rules, and refuses to participate in family activities. He has been caught on three occasions playing with matches and setting fires in his room. The fires have been with small pieces of paper, trash in his waste can, and books.

At school, Cory has been in fights with several of his peers in class. He reportedly threatens peers, runs around the classroom throwing crayons and pencils as if they were darts, spits, swears, and hits the teacher with various toys and supplies. Before coming for treatment, he was suspended from school for assaulting a classmate and choking him to the point that the child almost passed out. This is only one of several incidents and several suspensions that Cory has experienced within the last year.

HISTORY

There are several background events relevant to this case. Cory's mother is 27 years old. She stays at home with her children. She has experienced several stressful events in the last few years, including the death of her mother, a severely debilitating accident to her father, a change in residence, and custody disputes with her former husband (Cory's biological father). The biological father, who lives nearby, sees Cory about five or six times each year. The biological father physically abused Cory when he was young but apparently has not continued this practice during Cory's visits. However, the biological father engages in abuse of his live-in girlfriend, which Cory has observed on several occasions.

The family has suffered serious financial difficulties. The stepfather has been working in a steel mill but suffered a layoff for 12 months, a brief return to employment, and then a strike. Also, 1 year ago, there was a major financial loss when one of Cory's younger brothers set a fire when no one else was home. The damage was extensive and led to a loss of several pieces of furniture, clothing, and several other possessions. Most of the loss was not covered by any insurance and the items have yet to be replaced. The younger brother (8 years old) has begun to get into trouble at school and seems to be following Cory's pattern.

Although the mother and stepfather have expressed interest in working with Cory as part of treatment, they live in a relatively remote rural area that is 45 miles from the clinic where treatment is provided. With only one car, no access to public transportation, and no relatives or neighbors to assist, coming to treatment at the clinic on a regular basis poses practical restrictions.

ASSESSMENT

Initial Evaluation

The initial contact with the clinic was by phone, with Cory's mother indicating she wished him to be seen. An appointment was scheduled to provide an evaluation of the child and family. At that appointment the child and the parents were interviewed separately by a psychiatrist and a social worker. The purpose was to learn about the child's history, specific problems, and current functioning and pertinent parent and family information. On the basis of these interviews, and in consultation with the parents, the recommendation was made to admit Cory for a brief period to a child psychiatric inpatient unit where treatment might be initiated. The parents agreed and the child was scheduled to be admitted within the week, when an opening was anticipated. Four days later Cory was admitted to the hospital.

The facility was a children's inpatient unit that houses 22 children at any one time. The children (ages 5–13) are admitted for acute disorders, including highly aggressive and destructive behavior, suicidal or homicidal ideation or behavior, and deteriorating family conditions. When Cory and his family came to the hospital they received a brief tour of the children's unit. They also completed additional assessments at this time. The mother and the child were both interviewed to provide a more intensive evaluation of Cory's functioning at home, at school, and in the community. A semistructured diagnostic interview (Schedule for Affective Disorders and Schizophrenia for School-Age Children) was administered. The measure samples the full range of symptoms and can be used to provide a psychiatric diagnosis based on DSM-III criteria. On the basis of the interview, Cory was diagnosed as conduct disorder, undersocialized–aggressive subtype.[1]

Standardized Parent and Teacher Ratings

In addition to the interview with the child and the parents, other measures were administered to evaluate Cory's functioning. A standard parent rating scale, noted below, was completed to provide a profile of Cory's symptoms. In addition, a rating scale was sent to Cory's teacher to examine how he had been performing at school.

Cory's mother completed the Child Behavior Checklist (CBCL; Achenbach & Edelbrock, 1983). This measure includes 118 items each rated on a 0- to 2-point scale, depending on the degree to which the particular symptom or behavioral problem characterizes the child. The items constitute multiple behavior problem scales (first-order factors) derived from factor analyses completed separately for boys and girls in different age groups (e.g., 6- to 11- or 12- to 16-year-olds). Selected scales include aggression, delinquency, hyperactivity, social withdrawal, and depression. Broad-band scales (second-order factors) are also available that provide summary measures. Two scales are Internalizing and Externalizing, which reflect inwardly directed (e.g., depression) versus outwardly directed (e.g., aggression) problems. The Total Behavior Problem score includes items loading on the first-order factor plus items that do not load on specific scales. The total score reflects an overall summary of a broad range of symptoms.

In addition to the behavior problem scales, the CBCL includes three a priori scales pertaining to positive social behavior of the child. These include Activities (participation in activities), Social (interactions with

---

[1] In the DSM-III, four subtypes were recognized on the basis of classifying the child separately along two dimensions, aggressive versus nonaggressive and socialized versus undersocialized. *Aggressive* refers to whether there is any violence against persons or property (e.g., vandalism, fighting). *Nonaggressive* is restricted to other types of symptoms (e.g., running away, chronic lying). *Socialized* refers to evidence that the child has social attachments to others (e.g., feels remorse, has peer-group friendships). *Undersocialized* refers to the absence of such connections. The majority of conduct disorder youths on this system were of the undersocialized–aggressive type. In the revision of the diagnostic scheme (DSM-III-R), these subtypes have been abandoned. In their stead are two subtypes, namely, *group type* and *solitary aggressive type*. Cory would qualify as the aggressive type on this system.

others), and School (academic progress at school). These scales together yield a Total Social Competence score, which summarizes the child's overall prosocial functioning.

To evaluate Cory's performance at school, the School Behavior Checklist (SBCL; Miller, 1977) was sent to his teacher. The measure includes 96 items, each of which is rated as true or false. Factor analysis of the measure has yielded six scales, including Low Need Achievement (underachievement, low motivation), Aggression (fighting), Anxiety (fearful), Academic Disability (poor academic skills), Hostile Isolation (holding grudges, not respecting others' belongings), and Extraversion (self-centered, attracting attention). A summary score is provided by the Total Disability scale, which includes all of the symptoms of the six scales. The SBCL also includes 5 items that the teacher rates on a 9-point Likert scale: the child's intellectual ability, academic skills, performance, emotional adjustment, and personal appeal. These ratings can be summed to provide a global rating of school adjustment.

Selection and Administration of the Measures

The CBCL and the SBCL were selected as the primary measures to evaluate Cory's current functioning and changes over time. First, the measures sample a broad range of dysfunction. Antisocial behaviors were the reason for referral. However, it is also important to examine a much larger set of symptoms that may be evident. Second, the measures include facets of prosocial behavior. The CBCL includes three social competence scales and an overall summary scale. The SBCL includes the overall rating of school adjustment. Scales reflecting prosocial behavior are important because they are not simply the opposite of various symptoms. A child could show marked reductions in symptoms but still not gain appreciably in prosocial behavior. Finally, both the SBCL and the CBCL have been extensively evaluated with large samples of children at different ages. Scores can be discussed in relation to normative levels of performance among nonreferred ("normal") children.

The CBCL and the SBCL were administered at the beginning of hospitalization. They were readministered on two separate occasions after Cory had been released from the hospital. The first occasion was 1 month after he had been discharged. Cory had completed his treatment program in the hospital and returned home. One month was allowed to elapse to permit him to adjust to a routine at home and at school and to allow his parents and teacher to have a reasonable sample of performance before completing the rating scales. One year later, the CBCL and the SBCL were completed again. For the posttreatment and 1-year-follow-up assessments, the measures were mailed to the parents and teachers.

SELECTION OF TREATMENT

Background and Description

Several treatments have been implemented for conduct disorder, including diverse forms of individual and group therapy, behavior therapy, residential treatment, pharmacotherapy, and a variety of innovative community-based treatments (Kazdin, 1985). At present no treatment has been shown to ameliorate conduct disorder and to controvert its poor prognosis. One treatment that has been promising is cognitive-behavioral problem-solving skills training (PSST). This technique focuses on the child's cognitive processes (perceptions, self-statements, attributions, and problem-solving skills) that are presumed to underlie maladaptive behavior. The processes refer to the child's appraisals of the situation, anticipated reactions of others, and self-statements in response to particular events. Clinic and nonreferred children identified as aggressive show a number of maladaptive cognitive processes and deficits in relation to interpersonal situations (see Kazdin, 1985). Primary among these processes are deficits in the child's ability to generate alternative solutions to problems, means–end thinking, consequential thinking, and taking the perspective of others.

Many variations of PSST have emerged for conduct problem children. The variations share several characteristics. First, the emphasis is on *how* children approach situations. Although it is obviously important that children ultimately select appropriate means of behaving in everyday life, the primary focus is on the thought *processes* rather than the *outcome* or specific behavioral acts that result. Second, children are taught to engage in a step-by-step approach to solve interpersonal problems. They make statements (self-instructions) to themselves that direct attention to certain aspects of the problem or tasks that lead to effective solutions. Third, treatment utilizes structured tasks involving games, academic activities, and stories. Over the course of treatment, the cognitive problem-solving skills are increasingly applied to real-life situations.

Fourth, the therapist usually plays an active role in treatment. He or she models the cognitive processes by making verbal self-statements, applies the sequence of statements to particular problems, provides cues to prompt use of the skills, and delivers feedback and praise to develop correct use of the skills. Finally, treatment usually combines several different procedures, including modeling and practice, role-playing, and reinforcement and mild punishment (loss of points or tokens).

COURSE OF TREATMENT

PSST was the treatment administered to Cory. The treatment was scheduled while Cory was in the hospital because his parents said they could not bring him back for treatment on an outpatient basis once treatment had started. Cory received 20 individual sessions of PSST, with 2 to 3 sessions each week. The treatment was administered by a master's-degree-level social worker with special training in PSST.

The treatment sessions began by teaching Cory the problem-solving steps. These consist of specific self-instruction statements, with each statement representing a step for solving a problem. The steps or self-statements include the following:

1. What am I supposed to do?
2. I have to look at all my possibilities.
3. I have to concentrate and focus in.
4. I need to make a choice and select a solution.
5. I need to find out how I did.

In the first session of treatment, Cory was taught the steps so they could be recalled without special reminders or cues from the therapist. In the next several sessions, the steps were applied to simple problems involving various academic tasks (e.g., arithmetic problems) and board games (e.g., checkers). In each of these sessions, Cory's task was to find out what the goal was (e.g., to move his checkers without being jumped), what the choices were and the consequences of each, what the best choice was, and so on. In the session, Cory and the therapist took turns using the steps to work on the task. In these early sessions, the focus was on teaching the steps and training Cory to become facile in applying them to diverse but relatively simple situations. After session 8, the games were withdrawn, and the focus was on applying the steps to problems that were related to interactions with parents, teachers, siblings, peers, and others.

Cory was also given assignments outside of treatment. The assignments initially were to identify problems that emerged (e.g., with another child on the inpatient service) where he could use the steps. When he brought one of these situations to the session, he described how the steps could have been used. He earned points for bringing in such a situation and these points could be exchanged for small prizes. As the sessions progressed, he received points not only for thinking of situations outside of treatment but also for using the steps in the actual situations. His use of the steps could be verified by asking him exactly what he did, role-playing the situation within the session, and asking other staff on the ward if the events were accurate.

The majority of treatment consisted of applying the steps in the session to situations where Cory's aggressive and antisocial behaviors have emerged. To illustrate how this proceeds, portions of session 17 are provided below:

THERAPIST: Well, Cory, today we are going to act out some more problem situations using the steps. You have been doing so well with this that I think we can use the steps today in a way that will make it even easier to use them in everyday life. When you use the steps today, I want you to think in your mind what the first steps are. When you get to step four, say that one aloud before you do it. This will let us see what the solution is that you have chosen. Then, step five, when you evaluate how you did, can also be thought in your mind. We are going to do the steps in our heads today like this so that it will be easier to use them in everyday life without drawing attention to what we are doing. The same rules apply as in our other sessions. We still want to go slowly in using the steps, and we want to select good solutions.

O.K. today I brought in a lot of difficult situations. I think it is going to be hard to use the steps. Let's see how each of us does. I have six stacks of cards here. You can see the stacks are numbered from one to six. We will take turns rolling the die and take a card from the stack with the same number. As we did in the last session, we are going to solve the problem as we sit here, then we will get up and act it out as if it is really happening. O.K., why don't you go ahead and roll the die.

CORY: (rolls the die) I got a four.

THERAPIST: O.K., read the top card in that stack (therapist points).

CORY: (reads the card) "The principal of your school is walking past you in the hall between classes when he notices some candy wrappers that someone has dropped on the floor. The principal turns to you and says in a pretty tough voice, 'Cory, we don't litter in the halls at this school! Now pick up the trash.'"

THERAPIST: This is a tough one—how are you going to handle this?

CORY: Well here goes with the steps. (Cory holds his first finger up and appears to be saying step 1 to himself; he does this with steps 2 and 3 as well. When he gets to step 4—) I would say to him that I did not throw the wrappers down and I would keep walking.

THERAPIST: Well, it was *great* that you did not get mad and talk back to him. He was sort of accusing you and you didn't really throw the paper down. But, if you just say, "I didn't do it," and walk away, what might happen?

CORY: Nothing. Because I didn't do it.

THERAPIST: Yeah, but he may not believe you—maybe especially because you got into trouble before with him. Also, he asked you for a favor and you could help a lot by doing what he asked. Try going through the steps again and see if you can turn your pretty good solution into a great one.

CORY: (goes through steps 1, 2, and 3 again; at step 4—) I would say to him that I did not throw the wrappers down but that I would gladly pick 'em up and toss them in the trash.

THERAPIST: (with great enthusiasm) That's great—that's a wonderful solution! O.K. Go to step five. How do you think you did?

CORY: I did good because I used the steps.

THERAPIST: That's right, but you did more than that. You nicely told the principal that you did not do it *and* you did the favor he asked. What do you think he will think of you in the future? Very nicely done. O.K. Now let's both get up and act this out. I am the principal. Why don't you stand over there (pointing to the opposite corner of the treatment room). O.K. Let's start. Hey, Cory, pick up those wrappers on the floor, you are not supposed to litter in the halls; you know better than that.

CORY: (carries out steps 1, 2, and 3 in his head. At step 4 he acts out the step directly in face-to-face interaction with the principal [i.e., therapist] and—) Mr. Putnam, I didn't throw these on the floor but if you want I will pick them up and toss them in the trash.

THERAPIST: (acting as principal) Yeah, that would be great. Thanks for helping out; these kids make a mess of this place. (as herself) Well, Cory, how do you think you did?

CORY: Pretty good because I used the steps and got a good solution.

THERAPIST: (as herself) I think you did great.

The treatment session continues like this with a variety of situations. When the child does especially well, the situation may be made a little more difficult or provocative to help him apply the steps under more challenging circumstances.

TERMINATION

After completion of 20 sessions, Cory was discharged from the hospital. At three points during the hospitalization, the parents visited the hospital and met with the therapist. The therapist explained the goals and procedures used in treatment. In addition, the therapist described how the steps were used. When the parents came to take Cory home, the therapist spent 2 hours with the family to give them some hints to describe how they might help Cory use the steps. The therapist showed how the steps were used by modeling directly the procedures used in treatment. For part of the meeting, Cory came in and showed how he could use the steps in a problem situation at home with one of his brothers. Cory and his parents were encouraged to call the therapist whenever they wanted and informed that the clinic staff would be in contact with them.

FOLLOW-UP

Three weeks after Cory left, the CBCL was mailed home and the SBCL was mailed to Cory's teacher. The instructions were to complete

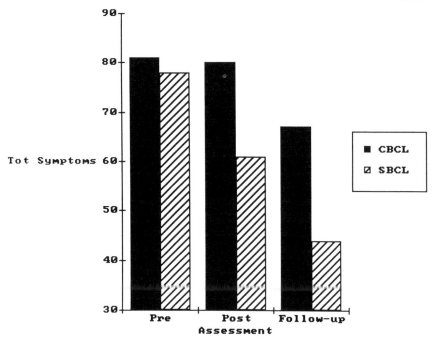

Figure 1. Total symptom scores for Cory on the CBCL (Total Behavior Problems) and SBCL (Total Disability) before (Pre) and after (Post) treatment and 1 year later (Follow-up). The CBCL and SBCL reflect home and school functioning, respectively. Reductions in scores on both measures reflect improvements in performance.

the measure to describe Cory's behavior and to return the materials in a return stamped envelope. This same procedure was followed 12 months later so that both posttreatment and 1-year follow-up data were available to evaluate the case.

The CBCL and the SBCL both yield scores for overall symptoms that cover the full range of problems. These scores are referred to as Total Behavior Problems (CBCL) and Total Disability (SBCL). Figure 1 plots these scores for Cory at each of the three assessment periods. As evident in the figure, Cory showed some improvements from pre- to follow-up assessment. Pre to post changes were not evident at home but were clear at school. Overall, for total symptoms, some improvements were evident.

The main reason for referring Cory to treatment was his aggressive behavior at home and at school. To see how Cory fared, aggression sub-scale scores from the CBCL and the SBCL are plotted in Figure 2. The pattern here is very similar to that of overall symptoms. In general, Cory's

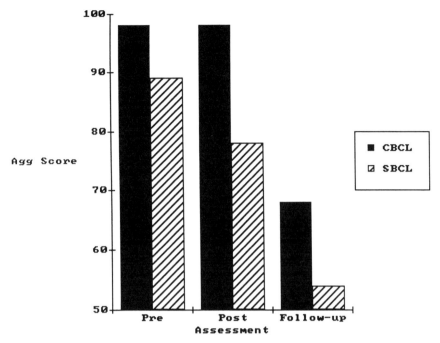

Figure 2.   Total aggression scores for Cory on the CBCL and SBCL before (Pre) and after (Post) treatment and 1 year later (Follow-up). The CBCL and SBCL reflect home and school functioning, respectively. Reductions in scores on both measures reflect improvements in performance.

aggression tended to decrease from pre- to follow-up assessment, and the improvements were greater at school than at home.

OVERALL EVALUATION

The improvements convey that there were changes. One cannot state without further information and experimental controls that the treatment was responsible for these changes. It is possible that Cory would have improved as a function of time owing to his own maturation or the period of separation from his parents. The reason for the change cannot be determined here.

Perhaps more relevant to this case is the information regarding the magnitude of the changes. Although Cory improved, the improvements did not place him within the range of his same-age peers. The level of behavior attained at follow-up was higher than most nonreferred children. Stated more simply, Cory was still having problems. He did not get suspended in the year since treatment, but he was considered by school personnel to be a problem in class and on the playground.

The case is rather typical in terms of the type of behavior that is evident and, given the current state of knowledge, what one can expect from treatment. Conduct disorder remains an extremely serious clinical problem. A great deal of research is under way to address critical diagnostic and treatment questions. The fact that change can be achieved in cases like Cory's generates considerable optimism. Yet the fact that treatment did not return his behavior to normative levels conveys the amount of research that remains to be accomplished.

What the case does not convey is the need for intervention with the entire family. Antisocial behavior has been associated with specific patterns of parent–child interaction (see Kazdin, 1987). Parents of antisocial youth often engage in behaviors that help foster antisocial behavior. One of the more viable treatments is *parent management training*, in which interaction patterns are altered directly. The approach is often the treatment of choice because the impact extends to other children in the home who are likely to show antisocial behavior as well. In fact, Cory's younger brother already had been identified as a troublemaker at school and had engaged in dangerous firesetting. A home treatment approach with a potentially broad impact would be highly desirable. The parent-based treatment was not executed with this family because they could not come to the treatment facility or continue on an outpatient basis for mainly practical reasons (e.g., transportation).

It is unlikely that a single technique such as parent management training or problem-solving skills training will address all of the problem areas that conduct disorder reflects. Such children often have severe and multiple deficits and come from families with a host of problems. An integrated treatment approach to focus specifically on a set of these problems seems reasonable, but as yet none has been shown to achieve the necessary changes. The case of Cory is poignant not because he is unique in the problems he shows and in the limited outcome of treatment but rather because his problems are shared by many and the outcome is rather typical.

ACKNOWLEDGMENT

Completion of this chapter was facilitated by a Research Scientist Development Award (MH00353) from the National Institute of Mental Health.

REFERENCES

Achenbach, T. A., & Edelbrock, C. S. (1983). *Manual for the Child Behavior Checklist and Revised Child Behavior Profile*. Burlington, VT: Author.

American Psychiatric Association. (1980). *Diagnostic and statistical manual of mental disorders* (3rd ed.). Washington, DC: Author.

American Psychiatric Association (1987). *Diagnostic and statistical manual of mental disorders* (3rd. ed., rev.). Washington, DC: Author.

Kazdin, A. E. (1985). *Treatment of antisocial behavior in children and adolescents*. Homewood, IL: Dorsey.

Kazdin, A. E. (1987). *Conduct disorder in childhood and adolescence*. Newbury Park, CA: Sage.

Miller, L. C. (1977). *School Behavior Checklist manual*. Los Angeles: Western Psychological Service.

CHAPTER 18

Firesetting

DAVID J. KOLKO and ROBERT T. AMMERMAN

DESCRIPTION OF THE DISORDER

The need for swift intervention to eliminate firesetting committed by children and adolescents is especially compelling given recent statistics indicating the prevalence and severity of this behavior (Kolko, 1985). Firesetting episodes are responsible for property damages in the millions, thousands of physical injuries, and hundreds of deaths each year. Associated consequences include, but are not limited to, significant insurance, unemployment, and firefighting costs, family and community apprehension and despair, and social repudiation. Often exacerbating the outlook for treatment is the difficulty in both detecting and assessing acts of firesetting, since they may be concealed from others. Although wide differences exist in the demographic characteristics, family backgrounds, and individual incidents of firesetters (Kolko, in press), recent controlled studies have found that firesetters exhibit more aggression, delinquency, and externalizing behaviors, and reside in environments characterized by more diffuse parental symptomatology and family discord than do nonfiresetters.

Intervention programs designed to reduce firesetting and its sequelae in children who evince psychiatric, behavioral, and emotional disturbances have been as diverse as the children for whom such services are provided (Kolko, 1985). The majority of psychosocial interventions have incorporated behavioral and social learning principles. Such programs

DAVID J. KOLKO and ROBERT T. AMMERMAN • Division of Child and Adolescent Psychiatry, Western Psychiatric Institute and Clinic, University of Pittsburgh School of Medicine, 3811 O'Hara Street, Pittsburgh, Pennsylvania 15213.

have included home-based contingency management, a work penalty threat for involvement with fire, and reinforcement for correctly answering fire safety questions and returning matches "planted" around the home. Satiation of fire interest by encouraging children to engage in match play by lighting matches repeatedly has applied separately and in conjunction with self-instructional training designed to alter the child's firesetting urges and substitute an alternative response, as well as special community activities and token reinforcement for appropriate behavior.

When the firesetter has been found to exhibit specific interpersonal and self-management deficiencies, training has been directed toward remediation of these deficits. Specific components have included social skills and fire safety training, as well as overcorrection during supervised firemaking and covert sensitization designed to reduce the appeal of fire play. Other procedures found useful have been relaxation training, response cost for firesetting, behavioral contracting, and the use of graphs to visually highlight the relationship involving the child's feelings, firesetting, and precipitating external stressors (Bumpass, Fagelman, & Brix, 1983).

As these case studies suggest, greater attention is now being paid to the youthful firesetter's individual behavioral excesses and deficits during treatment. Programs have been more firmly tied to treatment targets determined on the basis of functional analysis details. This direction is necessary in light of the broad clinical picture characteristic of these children. Consequently, the focus of treatment has expanded to include a more diverse range of problems and an emphasis upon skills training procedures, rather than contingency management alone. The present case description incorporates several cognitive-behavioral techniques to expand an adolescent firesetters repertoire and specific treatment outcome measures.

CASE IDENTIFICATION

The patient, B., was a 13.5-year-old white male who was referred to a child psychiatric unit of an urban teaching hospital from an out-of-state child welfare agency. B. was transferred from a children's psychiatric center where he had resided for 2 months. Placement in this setting called for specialized therapy, and one-on-one and small-group instruction. He had an extensive history of foster placements and psychiatric admissions for a broad range of conduct problems, which primarily began at the age of 8 years. Parental rights had been terminated since he was 10 years old.

B. was regarded as an appealing, handsome, and likable boy. He seemed to enjoy adult attention and was interested in learning about those in his environment, though he had a limited fund of knowledge for use in conversation. He enjoyed athletics, clothes, and video games. His general physical health was good, he was fully ambulatory, and he could easily complete activities of daily living and independent self-management tasks. He wore glasses owing to left esotropia. Neurological examination was normal. B. was in the sixth grade in a special classroom for emotionally disturbed children in light of delayed academic skill development and limited frustration tolerance.

PRESENTING COMPLAINTS

Primary problems identified upon referral reflected incidents of fire-setting and property destruction, oppositionality, and poor peer relations. The precipitating event for referral involved an episode in which he was observed holding a pack of matches and an aerosol spray can. It was alleged that he had been using the can as a "torch" to blacken the walls of his room. In a separate event, he had used a baseball bat to inflict extensive damage to the walls of his room and several pieces of furniture. A charge of malicious mischief was dropped contingent upon his voluntary admission to a local child psychiatric center for evaluation. Because this was B.'s second admission to the center, the staff of the center petitioned the children's services division to seek an alternative treatment facility.

In addition to firesetting and destructiveness, B. exhibited other behavioral and emotional symptoms worthy of mention. He was noted to steal from other children and to lie about his behavior, especially the reasons why he did certain things. Other conduct problems included throwing things, swearing, and tantrumming when he became upset or did not get his own way. Much of this particular behavior was deemed "passive–aggressive" by staff. Although he expressed a sincere desire to maintain friendships, he frequently provoked or teased peers, especially when he was able to determine their idiosyncratic faults or limitations. On occasion, he also had difficulty falling asleep and spoke about himself in a manner that lacked confidence and self-assurance. However, he denied various depressive symptomatology, including feelings of dysphoria, hopelessness, anhedonia, appetite change, or suicidal ideation. There was no evidence for manic or psychotic symptoms, or for drug and alcohol abuse.

HISTORY

B. was the product of a normal birth. He was the fourth of five children. His developmental milestones were reached at appropriate age levels. There was no apparent evidence of behavioral or emotional disturbance during infancy and toddlerhood. B.'s early home life was characterized by a disruption in caretakers and inconsistency. Specifically, his biological parents were separated when he was 3 years old. His mother had an extensive psychiatric history that involved one hospitalization for depression and two suicide attempts. Owing to oppositional behavior and lying, B.'s mother requested that he and his brother be offered for adoption when B. was 8 years old.

Between the ages of 8 and 10, B. was placed in three foster homes. He was in the first home for 4 months. Removal was requested because of various conduct problems, including defiance, lying, and stealing. B. resided in the second home for only 2 months owing to similar antisocial behaviors. He exhibited the same behaviors in the third home, where he stayed for 4 months. During this period, B. failed to develop any close friends and experienced poor peer relations in the home. At the same time, contact with his mother grew increasingly intermittent before parental rights were terminated.

Continued management difficulties in each of these settings resulted in a change to a more restrictive placement. B. was therefore placed in a group home where more consistent controls could be maintained and treatment initiated. An initial neurologic evaluation was negative. Individual therapy was therefore recommended for his conduct problems. He was then seen in weekly psychotherapeutic sessions designed to review his history of placement and possible rejection by his mother. B. also received special educational services and was closely supervised. Although his behavior was viewed as more adaptive, he continued to engage in negativistic and disruptive behaviors. He also was noted to provoke quarrels and to deny his responsibility for provoking peers. He was noted to argue frequently with his roommate. In general, he had difficulty following directions, preferring instead to do the opposite of what he was told.

It was in this setting that B. set his first fire. The fire was started following an altercation with his roommate. On a day when their mutual provocations had reached a peak, and after being reprimanded for a simple rule violation, B. set a fire to some paper in his roommate's dresser drawer. Shortly afterwards, he informed a staff member that he "smelled smoke." The fire department was then contacted to extinguish the fire. In general, B. was regarded by group home staff as displaying "little impulse control."

This firesetting incident precipitated B.'s first psychiatric hospitalization, which lasted for 10 months. His admitting diagnoses were conduct disorder: undersocialized–aggressive, and attention deficit disorder without hyperactivity. Significant clinical correlates included depressive symptoms and academic underachievement, although educational testing did not support a diagnosis of learning disability. A psychological evaluation upon admission described B. as "a depressed and angry boy who idealized a relationship between himself and his mother and father. He could not admit that his mother was rejecting him and appeared to have displaced this anger through firesetting and violent episodes."

Because of these psychological problems, B. was seen in individual psychotherapy. The primary focus of treatment was his perceived "abandonment" by his mother, as well as "masked" dysphoric affect. Emphasis was placed on forming a therapeutic alliance and sense of trust with a female psychologist. It was felt that these issues underlay B.'s acting-out and firesetting behaviors. B.'s therapist reported progress during treatment in terms of increasing trust in staff and self-confidence. However, increasing anger and frustration prevented him from relating more appropriately with peers and staff. Further, he was more insulting and aggressive toward adults. B. was subsequently discharged to a new foster home.

At his new foster home, B. continued to exhibit lying and oppositional behavior. After the first 4 months there he was found spreading kerosene around a neighbor's house. Although he denied any intention to actually burn the house down, the incident resulted in his removal from this home and subsequent placement in a temporary shelter. It was in this shelter that B. tried to ignite a deodorant can for use as a torch. Following this incident, B. was rehospitalized for several months. Inasmuch as his conduct problems continued and no other facilities would approve admission, B. was referred to the first author for treatment.

ASSESSMENT

Preliminary Evaluation

Preliminary observation based on unit staff reports revealed that B. was often noncompliant, defiant, and argumentative. Peer interactions typically were negative. Verbal altercations were common and usually included threats to both peers and staff. B. was involved in several physical fights that often would escalate because of his continued provocation. It was also noted that B. occasionally made cruel comments toward other children and staff, especially when he was angry. In several incidents, B. destroyed property (e.g., furniture, personal possessions) or concealed other children's possessions. In addition, he occasionally lied to peers about what others had said about them, seemingly in an attempt to instigate them to aggression. Not surprisingly, B. had no close friends on the unit and was generally disliked by almost all of the children.

A psychoeducational evaluation revealed that B. was functioning in the "low average" range of intelligence. Administration of the WISC-R yielded a Verbal IQ of 84, Performance IQ of 90, and Full Scale IQ of 85. He exhibited deficits in basic knowledge and complex problem-solving ability. His approach to many of the subtests was impulsive and poorly organized. Difficulties in making correct responses often elicited angry, self-critical reactions. Performance on the PIAT was consistent with his intellectual functioning, indicating a sixth-grade level in reading and language arts, and a seventh-grade level in mathematics. No evidence was found for a learning disability.

Behavioral Data

B.'s behavior on the children's unit or during structured activities was monitored by his primary worker or another nursing staff member. The staff recorded the daily frequency of timeouts for noncompliance and aggression during selected weeks. The frequencies were summed for the following 2-week periods: baseline, midtreatment, posttreatment/discharge, and follow-up.

Staff/Clinician Ratings

Staff or clinician ratings were obtained to provide an overall evaluation of B.'s unit adjustment and performance of prosocial behaviors. His primary therapist in the children's psychiatric setting in which he resided prior to hospitalization completed all of the baseline measures, whereas his primary therapist in the residential facility to which he was discharged after hospitalization completed all follow-up measures.[1]

Child Behavior Checklist. To examine general childhood dysfunction as perceived by unit staff, B.'s primary worker completed the CBCL, which assesses a variety of behavioral problems and social competencies. The measure includes 118 items covering individual symptoms that are

---

[1] References for all measures could not be included due to space limitations, but they can be obtained from the first author.

rated along 3-point (0–2) severity scales. Several factors are derived for behavior problems (e.g., aggressiveness, hyperactivity, depression, obsessive-compulsiveness). Social competence scales tap activities, social skills, and school performance. The CBCL provides a global and multidimensional assessment of diverse forms of child psychopathology and has been shown to possess good psychometric characteristics.

Firesetting Screen. The FS is a 12-item questionnaire that surveys one's firesetting history and repertoire. The questions that were selected to examine the nature and extent of the child's firesetting history were as follows: interest in fire, match play, firesetting, involvement in pulling alarms, possession of materials, and adult reports of community fireplay. Questions stated along 5-point scales (1 = not at all, 5 = very much) were included to survey the child's curiosity, knowledge, exposure to models, skill, and expression of negative affect. The time frame selected for this case study involved the 6 months prior to and following the present hospitalization.

Self-Report Assessment

The following self-report instruments and measures were collected to represent more accurately the nature of B.'s cognitive-behavioral repertoire and the impact of intervention. Selection of these and subsequent measures were guided by the history and above-mentioned findings indicating the presence of conduct problems, social competence and problem-solving deficiencies, and limited anger control.

Youth Self-Report Form. The YSRF is a 102-item questionnaire that surveys a broad range of individual symptoms. The measure serves as the child equivalent of the parent-rated Child Behavior Checklist. The YSRF is designed for youths 11 to 18 years old. Each item is rated along a 3-point severity continuum. The instrument assesses multiple areas of behavioral and emotional dysfunction (e.g., aggression, hyperactivity, anxiety).

Interview for Aggression. The IA consists of 30 items that are surveyed in a semistructured interview. The items represent the spectrum of antisocial behavior (e.g., fighting, threatening others, arguing, teasing). Each item is scored on a 5-point scale for severity of the behavior and on a 3-point scale for duration of the behavior.

Hostility–Guilt Inventory. The HGI consists of 38 items that are assessed in a true–false format. The instrument evaluates a broad spectrum of aggressive acts that are grouped into eight scales representing both direct (e.g., verbal aggression) and indirect (e.g., resentment, irritability) forms.

Matson Evaluation of Social Skills of Youngsters. The MESSY is a 92-item scale that samples diverse areas of social functioning, such as social isolation, expression of hostility, conversational skills, friendship making, and peer relationships. Each item is rated on a 5-point scale (1 = not at all, 5 = very much). Scores are derived for positive/prosocial behavior and negative/inappropriate behavior, as well as for overall social skills. The MESSY provide a comprehensive assessment of social skills, the quality of the child's interactions, and general social competence.

Children's Action Tendency Scale. The CATS evaluates child aggressiveness, assertiveness, and submissiveness. The measure consists of 50 items depicting interpersonal problem-solving situations. The child then endorses a particular response from alternatives presented in a forced-choice format. This measure provides an overall evaluation of response style in provocative or confrontational situations.

Trait Anger Scale. The Trait scale of the State-Trait Anger Scale (STAs) was administered to examine the child's generalized anger. The TAs measures general anger-proneness by evaluating the degree to which the respondent endorses specific characteristics or attributes associated with anger (e.g., quick-tempered, irritated, mad, frustrated). The measure consists of 15 items that are rated along 4-point scales (1 = almost never, 4 = almost always).

Children's Inventory of Anger. The CIA is a 71-item self-report instrument measuring anger arousal and reactivity in children. Each item is rated on a 4-point scale of anger intensity. The total score has been found to relate to peer and adult perceptions of anger control problems. Its inclusion in this case provides a more comprehensive assessment of anger responsivity.

Children's Depression Inventory. The CDI includes 27 items designed to assess affective, cognitive, and behavioral symptoms of depression. For each item, the child endorses one of three alternatives that best describes the child over the previous 2 weeks. The CDI provides an evaluation of the severity of depressive symptoms.

Bellevue Index of Depression-Modified.   The BID-M is a semistructured interview for children that includes 26 questions that tap depressive
symptoms (e.g., looks sad, cries easily, thinks about death). Each symptom is rated on a 5-point scale of severity and on a 3-point scale of duration. The sum of these ratings is used to assess the child's depression.

Coopersmith Self-Esteem Inventory.   The CSEI is a 58-item self-report measure of self-esteem as reflected in the child's attitudes about self,
parents and home, school, and peers. The score reported here did not
include the 8 Lie scale items.

Firesetting Inventory.   The child responded to the same questions
dealing with firesetting history as did the primary worker, with the exception of a series of questions about emergency responses.

SELECTION OF TREATMENT

B. exhibited a wide array of conduct problems and peer difficulties,
both historically and upon admission. The most serious problem may have
been his firesetting activities. Indeed, firesetting was sufficiently disturbing to his caretakers to promptly compel two psychiatric hospitalizations
and several changes in residence across state lines, even though he had
only three such episodes. He was considered to be a difficult child to
place in a foster home setting because of this past history with fire. An
analysis of these firesetting incidents revealed that B. was most likely to
commit them when he was extremely angry and frustrated. In fact, firesetting appeared to be his most extreme means of expressing anger,
albeit in an indirect manner. A similar formulation applied to his property
destruction and peer relationships.

However, given that B's firesetting and property destruction were
infrequent, it was virtually impossible to target these behaviors directly
by therapeutic contingencies. Therefore, the primary focus of intervention
was to alter the sequence of events that precipitated an escalation in
affective arousal (e.g., anger and frustration) and impulsive and explosive
behavioral reactions (e.g., breaking possessions), much in the same way
as other adolescents have been trained to control their anger or impulsivity
(Feindler & Ecton, 1986). Specifically, intervention was based on a cognitive-behavioral self-control model in which B. was trained to (1) recognize and identify self-statements that precipitated aversive emotional
states, (2) inhibit antisocial and counterproductive responses, and (3) replace these initial responses with more rational, adaptive, and construc-

tive self-statements and behaviors. This social-cognitive and problem-solving approach was designed to operate before B. reached the point at which he would consider setting a fire, destroying property, or engaging in related antisocial behaviors.

The intervention program was supplemented by an interpersonal skills training component. A modified version of social and assertion skills training was included to teach specific alternative responses to angry outbursts in challenging or provocative situations (cf. Kolko, Dorsett, & Milan, 1981). It was believed that B. would require explicit instructions and practice in the use of individual social behaviors that would maximize the likelihood of making his feelings or position known and altering the other person's behavior in a confrontive encounter without resorting to aversive tactics. The particular skills selected for training were also designed to promote and enhance more positive and reciprocal interactions with peers.

COURSE OF TREATMENT

Treatment sessions were approximately 45 minutes in duration and occurred on a twice-per-week basis. In general, each session began with a brief review of material and any homework from the previous session, and was followed by a discussion of salient events with which B. was involved before the next topic was discussed and practiced.

In the first session, an attempt was made to teach B. to identify those incidents or situations that typically elicited anger reactions and/or out-of-control behaviors. To facilitate this analysis, B. was asked to monitor the occurrence of each incident on a 3 × 5 card that he kept in his shirt pocket. The information he was asked to record was as follows: (1) who was involved in the incident, (2) the initial reason for the altercation or provocation, (3) the specific events preceding the altercation, (4) the thoughts and feelings he had during the incident, (5) his behavior during and after the incident, and (6) the outcome(s). Unit staff were informed that he would be recording such information and reminded him to do so on several occasions. B.'s initial compliance with this self-monitoring procedure was moderate at best. He frequently complained about the difficulty of recalling and then recording specific details after the incident, although he could do so upon being prompted and encouraged. With repeated interviewing during sessions, B.'s self-monitoring and accuracy improved considerably, to the point where details were described in all categories. A side effect of this procedure was his improved ability to relate his other experiences (e.g., actions, thoughts) in greater detail.

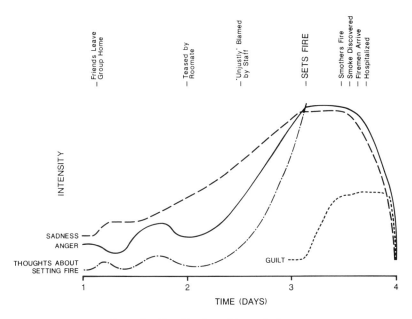

Figure 1. Results of graphing technique.

During the next three sessions, B.'s developing skill in self-monitoring the details of significant events was used to teach him the causal interrelationship among specific feelings, self-statements, and behaviors. This was accomplished by using the graphing technique described earlier that has been used effectively with firesetters (cf. Bumpass *et al.*, 1983). Graphing consists of charting a particular event on a graph that represents time on one axis and intensity of affect on the other axis. Changes in the patient's feelings and thoughts are drawn along with the sequence of activities associated with the event itself. B.'s first firesetting incident was graphed initially. As noted previously, this particular fire followed prolonged difficulties with his roommate, which culminated in a heated argument and then his being reminded by a staff member. The escalation of feelings of anger and frustration apparently served as the precipitant or the motivation to "get even." This motive was resolved or mediated by setting the fire. Figure 1 shows the graph depicting the interplay among these variables that was developed during these sessions.

The first graphing session proceeded slowly since B. provided very few details of the incident and seemed to have difficulty recalling what had happened. He was apparently reluctant to acknowledge responsibility for the fire, even though he realized that his culpability was a matter of record. However, by the end of the second session, almost all of the details had been discussed in an attempt to demonstrate the personal and situational context in which the fire took place. Specific emphasis was placed upon recalling major precipitants and consequences, including the person who noticed and reported the fire, the reactions of his peers to the fire, and his feelings immediately following the fire.

B.'s willingness to review the incident during the fourth session facilitated an understanding of his role in the event, as well as his reactivity in that situation. The rigorous manner in which the graph was developed lent credibility to the therapist's proposition that B.'s response to different events could be described and predicted in a lawful, systematic manner. In addition, use of the graphing procedure strongly supported the rationale for proceeding with a skills-based approach in which he was trained to employ specific cognitive and behavioral responses to facilitate self-control and more prosocial reactions to stressful interactions.

The focus of the next four sessions was attributional retraining through the use of self-statement instruction and general problem solving designed to reduce impulsive acts (cf. Kazdin, 1985; Milan & Kolko, 1985). Attributional retraining proceeded with a discussion of six self-statements that he frequently made in confrontive situations. As determined by a review of his self-monitoring cards, such statements were found to consistently escalate interpersonal altercations and increase anger arousal. Training was therefore directed toward substituting more prosocial and reflective self-statements for these antagonistic ones. At first, B. had difficulty grasping the intent of this technique since the idea of using "replacement thoughts" was foreign to him. With persistent inquiry, encouragement, and modeling, though, he actively participated in the process of developing more functional self-statements. Two examples of these statements were "It's not worth getting into trouble over this" and "I can stay in control even if he isn't."

Once identified, the function of these phrases was discussed by demonstrating their likely impact on the outcome of everyday encounters. Next, the therapist modeled both appropriate and inappropriate self-statements in order to sharpen B.'s ability to discriminate among types of self-statements. The therapist first verbalized them aloud but later said them quietly before simply pausing to say them to himself. B. was also required to practice using the prosocial/coping self-statements that he had identified. Several incidents that had occurred during hospitalization were incorporated into these scenarios. To facilitate generalization and maintenance, novel scenarios generated by the therapist were introduced in training. Many of these scenarios dealt with common types of provocation, including insults, intimidation, hostile comments, and criticisms (cf. Kolko *et al.*, 1981).

A necessary modification in this procedure involved the use of "cue cards" containing his self-statements to which B. would refer whenever he needed to bolster a response to a challenging interaction. It was felt that the cards would not only provide him with a concrete visual aid that would deter impulsive responding but would also provide peers and staff with an explicit behavior that could be reinforced. Accordingly, unit staff were instructed to praise and then document his use of the cards and self-statements. Indeed, both he and the staff confirmed their application in several problematic interactions.

In order to address B.'s interpersonal difficulties, a modified social skills training program was implemented over the next six sessions. Treatment emphasized situations involving assertion and appropriate expression of anger. Staff observations on the unit and role-plays enacted during treatment sessions were used to target specific interpersonal contexts and behaviors. B. generally responded passively in situations requiring assertion, such as a confrontive encounter. Specifically, he would allow intrusive and provocative peers to treat him unfairly by cutting in front of him in line, stealing his toys, or making unreasonable demands. In some instances, he would respond with physical aggression, while in others he would "get back" at them by stealing, destroying, or hiding their personal property.

The following sequence was used during each session: (1) selection of a problematic interpersonal event, (2) rationale for the skill, (3) initial role playing, (4) live modeling by the therapist, (5) practice, (6) review and feedback (cf. Kolko *et al.*, 1981). The situations used for training were first developed after extensive discussion of B.'s peer relationships. Role-play narratives were either derived by the therapist from commonly occurring situations on the unit or adapted from a set of social skill scenarios previously used with adolescent patients. The role-play paradigm consisted of reading a scene description of background context (e.g., "you're in class and someone calls you a jerk"), followed by an enactment of the scene with the therapist playing the role of another child or adult. Up to five interchanges were permitted before the termination of each scene in order to enhance the provocative and real-life quality of the role-play and to increase the difficulty in making continued socially appropriate responses.

Following the initial role play, specific components of social skill in which he was noted to be deficient were identified. These included assertive verbal content, gaze, voice volume, and affective expression. A rationale was offered to highlight the potential benefits accruing to the

Table 1
Results of Short-Term Outcome Assessment

Measure	Baseline	Posttreatment
Children's inventory of anger	166	129
Trait anger inventory	33	25
Interview for aggression	46	41
Hostility-guilt inventory		
Assaultiveness	4	0
Indirect aggression	3	2
Irritability	2	3
Negativism	1	0
Resentment	1	1
Suspiciousness	3	1
Verbal aggression	2	1
Guilt	1	0
Children's action tendency scale		
Aggression	2	0
Assertiveness	18	27
Submissiveness	10	3
Matson evaluation of social skills of youngsters		
Positive	166	158
Negative	69	46
Total	97	112
Children's depression inventory	7	10
Bellevue inventory of depression–modified	90	80
Coopersmith self-esteem inventory	29	41

use of each skill. In the initial role-play, the therapist and B. reversed roles to allow the therapist to clearly demonstrate the nature and impact of B.'s typical response to the situation. Variations in correct responding were then modeled by the therapist before B. was asked to practice the appropriate skill. The role-play was repeated three or four times so that feedback regarding improvements could be incorporated into subsequent performances. In addition, repeated practice enabled B. to attempt alternative verbal responses and discuss their relative effectiveness.

In vivo unit assignments were given to encourage the generalization of appropriate responses with peers and adults. Situations that were similar to those used during role-plays were developed and prepared for enactment outside of the session. Written guidelines specified the context and skills to be addressed. As monitored by staff, B. complied with almost all of these assignments.

The results of assessment conducted during baseline and following treatment are presented in Table 1. In terms of child report measures, several improvements were noted on the FRS. Specifically, B. acknowledged less general curiosity about, and attraction to, fire. He also exhibited greater skill in responding to role-plays involving fire safety and prevention. He was generally knowledgeable about the hazards of fire and appropriate emergency responding before training was initiated.

B. also showed an improvement on measures of affective arousal. Specifically, a decrease in the degree of anger elicited by common interpersonal situations was found on the CIA. A modest reduction in generalized anger was also apparent on the TAI, suggesting that B. characterized himself as a less anger-prone person, in general. Such findings may suggest that B. could exert greater control over a subjective reaction likely to be associated with firesetting and property destruction. B.'s scores on the IA scale did not represent a change in the severity of his general antisocial and noncompliant behavior. However, he acknowledged a substantial reduction in specific forms of verbal and physical aggression on the HGI. The most dramatic improvement in HGI scores was found for the assault scale.

Measures of social skill and interpersonal response style were in accord with these improvements. On the CATS, B. made fewer aggressive and submissive responses, and selected more prosocial or assertive responses in response to provocative situations at posttraining than baseline. B. also received a slightly higher score on the MESSY following treatment. Interestingly, improvement on this measure primarily reflected a greater reduction in negative behavior, rather than an increase in prosocial behavior.

In contrast, individual measures of depression remained quite stable across the two assessment conditions. Whereas B.'s CDI score was somewhat higher following treatment, his score on the BID was somewhat lower at posttreatment. The scores for both measures remained in the average range. Treatment was associated with an increase in self-esteem, as noted on the cSEI. This outcome may represent an improvement in general self-efficacy as a consequence of his becoming more effective in interpersonal interaction.

TERMINATION

The primary goal of termination was to prepare B. for future incidents that might precipitate an inappropriate response to an angry situation. Scenarios likely to be encouraged were generated, role-played, and practiced. B. was also given a list of alternative self-statements developed during treatment for use in his new placement. B. asked appropriate questions about the impact of certain behaviors exhibited during the role-plays.

Finding a placement proved to be difficult owing to B.'s history of firesetting. Indeed, he was quite upset about the ambiguity surrounding disposition, since he had spent 5 years being moved from one setting to another and he viewed his current situation as one more adult rejection. His anger led to increased disruption on the unit in the form of aggression toward peers and, to some extent, noncompliance close to the time of discharge. Termination occurred shortly before discharge (see next section). B.'s concerns about his future placement, as well as his chances for being adopted by another family, were explored in the final two sessions. Repeated emphasis was placed upon reminding him that the likelihood of adoption was higher if he demonstrated greater self-control in subsequent weeks.

FOLLOW-UP

Following inpatient treatment, B. was discharged to a long-term residential treatment facility for emotionally disturbed children. A short-term follow-up was conducted at 6-months. At that time, both B. and his primary therapist were asked to complete several of the self-report measures. In addition, the therapist recorded specific incidents of time-out.

Table 2 presents follow-up data based on child- and staff-reported measures obtained at baseline and 6-month follow-up. In terms of child report, the findings from the SA indicated that B. endorsed an interest in fire and a recent history of firesetting at baseline but denied either of these characteristics at follow-up. A similar pattern of improvement was noted for pulling fire alarms and hiding matches in his room. More extensive inquiry of his involvement with fire revealed that he had not considered engaging in any form of fire-related activity since treatment had been discontinued. As to the level of general dysfunction, B.'s scores on the YSRF were comparable for all scales at both assessment phases. The highest scores were reported for the internalizing syndromes, such as somatic complaints and obsessive–compulsive behavior.

Screening assessment by his primary worker revealed that B. showed an interest in fire and had set two fires during baseline, whereas no such interest or involvement in fire was acknowledged after treatment. Completion of the FRS indicated that B. showed an improvement in his ability to appropriately express "negative" emotions and, to a lesser extent, in fire safety skill. The staff also noted that B. received more frequent discipline in the form of feedback regarding positive and punishment for

Table 2
Results of Follow-up Assessment

Measure	Baseline	Follow-up
Child		
Firesetting history		
Likes fire	Yes	No
Plays with matches	No	No
Sets fires	Yes	No
Pulls fire alarms	Yes	No
Possesses incendiary materials	Yes	No
Reported for fire play by adults	No	No
Firesetting repertoire		
Curiosity/attraction	15	8
Knowledge	21	21
Models/exposure	6	4
Skill	18	25
Emergency response	23	23
Youth self-report form		
Externalizing symptoms	3	19
Internalizing symptoms	15	25
Staff		
Firesetting history		
Likes fire	Yes	No
Plays with matches	No	No
Sets fires	Yes	No
Pulls fire alarms	Yes	No
Possesses incendiary materials	—	—
Reported for fire play by adults	Yes	No
Firesetting repertoire		
Curiosity/attraction	8	11
Knowledge	14	13
Models/exposure	4	8
Skill	9	15
Ability to express negative affect	10	17
Child behavior checklist		
Externalizing symptoms	72	59
Internalizing symptoms	57	70
Social activities	36	46
Social skill	23	31
School performance	33	37

Table 3
Frequency of Time-Out for Noncompliance and Aggression

Time period (3-week blocks)	Noncompliance	Aggression
Baseline	4	2
Midtreatment	0	1
Posttreatment/discharge	4	7
Follow-up	0	1

undesireable behaviors. No change was evident in his knowledge of fire emergency responses. Interestingly, it was reported that he was somewhat more curious about fire and had more exposure to firesetting models/ materials after treatment. In contrast to baseline, B. had not pulled any fire alarms, nor had he been accused by any community agency officials of having been involved with fire.

An examination of the severity of B.'s general psychopathology on the CBCL at follow-up was conducted. Consistent with B.'s self-report, the staff indicated an increase in internalizing symptoms at follow-up. However, in contrast to his self-report, the staff noted a decrease in externalizing symptoms at follow-up. A corresponding increase was obtained in social competence ratings of his involvement in social activities, social skill, and school achievement. The staff reported that B. engaged in several recreational activities, such as swimming, skating, and soccer. He had also developed an interest in cooking, while maintaining his creative pursuits in writing and drawing. Although his peer relationships were generally provocative, they were reciprocal and pleasant with the three children with whom he had developed close friendships.

Table 3 also shows the number of time-outs occurring in response to noncompliance and more serious aggressive behaviors on the unit. The findings suggest that B. had fewer time-outs for noncompliance and, to a lesser extent, for aggression by midtreatment. Follow-up in another residential setting indicated that B. required very few visits to the time-out room.

At 15-months, a long-term follow-up was conducted by contacting the director of the residential treatment facility to which B. was discharged following his inpatient treatment program. At the time, it was learned that B. had remained on the intensive treatment unit for 12 months where, among several improvements, he exhibited a reduction in aggressive behavior and an increase in inappropriate social and self-care behaviors. Before discharge, B. had been allowed to visit his mother and had spent a week with one of his previous foster families. Upon discharge from the unit during a period of some escalation in provocativeness, B. was returned to his foster family in light of the general progress that he had made and their willingness to accept him back. The director also reported that B. had not engaged in any firesetting during the entire follow-up period and that he had been doing well in his foster home.

OVERALL EVALUATION

The general outcome of the present case study application appears positive inasmuch as B. actively participated in treatment, reported and exhibited no involvement with fire and less attraction to fire, and achieved specific affective and social improvements likely to mediate therapeutic maintenance. Accordingly, training was associated with an increase in appropriate assertion and social skill, and a decrease in hostility and anger potential or responsivity. Although there were some changes in externalizing symptoms based on staff ratings, little or no improvement was evidenced in most areas of behavioral or emotional dysfunction. Thus, B. continued to exhibit various symptoms of an internalizing nature and certain provocative or antagonistic behaviors.

From a therapeutic perspective, then, it is plausible that B.'s tendency to resort to firesetting and property destruction was diminished by developing an interpersonal repertoire that could more efficiently express his needs and motives. Of course, this treatment program was fairly limited in scope and duration by comparison with a full complement of additional procedures that might have been included, such as relaxation training, stress inoculation training, and problem-solving instruction. Although novel cognitive-behavioral techniques have shown promise with firesetters and other antisocial children, their systematic application with various children has yet to be documented (see Kolko, 1985). Therapeutic outcomes with this population might be enhanced by comparing these and other alternative procedures, including fire safety training, covert sensitization, and restitution. The fact that B. continued to evince generalized dysfunction speaks to the need for comprehensive and diverse interventions with psychiatrically disturbed firesetters.

In terms of empirical evaluation, it should be noted that B. was primarily treated and assessed in residential facilities. A primarily controlled setting permitted exposure to complementary contingency management procedures that increased compliance and reduced inappropriate behavior, and, understandably, minimized opportunities for involvement in various deviant activities, not limited to firesetting. Assessment of therapeutic efficacy would have been more rigorously documented if B. had demonstrated his improvements in more naturalistic community settings. Staff reinforcement of program improvements may also have influenced the progress he achieved during training. The examination of outcome across settings was likewise complicated by the need to use of ratings from a different staff member at each assessment point. Nevertheless, the present case study provides additional technical and procedural details that will, one hopes, facilitate therapeutic application of cognitive-behavioral procedures with disturbed youths whose antisocial behaviors include firesetting behavior.

REFERENCES

Bumpass, E. R., Fagelman, F. D., & Brix, R. J. (1983). Intervention with children who set fires. *American Journal of Psychotherapy, 37,* 328–345.

Feindler, E. L., & Ecton, R. B. (1986). *Adolescent anger control: Cognitive-behavioral techniques.* New York: Pergamon Press.

Kazdin, A. E. (1985). *Treatment of antisocial behavior in children and adolescents.* Homewood, IL: Dorsey Press.

Kolko, D. J. (1985). Juvenile firesetting: A review and critique. *Clinical Psychology Review, 5,* 345–376.

Kolko, D. J. (in press). Firesetting. In C. G. Last & M. Hersen (Eds.), *Handbook of child psychiatric diagnosis.* New York: Wiley.

Kolko, D. J., Dorsett, P. G., & Milan, M. A. (1981). A total-assessment approach to the evaluation of social skills training: The effectivenss of an anger control program for adolescent psychiatric patients. *Behavioral Assessment, 3,* 383–402.

Milan, M. A., & Kolko, M. A. (1985). Social skills training and complementary procedures in anger control and the treatment of aggression. In L. L'abate & M. A. Milan (Eds.), *Handbook of social skills training and research* (pp. 101–135). New York:Wiley.

CHAPTER 19

Anorexia Nervosa

DAVID M. GARNER

DESCRIPTION OF THE DISORDER

Anorexia nervosa is an increasingly common eating disorder that is characterized by self-imposed starvation to the point of emaciation. Recent theories have stressed the multidetermined nature of anorexia nervosa with an emphasis on cultural, individual, and familial predisposing factors (Garfinkel & Garner, 1982). The disorder usually begins with simple dieting, which becomes crystallized around issues related to control or autonomy within the individual or the family. Weight loss sets into motion a host of physiological, psychological, and environmental perpetuating mechanisms that make the disorder exceptionally resistant to treatment.

Much of the clinical thinking related to the development of anorexia nervosa in late childhood or early adolescence has been influenced by the formulations of Crisp (1980) and Minuchin, Rosman, and Baker (1978). Crisp (1980) has provided a compelling developmental view, which presumes that the central psychopathology of anorexia nervosa is rooted in the biological and psychological demands that accompany the emergence of puberty. Dieting and consequent starvation become the mechanisms by which the adolescent attempts to cope with developmental fears and family conflicts. Weight loss to a subpubertal level produces shape, hormonal, and experiential "regression" that enables the patient and family to avoid sources of developmental apprehension. Renourishment reevokes these concerns, and treatment must be aimed at helping both the

DAVID M. GARNER • Department of Psychology, University of Toronto, Toronto, Ontario, Canada M5A 1S1.

individual and the family traverse these emergent maturational demands. Minuchin *et al.* (1978) recommend family therapy as a means of challenging certain overprotective and enmeshed interactional patterns that have come into conflict with developmental pressures for change. An overprotective family life may have discouraged independence seeking and possibly magnified the concerns that normally occur with adolescence. In many instances, the child has become "overvalued" in the sense that she has become the exclusive source of parental self-validation. Sessions are aimed at examining the assumptions implied by excessive intrusion and supporting the parents in appropriate limit setting.

In some cases, inpatient treatment is necessary to normalize eating and weight, to interrupt bingeing and vomiting, to treat complications, and occasionally to disengage the patient and the family from destructive interactional patterns. Drawing from the principles described earlier, Strober and Yager (1985) have presented a thoughtful approach to inpatient treatment that is specifically designed to meet the developmental needs of the adolescent with an eating disorder.

Throughout all stages of treatment, we recommend a cognitive-behaviorally oriented, "two-track" approach that is aimed at achieving a balance in attending to salient psychological themes while not neglecting or underestimating the impact of biological changes brought about by disturbed eating patterns (Garner & Bemis, 1985; Garner, Rockert, Olmsted, Johnson, & Coscina, 1985). It relies on the developmental and family therapy formulations described earlier but does so within the overall framework of the cognitive-behavioral model. Cognitive restructuring is aimed at challenging distorted attitudes toward weight and shape that may be tied to cultural values as well as helping the patient de-couple self-esteem from social and familial expectations. Cognitive and behavioral methods are viewed as interdependent in that correction of distorted beliefs within the individual or family system may prepare individuals to engage in feared behavior, which provides data that may be used to challenge fundamental assumptions. The use of behavioral methods such as meal planning, gradual introduction of avoided foods, self-monitoring, and stimulus control techniques presuppose a trusting therapeutic relationship. Moreover, they are facilitated by cognitive methods designed to deal with the patient's resistance to surrendering symptoms that provide considerable gratification (Garner & Bemis, 1985).

CASE IDENTIFICATION

Lisa is a 13-year-old single white female eighth-grade student who lives with her parents and one of two older sisters in an upper-middle-class urban area. She presented with primary amenorrhea at a weight of 76 pounds and a height of 5 feet 0 inches. She was pale and emaciated and looked much younger than her actual age. She had been hospitalized eight times since the age of 11 and had not been able to maintain an appropriate weight as an outpatient. Lisa's father is a 58-year-old vice-president of a small business and her mother is a 57-year-old homemaker. Lisa is her parents' only natural child; her two older sisters were adopted when they were infants.

PRESENTING COMPLAINTS

Lisa did not offer any presenting complaints. She knew that she had anorexia nervosa and was adamant that she did not want to recover if it meant gaining weight. Her parents were extremely distressed about their daughter's condition and reported that they had received so many contradictory recommendations during the course of treatment that they did not know what to do. They reported that Lisa complained of "feeling fat" and appeared to be terrified at the prospect of weight gain. She had gained weight on numerous occasions while in the hospital but would lose it rapidly upon discharge. She accomplished this primarily by consuming very small amounts of food but would resort to self-induced vomiting if forced to eat larger quantities. Vomiting occurred in the absence of episodes of bulimia. Lisa avoided being around food because she reported believing that her body "could absorb calories from smells." Lisa also reported certain obsessive and compulsive rituals. Most were superstitious measures to ensure that her weight would not increase or that "calories would not turn to fat." These included foot tapping, running up and down stairs a set number of times, eating foods in a specific order, and sit-ups.

HISTORY

Lisa began to diet in April of 1983 with the approval of her pediatrician. Within 2 months her weight had dropped to 83 pounds, and her pediatrician referred her to a social worker for outpatient family therapy. The treatment focused on Lisa's weight loss as part of a struggle for autonomy, and the parents were discouraged from intervening in the areas of food or weight. By August of 1983, Lisa weighed 75 pounds and was admitted to the psychiatry ward of a general hospital. She was on a strict behavioral program in which privileges, such as television and telephone use, were contingent upon weight gain. She was discharged 6 weeks later at 83 pounds and was referred back to the outpatient therapist with the understanding that she would be readmitted if her weight fell below 80 pounds. By January of the following year, Lisa's weight had dropped to 71 pounds, and she was readmitted to the same psychiatry unit. She was discharged seven weeks later at 84 pounds, with a readmission weight set at 82 pounds. Conflict intensified at home with Lisa's emergent fears that she would absorb calories through smells. She insisted that her parents and sisters not cook certain foods and refrain from using perfumes or other odorous substances. In May of 1984, Lisa's parents and her therapist coincidentally went on three-week vacations. Within a week, Lisa was down to 79 pounds and was readmitted to psychiatry, but she was discharged after 1 week because of insurance constraints. Lisa spent most of the next year in inpatient or residential treatment. This included almost 4 months in a residential program in which various pharmacological approaches were applied; however, her weight and eating behavior continued to deteriorate. Again, she was admitted to psychiatry for weight restoration and discharged to the care of a psychoanalytically oriented psychiatrist who saw her as an outpatient and did not weigh her in the office. Lisa entered seventh grade and, despite excellent academic performance, her weight dropped to 62 pounds, whereupon she was admitted for refeeding. After weight restoration to 76 pounds, she was referred for consultation. She reported feeling safe in the hospital and stated that she would not mind if she had to spend the rest of her life in institutions. She reported that she had become less dependent on her parents by spending so much time in the hospital but that she now felt dependent on the hospital staff.

Social and Developmental History

According to her parents' report, Lisa had normal development until the age of 4 or 5 when she reported recurrent nightmares and fears of being kidnapped. When Lisa was 6 there were several deaths and illnesses among extended family and friends. At about this time Lisa began waking in the middle of the night feeling frightened and began sleeping with her parents for the remainder of the night. This behavior occurred every night until Lisa was 9 years old and intermittently until she was 12. She reported intense fears that her parents would be harmed and stated that she would rather die than have anything happen to them. She reported feeling guilty when she went out with friends and stated that she would rather stay home with her parents. She developed uncontrollable jealousy toward anyone who became close to her parents and threatened to lose weight if her sisters received too much attention. Until the development of her disorder, Lisa seemed to demonstrate adequate social and excellent academic performance. She reported that many of her academic and artistic pursuits were done more for her parents than for herself.

ASSESSMENT

The general format for assessing the eating disorder patient has been outlined elsewhere (Garner & Davis, 1986) and involves evaluation of several key areas, including (1) abnormal attitudes toward weight and shape, (2) the presence, frequency, and duration of bingeing and vomiting, (3) weight-losing behaviors such as dieting, exercise, and diuretic and laxative abuse, (4) complications such as swollen parotid glands, edema, paresthesias, erosion of the dental enamel, and others (cardiac and metabolic functioning should be evaluated by a physician familiar with the complications of eating disorders), (5) psychological state with particular reference to depression and anxiety, (6) social and family functioning with an emphasis on potential maturational fears, (7) personality features, (8) body image disturbances, (9) impulse-related behaviors, and (10) motivation for change. Although much of this information is gathered through interview, psychometric evaluation with instruments such the Eating Disorder Inventory (EDI) or the Eating Attitudes Test (EAT) provides standardized scores on dimensions relevant to the eating disorder patient.

Lisa's scores on the EDI and the EAT revealed typical profiles for the "restricting" subtype of anorexia nervosa. She reported a marked drive for thinness, a morbid fear of weight gain, and moderate dissatisfaction with her shape at presentation. Other subscales of the EDI indicated extreme perfectionism and poor self-esteem. Standardized measures of overall psychological distress indicated marked obsessionality, depressed affect, interpersonal sensitivity, and sad mood. On a self-report measure of family functioning, Lisa's profile revealed an idealized perception of her family.

SELECTION OF TREATMENT

Hospitalization

It should be emphasized that in many cases hospitalization in a program with a cognitive-behavioral orientation plus family therapy would have been considered as a treatment option. Although it was concluded from the initial interviews that there would be benefits to an inpatient treatment designed to normalize eating and weight, Lisa's growing dependence on the ward milieu and the repeated hospital failures led to the decision to begin with a structured outpatient program in which the family would be heavily involved in management of food intake. For most patients, hospitalization also serves a negative reinforcement function in that they can be persuaded to gradually increase their weight to avoid what they perceive as a potentially unpleasant experience. This was not the case for Lisa, who viewed hospitals very positively. If the outpatient approach failed with Lisa, hospitalization would be considered necessary, with a heavy emphasis on continuity between the inpatient and outpatient management. In my opinion, one of the reasons for previous failures in this case was the lack of coordination between these two components of treatment.

Family Involvement

The first treatment hypothesis tested was that ineffective parenting (reinforced in Lisa's case by early treatment recommendations prohibiting parents from being involved in the area of food) may have played a role in maintaining the disorder. It was explained to Lisa and to the family that Lisa had experienced a "developmental arrest" and had not moved much beyond the age of 11. Moreover, it was indicated that, although Lisa might have competence in other areas, she was incompetent in the domain of food intake. Therefore, until she was able to manage this basic bodily function responsibly, the family must take charge of ensuring that she consumed an amount of food that would be agreed upon in advance. Sessions were structured so that Lisa was met with individually for 20 to 30 minutes (to help foster her sense of autonomy from the family) and the family met as a group for 20 to 40 minutes to deal with issues that related to the family unit.

Weight

In line with the educational approach outlined elsewhere (Garner *et al.*, 1985), it was explained to Lisa that she was unquestionably suffering from numerous symptoms of starvation and that it was quite possible that her "hyperacuity" to smells could be related to this starved state. She would not be allowed to gain more than 2 pounds per week, and a number of calories would be "prescribed" to achieve this end. A weight gain of less than 1 pound per week would be unsatisfactory and would lead to changes in her eating regimen or other aspects of her life to produce a gradual increase in weight. A target weight was set in two stages. The first was 95 pounds, which was not as high as would have been desirable to meet her projected menstrual threshold (Garfinkel & Garner, 1982), but which was the highest weight to which she would agree. It was stated that she would be allowed to level off at this weight for an unspecified period and then stage two would involve gaining to a weight that would be several pounds over her menstrual threshold. Renutrition in the hospital would have proceeded faster without the differentiation between the two stages. Weighing was to be done only at the office, and she and her parents were instructed to dispose of their scale at home. This was designed to stop Lisa from weighing herself (which occurred over 50 times daily) and to reduce the struggles between Lisa and her parents that followed their weighing her. Lisa expressed a strong desire to go to school and was informed that this would be possible only if she made improvement with her weight. This and other obvious behavioral contingencies described throughout this case were not presented as arbitrary goals but were supported with a rationale that made sense within the context of Lisa's living arrangements and her overall progress. For example, she could not go to school at her current weight because she was physically vulnerable and needed first to demonstrate that she was making some progress with her life-threatening disorder. This approach was the opposite of that which the parents had used; they had agreed to most of Lisa's demands in order to avoid threatened weight loss.

Food and Eating

A detailed examination of Lisa's current eating revealed that she was probably consuming about 800 calories per day. The first week, the therapist stated that the level would be increased to 1,500 calories per day, and then to approximately 2,000 calories daily thereafter. Initially, Lisa refused to eat this amount but relented when it was made clear that this was a nonnegotiable aspect of treatment. If she disposed of food or vomited after eating, this would have several disadvantages. First, she would be left with great uncertainty about how many calories she really needed to maintain a particular weight. Second, an inevitable escalation would occur, with her having to dispose of an ever-increasing amount of food since her calories would be increased each week owing to her failure to meet the weight gain requirements. Third, failure to gain weight would lead to increasing environmental controls, which would ultimately lead to her having to consume the specified number of calories. Fourth, she would not be able to begin school until she made some initial progress with eating.

The exact foods to be consumed each day were to be written out in advance to make sure that they met the calorie requirements. Lisa could specify the types of foods, and her parents were to check that the calorie values were correct. Again, once the menu had been established, there was to be no negotiation or change in the plan. At mealtime Lisa's parents were instructed to make sure that all food was consumed and to assume that she would try to dispose of food if she had the opportunity. This was interpreted as a sign of her understandable anxiety rather than her attempts to "manipulate" them. The detailed attention to removing the option of disposing of food actually had the effect of reducing Lisa's guilt and anxiety since, as she stated it, "if I have the 'choice' whether or not to complete a meal, and if I do eat everything, I feel terribly guilty."

Lisa's previous hospitalizations had depended heavily on the use of liquid supplements to facilitate weight gain. She reported feeling relatively comfortable consuming her calories by liquid supplement but was terrified taking in any other form of nourishment. This was because she would become overwhelmed by anxiety if she thought that she might have inadvertently overestimated the caloric content of a particular food by even 1 calorie. Therefore, initial management involved her continuing supplements, which amounted to approximately 1,000 calories per day, plus another 1,000 calories of a solid food. The use of supplements is contrary to standard practice but illustrates a recurrent theme in therapy with these patients—namely, bending in some areas that the patient views as important while remaining absolutely firm in other objectives, such as meal completion and weight gain.

COURSE OF TREATMENT

Initial Interviews

In the initial interview, a directive style was used in describing the effects of starvation, assessing current eating behavior, eliciting motivation for recovery, reviewing principles related to eating and weight, as well as determining the ability of family members to carry out the details of the protocol. This provided the opportunity to evaluate the beliefs and assumptions of each of the family members, as well as to challenge salient misperceptions and distortions (Garner & Bemis, 1985). Goals related to change in eating behavior were placed within the context of global positive functioning. Weighing always occurred at the beginning of the session since it formed the context of the report on symptoms. The following illustrates the initial difficulties around weighing and the need to know weight in assessing other areas of functioning:

THERAPIST: How did things go last week in the area of eating?

PATIENT: I am still terrified about gaining weight but I was able to follow through in eating and now I feel better.

THERAPIST: Well, let's check your weight.

PATIENT: I don't want to.

THERAPIST: It is absolutely necessary since I have to know all of the details of eating and weight in order to help you.

PATIENT: I still don't want to.

THERAPIST: If you are really anxious, you do not have to look, but I must know in order to keep a precise record of the change from week to week. If you gain too much weight, I must know so that I can cut your calories. By weighing yourself many times each day, you have been making repeated corrections in your eating based upon relatively meaningless fluctuations in weight. You have been haunted by the scale, and rather than reassuring you, it has just created anxiety. That won't happen with me since my interests are to protect you from losing weight as well as from gaining inappropriately. Finally, knowing your weight change in response to gradually increasing calories will give us an idea of changes in your metabolic rate, which is your real protection against inappropriate weight gain.

PATIENT: O.K., I will get on the scale. (weight dropped 2 pounds)

THERAPIST: Well, I guess you have not been following through or you have totally misperceived the number of calories eaten.

PATIENT: I have eaten but I have been so frightened that I have been throwing up some meals.

The therapist then obtained the details of the vomiting behavior and instructed the parents to monitor Lisa for 2 hours after every meal, and showers were allowed only before breakfast in the morning.

Lisa began therapy with very little motivation to change her symptoms, and considerable time was spent eliciting beliefs that she had about the disorder and then challenging distortions. The following illustrates one typical interchange designed to increase motivation:

PATIENT: It really is everyone else that thinks I should change; I don't want to give up the disorder.

THERAPIST: You know what you are opting for, don't you? Anorexia nervosa is a disorder that leaves you very little else. It puts a very low ceiling on your social and vocational functioning and it virtually guarantees chronic anxiety and depression. Nevertheless, you have your reasons—maybe you could go over some of the pros and cons of the disorder and write them down on the blackboard? (If the patient had been unable to generate these on her own, it might have been necessary to help)

PATIENT: On the con side, I might die. (long pause) I can't think of any others.

THERAPIST: Maybe we can come back to these; what about the pros?

PATIENT: I will be thin, I will be in control, people will care about me.

THERAPIST: How is it that people care more about you with the disorder?

PATIENT: It is just a feeling that I have. I am afraid to get better because it will mean that my parents will not care about me anymore—not in the same way. In fact, I hate it when people say that I look better; I like it when I look sickly.

THERAPIST: What evidence do you have that your parents care more when you are ill?

PATIENT: They say that they care for me when I am well, but I just don't believe them. It is not the same type of caring.

THERAPIST: Can you explain the different types of caring?

PATIENT: Well, one is what every parent feels for their child but when I am sick or suffering, the caring is more intense.

THERAPIST: Is it true that as you have become more ill, your parents have given you more caring of any type?

PATIENT: I don't really think that I have thought about it in this much detail.

THERAPIST: It seem to me that in this last year your parents have seen less of you and perhaps have become resigned to your disorder. Maybe what you say was true initially, but is it true now?

The therapist went on to illustrate that Lisa's thinking was flawed in that (1) it was a form of selective abstraction, (2) it was based on historical information that was not relevant now, and (3) even if she did receive caring for being ill, it was a terribly self-defeating system.

In individual meetings with Lisa, a great deal of time was spent helping her identify the disadvantages of placing supreme importance upon thinness and self-control as barometers of self-worth (Garner & Bemis, 1985). Gradually she was encouraged to construe herself in a more multidimensional fashion based less on approval from others.

Crisis Intervention

Early in treatment, both Lisa and her parents had difficulty in sustaining adherence to rules around food intake, so they were instructed to telephone if there was any breakdown in the plans outlined in the meetings. This was done to minimize the rapid deterioration in Lisa's eating following conflicts over the interpretation of a rule. All family members involved in the contentious issue had to be available to talk if a call was initiated. In one instance, the mother was surreptitiously adding food to the agreed-upon portions because of her anxiety about Lisa's progress.

In other cases, the parents called because they required support when their insistence that Lisa comply was met by refusal or even violent tantrums. Their firmness led to fewer altercations and an increased sense of effectiveness on their part.

Midtreatment

As in earlier meetings, each interview focused initially on "track one" issues related to food management problems experienced by Lisa. For example, Lisa's refusal to incorporate avoided foods into her diet was met with the following:

PATIENT: If I begin eating foods that I don't eat now, I am afraid that I will lose complete control and become fat.

THERAPIST: This is a fear that most patients express. First you must remember that you are arguing from the standpoint of being starved. Once you have reached a healthy weight and have sustained it for some time, you will simply not have the urge to eat uncontrollably.

PATIENT: But I can't take that chance.

THERAPIST: I understand your feelings, but it will not happen. The only way that you will learn that your fear won't materialize is to eat these foods in prearranged amounts and see that they do not lead to uncontrollable weight gain. Nevertheless, you deserve some protection. If you do find yourself losing control, every action will be taken to interrupt it. You would be hospitalized immediately and protected from overeating if it was required.

Subsequently, Lisa began eating specified amounts of previously avoided foods, and this behavior led to a shift in the belief: "I can't eat these foods without losing control."

The mother required help in becoming less intrusive in areas such as demanding too frequently to know how Lisa felt, or making plans for her at school and with friends. This was done by examining various examples related to the assumption held by the mother that her own self-esteem was directly related to her daughter's approval. This assumption was reflected by the mother's scrupulous avoidance of criticism of her daughter's behavior and by statements such as "I am nothing if Lisa is not happy," "Lisa is my entire life," "I could not live without my daughter." Lisa met this expectation by continual reassurance of her mother and by avoidance of any expression of independence except for debate around food intake. Lisa's refusal to eat was a means for her to assert herself while denying any aggressive intent since it was assumed that her behavior was caused by "an illness." By means of the therapist's establishing all

rules regarding food intake and strongly urging the parents to be un-
bending in enforcing these rules, the parents became more effective and
less anxious in this area. Gradually, the fighting in the family moved from
food to other more typical areas of adolescent conflict. Increasingly, Lisa
resented her mother's monitoring of her food intake and was reminded
that this would end as soon as she could monitor it successfully on her
own. In this way, the mother's monitoring served the role of a negative
reinforcer for Lisa's normal eating.

Lisa's weight gradually increased over 5 months to 90 pounds. Several times over this period she requested to have more control over her
intake and was allowed to plan and consume her meals for 1 week or less
without her parents' monitoring. The first three attempts resulted in
weight loss and return to rigid monitoring by her parents. On the fourth
occasion she was successful but could not eat in front of her parents. She
was told that as long as she was dealing with eating and weight responsibly, it would be inappropriate to have her parents intrude. Her parents
had to be assisted in overcoming panic that resulted from relaxing their
control over Lisa's food intake. After 6 months, the liquid supplement
was phased out of the meal plan and foods without a dietetic connotation
were introduced. After 8 months, Lisa reported that the smell of food no
longer bothered her and she did not feel that she had to engage in superstitious rituals related to feared weight gain.

TERMINATION

As eating and weight normalized, family meetings became shorter
and, finally, were discontinued. Although there was some discussion
about eating and weight in every meeting with Lisa, the content shifted
to themes that reflected concerns about peer relationships, sexuality, self-
esteem, perfectionism, and unrealistic parental expectations. These issues
were addressed in weekly meetings for approximately 1 year, and then
meetings were gradually tapered to once per month for the next 6 months.
Meetings were occasionally scheduled around a specific concern, such as
a disagreement with parents or a disappointment at school. At this time
the therapist recommended that meetings no longer be regularly scheduled
but rather be initiated by Lisa on the basis of her needs. Either the parents
or Lisa could call if they felt that there was a deterioration in eating or
weight. Meetings occurred periodically during the next 4 months and then
ceased until a follow-up interview by telephone 1 year later.

FOLLOW-UP

At follow-up, Lisa had just completed 12th grade and was making plans to work for at least 1 year before deciding to attend a university. Lisa was 5 feet 4 inches tall and weighed 117 pounds. There was no evidence of a disturbed eating pattern according to both Lisa and her parents. Lisa indicated that she was generally satisfied with her weight and shape but reported periodically feeling "too fat." She resisted acting on this feeling and found that it dissipated with time. She completed a battery of psychometric instruments including the EAT and the EDI. These corroborated her verbal report and also revealed that she no longer held an idealized view of her family. She recognized that her parents had wanted her to attend a university and she felt very positively about her decision to resist their expectations.

OVERALL EVALUATION

In many respects this case was typical of treatment of the child or adolescent with anorexia nervosa. The prognosis for younger patients is very good, with approximately 80% recovering from the disorder (Garfinkel & Garner, 1982). The treatment in this case was complicated by the relatively long duration of illness and the multiple treatment failures. The initial stages involved education, establishing a trusting relationship with the patient, defusing parental guilt, and developing a clear plan related to food management that enabled more effective parenting to occur. Hospitalization was not necessary in this case but is required when the child's physical state is deteriorating or when the parents are incapable of taking sufficient control in the area of food management. The overall treatment orientation was cognitive-behavioral, but principles were integrated from several family and individual theorists. The format began with family meetings and progressed toward individual sessions in the later stages. A "two-track" approach was taken in which issues related to food, weight, and shape were initially the primary focus, with other psychological themes predominating as therapy progressed. In cases in which binge eating, vomiting, and laxative or diuretic abuse complicate the disorder, other specific methods must be implemented (see Garner & Bemis, 1985; Garner et al., 1985).

REFERENCES

Crisp, A. H. (1980). *Anorexia nervosa: Let me be.* New York: Grune and Stratton.
Garfinkel, P. E., & Garner, D. M. (1982). *Anorexia nervosa: A multidimensional perspective.* New York: Brunner/Mazel.

Garner, D. M., & Bemis, K. M. (1985). Cognitive therapy for anorexia nervosa. In D. M. Garner & P. E. Garfinkel (Eds.), *Handbook of psychotherapy for anorexia nervosa and bulimia*. New York: Guilford Press.

Garner, D. M., & Davis, R. (1986). The clinical assessment of anorexia nervosa and bulimia nervosa. In P. A. Keller & L. Ritt (Eds.), *Innovations in clinical practice: A source book* (Vol. 5, pp. 5–28). Sarasota, Florida: Professional Resource Exchange.

Garner, D. M., Rockert, W., Olmsted, M. P., Johnson, C. L., & Coscina, D. V. (1985). Psychoeducational principles in the treatment of bulimia and anorexia nervosa. In D. M. Garner & P. E. Garfinkel (Eds.), *Handbook of psychotherapy for anorexia nervosa and bulimia*. New York: Guilford Press.

Minuchin, S., Rosman, B. L., & Baker, J. (1978). *Psychosomatic families: Anorexia nervosa in context*. Cambridge: Harvard University Press.

Strober, M., & Yager, J. (1985). A developmental perspective on the treatment of anorexia nervosa in adolescents. In D. M. Garner & P. E. Garfinkel (Eds.), *Handbook of psychotherapy for anorexia nervosa and bulimia*. New York: Guilford Press.

CHAPTER 20

Bulimia Nervosa

L. K. GEORGE HSU and BETTY E. CHESLER

DESCRIPTION OF THE DISORDER

Bulimia (Greek for "ox appetite") occurring in the context of anorexia nervosa has been recognized for many years (Bliss & Branch, 1960, p. 37). In 1977, Nogami and Yabana used the term *kiberashi-gui* ("binge eating with an orgiastic quality") to distinguish the bulimic disorder from anorexia nervosa. Subsequently, the terms *bulimarexia* (Boskind-Lodahl & White, 1978), *dietary chaos syndrome* (Palmer, 1977), *bulimia nervosa* (Russell, 1979), and *abnormal normal weight control syndrome* (Crisp, 1979) have been proposed by various authors to distinguish the bulimic syndrome from anorexia nervosa. In 1980 the DSM-III used the term *bulimia* to delineate the syndrome. Unfortunately, using the term *bulimia*, which is a symptom, to describe the syndrome created much confusion. In 1987, the DSM-III-R used Russell's term *bulimia nervosa* for the syndrome, and the diagnostic criteria are listed in Table 1.

The cardinal feature of bulimia nervosa is the occurrence of episodes of binge eating, which may last from a few minutes to 2 hours. The food that is consumed in a binge is usually high in carbohydrate and fat content, which may amount to several thousand calories and which the patient normally forbids herself to eat. At the onset of the binge she often feels a sense of relief, pleasure, liberation, oblivion, or comfort. Binges are most often triggered by feelings of depression, anxiety, boredom, or anger. They almost always occur when she is alone or if she is surrounded

L. K. GEORGE HSU and BETTY E. CHESLER • Outpatient Eating Disorder Clinic, Western Psychiatric Institute and Clinic, University of Pittsburgh School of Medicine, 3811 O'Hara Street, Pittsburgh, Pennsylvania 15213.

Table 1
Diagnostic Criteria for Bulimia Nervosa

A. Recurrent episodes of binge eating (rapid consumption of a large amount of food in a discrete period of time)
B. A feeling of lack of control over eating behavior during the eating binges
C. Regular engagement in either self-induced vomiting, use of laxatives or diuretics, strict dieting or fasting, or vigorous exercise in order to prevent weight gain
D. A minimum average of two binge eating episodes a week for at least 3 months
E. Persistent overconcern with body shape and weight

---

by plenty of food. They tend to occur in the late afternoon or evening when she comes home from school or work, having fasted all day. As the binge continues, the sense of pleasure is replaced by a feeling of guilt and anger at herself. However, she often feels powerless to stop the binge since after taking the first bite she will say to herself, "Now that I have started I might as well go all the way and finish it." When the sense of fullness becomes intolerable, she will self-induce vomiting or else take a large amount of laxatives. Diuretic abuse and diet pill abuse are also common. Some patients will find it hard to self-induce vomiting and may resort to the use of syrup of ipecac, which is a skeletal muscle poison. Most patients do not enjoy the purge and they do it only to prevent weight gain, although about 10% of the patients may feel that vomiting has a cleansing and calming effect on them.

Bulimia nervosa always occurs in the context of dieting to lose weight. About 50% of the patients developed their first binge in the context of anorexia nervosa, while the remaining 50% would have lost some weight although not enough to qualify for a diagnosis of anorexia nervosa. Bulimics are often torn between a need to gain control by fasting and a need to discard all control by bingeing. Dysphoria is common, and perhaps one-third of the patients qualify for a diagnosis of major depression. Social anxiety, obsessive compulsive features, and borderline personality features may also occur. Other concurrent psychiatric diagnoses are rare.

Currently, there are several promising treatment approaches for this distressing disorder. In the following case, an adolescent bulimic patient was treated with weekly cognitive behavior therapy, an approach based largely on the principles outlined by Fairburn (1981).

CASE IDENTIFICATION

Ann K. was a 16-year-old, 5-feet 5-inch, 113-pound white female residing with her mother and father (43 and 44 years old, respectively).

Her mother worked as a secretary and real estate agent; her father operated a family insurance business. Ann had an older brother, 19, who attended college in another state. She was in the appropriate grade for her age and was an A student. She participated in her high school's track team and cheerleading squad. She worked part time 1 day a week after school. Although she had a few female friends, Ann stated that she "did not trust girls." She had a boyfriend, age 17, whom she had dated steadily for 10 months. She regarded him as her best friend, and told him about her bulimia before anyone else. When Ann was in seventh grade her favorite uncle was killed while driving under the influence of alcohol. She felt a strong attachment to him because he made her feel special. She said, "It's a big thing that I lost him." This uncle had caused great turmoil in the family because of his affair with a much younger woman, an event that coincided with Ann's effort to control her weight by dieting. More recently, Ann's older brother also caused the family some anxiety because, although always an A student, he suddenly developed difficulties in college. No psychiatric disorders were reported in either the immediate or extended family. Both parents accompanied Ann to the initial assessment; subsequently, her father brought her to sessions.

PRESENTING COMPLAINTS

Ann began treatment in December of 1986. Her presenting symptomatology included binge eating and self-induced vomiting three to four times a week, fear of fatness, irregular menstrual periods, initial insomnia, crying spells three times a week, and mood changes from sad to happy several times a day.

HISTORY

Ann began binge eating and self-induced vomiting in July of 1986, although her dieting had begun 18 months earlier. She adopted this eating pattern when she saw it portrayed in a movie. Her friends responded similarly to the film. Initially, Ann engaged in binge eating and self-induced vomiting once a week for 2 consecutive weeks. She accelerated this pattern to twice a week for 1 to 2 weeks. At this point, she stopped binging and vomiting for 1 month. This hiatus was followed by a pattern of binge eating and vomiting once a week for 1 month. For the next 3 months, the patient engaged in binge eating and vomiting three to four time a week.

At the onset of the bulimic eating pattern, Ann binged on junk food. However, in the 3 months prior to treatment her binges consisted of anything that was available. A typical binge included 30 "Gobs"; three pieces of toast, a bowl of cereal; two glasses of milk and fruit. When bingeing and vomiting three to four times a week, the patient typically skipped either breakfast or lunch and ate dinner with her parents from time to time.

SELECTION OF TREATMENT

An initial session with the family was held to provide information on bulimia and its treatment and to address parental and patient concerns. A cognitive-behavioral treatment plan was developed that focused on the establishment of a regular eating pattern, cessation or reduction of binge eating by at least 50%, and cessation or reduction of vomiting by at least 50%.

To establish a regular eating pattern, the patient was advised that skipping meals, restricting food intake, or eating inappropriately resulted in food deprivation that inevitably led to bingeing. A consultation with the hospital dietician was arranged in which Ann received guidelines for the establishment of a daily eating plan that encompassed three to four nutritionally and calorically balanced meals plus a snack. She was instructed to record her daily food intake, identifying food consumed as binges, regular meals, or snacks. She was also asked to record urges to binge/vomit and active binge/vomit episodes. This information was reviewed at each therapy session.

Strategies designed to combat urges to binge and vomit encompassed psychoeducation, alternative behavior, cognitive restructuring, and coping with and monitoring anxiety based on the anxiety reduction model for treatment of bulimia developed by Leitenberg, Gross, Peterson, and Rosen (1984).

The patient was provided with a handout identifying the physiological dangers associated with bulimia. Additionally, she was advised that (1) stress frequently triggers bingeing and vomiting; (2) bingeing and vomiting are mechanisms for coping with uncomfortable feelings or anxiety; (3) anxiety is time-limited, reaches a certain level, and begins to dissipate in 30 to 40 minutes; (4) repeated toleration of anxiety without bingeing or vomiting results in decreasing initial anxiety levels, and generally, decrease in the amount of time for anxiety to dissipate; (5) anxiety or uncomfortable feelings are a function of irrational thoughts.

Ann was informed that she could combat urges to binge and vomit

Date	Situation	Emotions	Automatic thoughts	Anxiety level before response 1–10	Rational response or activity till feeling comfortable. Time spent.	Anxiety level before response 1–10	Result: Did I binge or vomit? How do I feel?

Figure 1. When I have the urge to vomit.

in two ways: (1) She could engage in a pleasurable activity (e.g., talking to a friend, bathing, exercising) or record the pros and cons of bingeing or vomiting for 20 to 30 minutes; (2) she could learn how to combat irrational thoughts. Treatment provided for the incorporation of both of these strategies, facilitated through the cognitive behavioral chart (Figure 1), based on the work of Burns (1980) and Leitenberg et al. (1984).

Chart reviews at each session served as a vehicle for teaching the patient how to combat irrational thoughts, and as an indication of progress. The client was encouraged to record her positive feelings after successfully combating urges to binge and/or vomit. It was hoped that this would promote internal attributions for coping and improvement, a process theorized to be an essential step in working toward maintenance of coping skills and relapse prevention (Greenwald, 1987; McKay, Davis, & Fanning, 1981). Additionally, *Feeling Good* (Burns, 1980), a book outlining cognitive techniques for coping with unpleasant situations and feelings, was recommended and referred to during treatment.

COURSE OF TREATMENT

Over the course of 23 weeks, Ann met in 60-minute weekly sessions with a female therapist. Therapy progressed in the following way: The patient exhibited motivation to get well, as reflected in a desire to be healthy for athletic endeavors and in the conscientious fulfillment of homework assignments. Using the strategies outlined previously, treatment subsequently assumed a specific pattern. She identified the situations, feelings, and thoughts that triggered urges to binge and/or vomit as well as actual episodes of bingeing and vomiting. She recorded her anxiety level. Early in treatment she combated binge/vomiting urges by engaging in pleasurable activities until her anxiety receded to a comfortable level. In later sessions she combated urges to binge and vomit cognitively as well as behaviorally. Her ability to successfully cope with binge/vomit urges, along with the positive self-statements accompanying these efforts, was regularly reinforced by the therapist. Episodes of bingeing and/or vomiting were associated with the nonutilization of coping strategies. Therapy sessions focused on exploring the situations, feelings, and thoughts preceding urges or episodes of bingeing and vomiting. Specifically, the therapy dealt with two principal areas: (1) vomiting urges or episodes associated with feelings of fullness and fear of fatness, and (2) binge/vomit urges or episodes corresponding to interpersonal relationships. Ann's feelings of fullness and fear of fatness occurred primarily in conjunction with the prescribed regimen of eating regular nutritionally balanced meals, which often left her feeling sick. This feeling of "sickness" was reinterpreted as the normal feeling of "fullness" that accompanies the ingestion of complete meals. She was told that this fullness ordinarily disappears in about 20 minutes. She was informed that the new eating plan might entail some weight gain but would not lead to obesity.

Utilizing the coping strategies outlined previously, Ann successfully learned to combat urges to vomit related to feeling of fullness and fear of fatness over 23 weeks of treatment. Vomiting episodes associated with nonutilization of coping strategies occurred only during the first 4 weeks of treatment, and subsequently once in the 17th week of treatment. The latter episode corresponded to a 5-pound weight gain and fear of fatness. The balance of this case study will deal with antecedents of binge/

vomit urges and episodes associated with interpersonal relationships. The following is a portion from the first treatment session, during which Ann was made aware of the connection between binge/vomit behavior and situations, feelings, and thoughts. This dialogue, focusing on the antecedents of one binge/vomit incident reported from the previous week, revealed Ann's desire to establish a close relationship with her father. This theme continued to be important throughout therapy and proved to be a major stressor contributing to the patient's eating disorder.

THERAPIST: Let's see what was happening when you binged and vomited that day.

PATIENT: Nothing was going on.

THERAPIST: Where were you prior to the binge?

PATIENT: I was in my bedroom.

THERAPIST: Imagine yourself in your bedroom now, and try to recall what you were thinking about.

PATIENT: I was thinking about the family session we had, and I realized that I'm not special to anyone in my family.

THERAPIST: So you believe that neither your mother, father, or brother thinks you are special?

PATIENT: No, I guess it's that I'm second-best to my father.

THERAPIST: How do you know that?

PATIENT: My father talks less to me than my brother, and does more things with my brother.

THERAPIST: What kinds of things do your father and brother do together?

PATIENT: They hunt and fish.

THERAPIST: Do you like to do these things?

PATIENT: No.

THERAPIST: Is it possible that your father spends more time with your brother because he's male, and they both enjoy doing the same things? Is it possible that your father thinks you are special, but doesn't know how to relate to a female child or what to do with her?

PATIENT: I don't know.

THERAPIST: How about making an experiment? Ask your father to join you in one activity for an hour or two in the coming week. (Both the patient and her father have exceedingly busy schedules.)

PATIENT: I would resent doing that.

THERAPIST: Why?

PATIENT: My father should ask me. He should know how I feel.

THERAPIST: It would be great if he did, but no one can read another person's mind, not even a parent. What would happen if you asked your father to spend an hour or two with you this week?

PATIENT: (The patient was thoughtful and paused a minute or two before speaking.) I guess he would do it. He's a nice guy.

The patient agreed to ask her father to engage in an activity for 1 to 2 hours in the coming week. She was advised to check her thinking when she felt upset. Specifically, she was instructed to ask herself if her thoughts were true (based on what evidence), and if true, what they meant. Was it something she could change?

Although Ann and her father established a pattern whereby he brought her to the clinic and spent time with her afterward, she continued to experience a troubled relationship with him. Early in treatment, it was revealed that father was going through a midlife crisis and was spending less time at home, and that Ann and her mother feared he would seek a divorce. Ann reported at least one binge/vomit episode connected with feelings of being abandoned by her father. On one occasion she expressed concern that she might be the cause of her parents' marital difficulties. Therapy focused on challenging the validity and rationality of these beliefs.

It became evident in later sessions that Ann's relationship to her father reflected one aspect of a coping style in which she assumed the role of nurturer. Specifically, she was protective of her mother. She believed that the establishment of a close relationship with her father constituted a betrayal of her mother. She showed nurturance in her relationship with her boyfriend, also watching out for his safety when he became drunk at a party, and sharing his problems. Similarly, she was a problem-solver for her girlfriends. From time to time she stated that she felt alone. She came to recognize that although she listened to others, she did not share her own feelings with them. She was encouraged to begin to take risks in self-disclosure.

This maladaptive pattern of relating to others and the conflict and stress it caused her became the focal point of the eighth therapy session, when the patient reported a week of turmoil associated with a fight with her boyfriend, an argument with her mother, and feelings of estrangement from her father. Through discussion, the patient became aware of her role as nurturer. She realized that her feelings of estrangement from her father resulted more from her concern about betraying her mother than from the father's lack of interest in her. Additionally, she acknowledged for the first time that she had a female friend who potentially could become an intimate friend. However, she continued to feel distrustful of females. Further, she stated that in her crowd, going steady meant spending all of one's free time with one's boyfriend. The therapist pointed out how the patient's role as nurturer with respect to her mother and boyfriend served to cut her off from developing other potentially satisfying relationships. She was encouraged to seek greater closeness with her father and her girlfriend in the coming week. This was proposed as an experiment, to see if, in fact, she continued to perceive these relationships as evidence of disloyalty to her mother and boyfriend.

Over 23 weeks of treatment, Ann periodically worked to strengthen ties with her peers, while maintaining a close relationship with her boyfriend. This effort produced stress and conflict, and she frequently questioned whether she wanted to maintain the relationship with her boyfriend, which failed to provide for her emotional needs. Her role as nurturer in the family constellation was exacerbated as her parents' marital relationship worsened and her father left home. Even so, father continued to bring Ann to the clinic and spend time with her afterward. Initially, Ann worried that she might be the cause of her father's leaving home. Through cognitive exploration Ann came to realize that she was not responsible for the state of her parents' marriage or for her father's behavior. Ann's father, invited to join one session, told his daughter, "It's not your fault. You have to know that." Subsequent sessions dealt with Ann's anguished feelings about her parents' separation, their complaints to her about each other, and her belief that she was betraying her mother by spending time with her father. Therapy focused on accepting the reality of her parents' situation while recognizing she was not to blame. It was pointed out that her father did not leave her, and the importance of establishing a relationship with each of her parents was emphasized. Ann was instructed to politely inform her mother and father that she did not wish to hear complaints about the other parents' behavior. Through cognitive exploration Ann began to separate feelings of love and loyalty for her mother and her right to pursue a relationship with her father.

Ann's boyfriend brought her to the clinic for her 20th session. Ann announced that during the past week she had learned that her father had been intimately involved with a 25-year-old woman for the past year. She did not assume responsibility for her father's behavior. Rather, she stated angrily that he had lied, betrayed her, made a fool out of her, and that she hated him. Therapy focused on separating feelings of hatred and anger about her father's behavior from her feelings of love for him. The patient commented that if her father died now, she knew she would feel guilty about hating him. Through discussion, Ann came to realize that her father had not betrayed her by not telling her about his extramarital affair. He had kept silent in the hope of not losing his family entirely. At the end of the session Ann felt a little better. She acknowledged that although she hated what her father had done, it did not change the fact that he brought her to clinic sessions and spent time with her. She recognized that he was not the "perfect" father, but neither was he completely uncaring. Ann was encouraged to think about resuming her relationship with her father in the near future. She was advised that this would be a painful time, but that people were not made out of paper and could tolerate pain without resorting to self-destructive behavior.

Over the next 3 weeks the therapy focused on Ann's feelings, thoughts, and behaviors connected with processing the fact of her father's extramarital relationship. She was torn between wanting to know more about his lover and wishing that she did not exist. Initially, Ann angrily pressed her father for information. When he refused to comply, Ann hit him. Subsequently, she tended to cope cognitively with feelings of anger and pain. She stated that she realized she could handle painful emotions cognitively, and felt good about herself when she did. She used these coping skills when she accidentally saw her father's lover in his car. Feeling angry, hurt, and disgusted she told herself, "Life isn't fair. This is what my father wants to do. This is his problem. I won't feel this way forever." She spoke to herself in this vein until she felt comfortable. On another occasion she was unable to utilize these strategies and resorted to vomiting when overwhelmed with feelings of sadness about her father, irritation with her mother, and anger at her boyfriend, and feeling out of shape and fat.

Over the course of 23 therapy sessions Ann came to recognize and live with her angry feelings. That is, she grew to to externalize hurtful feelings expressed as anger as opposed to internalizing anger expressed as self-blame. This process became particularly evident to Ann after her father left home. She reported experiencing intense feelings of anger, and stated that she had never felt this way before. It was explained that recovering from an eating disorder entailed coming to grips with emotions that had been covered up by bingeing and vomiting. Initially, Ann coped with feelings of anger by going to her room and punching a pillow for 10 minutes. In the sessions, she was encouraged to probe the situations and cognitions that elicited angry feelings. She utilized this tactic from time to time. At other times she expressed her rage verbally or sought to soothe it through bingeing and vomiting or drinking alcohol (Ann's use of alcohol will be addressed later). The evolution of feelings of anger as a response to stressful events as opposed to feelings of self-blame may be evidenced by Ann's reactions to her father's withdrawal while living at home, his leaving home, and her learning about his romantic involvement with a 25-year-old woman.

Despite sustained family turmoil, Ann made marked progress in reducing bulimic behavior associated with interpersonal problems. From session 5 through session 20, weekly assessments indicated that incidents of bingeing and vomiting ranged from none to two vomits and one binge. Utilizing the coping strategies outlined previously, she successfully combated about four to six urges to binge and vomit per week. At times she

Table 2
Assessment Data

Assessments[a]	Pretreatment	Week 8	Week 12	Week 16	Week 20	Week 23
Weight (lb.)	113	114	116	114	114	115
B/V episodes	3 b.,	No b.,	1 b.,	No b.,	No b.,	No b.,
per week	4 v.	no v.	no v.	no v.	no v.	no v.
BDI	19	19	8	9	11	9
SAD	16	22	20	23	23	23
FNE	5	14	17	12	14	12
EDI	58	47	15	40	27	28
SCL-90	149	148	95	133	147	128
EAT	20	5	3	6	3	2
WLAS	41	41	48	39	43	41
Alcohol	None	None	None	None	2 drinking	None
consumption					episodes	

[a] BDI = Beck Depression Inventory, SAD = Social Anxiety and Distress Scale, FNE = Fear of Negative Evaluation Scale, EDI = Eating Disorder Inventory, SCL-90 = Symptom Distress Checklist, EAT Eating Attitude Test, WLAS = Wolpe-Lazarus Assertiveness Scale.

tolerated high anxiety levels for 1 to 3 hours. However, shortly before her father left home, at session 11, the weekly assessment revealed her use of alcohol as a mechanism for relieving tension. At that time, the therapist explained that drinking served the same purpose as bingeing and purging since it functioned to camouflage painful feelings. The patient was advised to utilize the same strategies for urges to drink as she used when she felt like bingeing and vomiting. Subsequently, Ann successfully combated from two to five urges to drink per week over 3 weeks. Between the 11th and 20th sessions Ann drank excessively once or twice a week for 5 weeks, and sometimes vomited afterwards. During the weeks when Ann drank, she did not binge and vomit. The last drinking episode occurred before the 20th session and followed fighting with her boyfriend and learning about her father's romantic relationship. Assessment for weeks 21 through 23 indicated no incidents of drinking. One vomiting episode was reported for week 23. A summary of the assessment data during treatment is presented in Table 2.

OVERALL EVALUATION

This case illustrates that cognitive behavioral therapy can be effective even when severe stresses are present. In such cases, therapy may require more time because more issues need to be worked through. This patient achieved a reduction in binge/vomit behavior over a relatively short treatment period despite significant concurrent family trauma. However, her utilization of alcohol in the latter half of treatment suggests the possibility that consumption of alcohol could replace bingeing as a means of relieving tension. Continued treatment will aim at maintaining her improvement by cognitive behavioral techniques. Intensive exploration of interpersonal and family issues will also be necessary. A further theme may be the issue of sexuality, in view of the fact that her illness seemed to have been precipitated by the uncle's affair and also exacerbated by her father's affair. Emphasis will be placed on cognitive coping strategies and risk-taking behavior.

The patient is currently doing well. If there is a relapse it will probably be advisable to add an antidepressant, which has been shown to be effective in the treatment of bulimia nervosa (Hughes, Wells, & Cunningham, 1986; Walsh, Stewart, Roose, Glandis, & Glassman, 1984). Individual therapy for the mother, who has become quite depressed, may also be indicated. Family therapy is unfortunately not feasible since the father has moved out of the house and has no intention of working on the marriage.

REFERENCES

Bliss, E. L., & Branch, C. H. H. (1960). *Anorexia nervosa—Its history, psychology and biology*. New York: Paul B. Huber.

Boskind-Lodahl, M., & White, W. C. (1978). The definition and treatment of bulimarexia in college women—A pilot study. *Journal of American College Women Health Association, 27*, 84–97.

Burns, D. D. (1980). *Feeling good: The new mood therapy*. New York: New American Library.

Crisp, A. H. (1979). Fatness, metabolism and sexual behavior. In L. Carenza & L. Zichella (Eds.), *Emotion and reproduction*. London: Academic Press.

Fairburn, C. G. (1981). A cognitive behavioral approach to the management of bulimia. *Psychological Medicine, 11*, 707–711.

Greenwald, M. A. (1987). Programming treatment generalization. In L. Michelson & L. M. Ascher (Eds.), *Anxiety and stress disorders: Cognitive-behavioral assessment and treatment*. New York, London: Guilford Press.

Hughes, P. L., Wells, L. A., & Cunningham, C. J. (1986). Treating bulimia with desipramine: A double-blind, placebo-controlled study. *Archives of General Psychiatry, 43*, 182–186.

Leitenberg, H., Gross, J., Peterson, J., & Rosen, J. C. (1984). Analysis of an anxiety model and the process of change during exposure plus response prevention treatment of bulimia nervosa. *Behavior Therapy, 15*, 3–20.

McKay, M., Davis, M., & Fanning, P. (1981). *Thoughts and feelings: The art of cognitive stress intervention*, Richmond, CA: New Harbinger Publications.

Nogami, Y. & Yabana, F. (1977). On kibarashi-gui. *Folia Psychiatrica et Neurologica Japnica, 31*, 159–166.

Palmer, R. L. (1977). The dietary chaos syndrome: A useful new term? *British Journal of Medicine Psychology, 52*, 187–190.

Russell, G. (1979). Bulimia nervosa: An ominous variant of anorexia nervosa. *Psychological Medicine, 9*, 429–448.

Walsh, T., Stewart, J. W., Roose, S. P., Glandis, M., & Glassman, A. H. (1984). Treatment of bulimia with phenelzine: A double-blind, placebo-controlled study. *Archives of General Psychiatry, 41*, 1105–1109.

CHAPTER 21

Atypical Eating Disorder

STEVEN A. HOBBS and DON P. WILSON

DESCRIPTION OF THE DISORDER

Selective eating and food refusal are patterns of behavior commonly observed in toddlers and young children. By the second year of life, most children demonstrate a relatively erratic appetite characterized by frequent shifts in food preferences along with a general tendency to assert their independence. In most cases, parents are informed that this pattern is normal, and that for children ages 1 to 5 years, eating at each meal is not necessary to achieve a normal weight gain of about 5 pounds per year (Smith, 1977). However, selective eating and food refusal in an infant or a young child with a predisposition for hypoglycemia can produce devastating effects.

In general, hypoglycemia is usually significant when the blood glucose concentration is less than 40 mg/dL. Especially during the period of active brain growth, depriving the brain of glucose, its primary fuel, can result in permanent neurological sequelae. Although sometimes asymptomatic, many children with hypoglycemia exhibit pallor, sweating, irritability, weakness, and mental confusion. Prolonged or severe episodes may result in convulsions or coma (Cornblath & Schwartz, 1966). When the onset of hypoglycemia is first noticed after the first 18 months of life, it is commonly due to the child's inability to adapt to prolonged fasting,

STEVEN A. HOBBS • Department of Pediatrics, Children's Medical Center, and University of Oklahoma Tulsa Medical College, 5300 East Skelly Drive, Tulsa, Oklahoma 74135. DON P. WILSON • Section of Endocrinology, Diabetes, and Metabolism, Chapman Institute of Medical Genetics, and University of Oklahoma Tulsa Medical College, 5300 East Skelly Drive, Tulsa, Oklahoma 74135.

a condition referred to as ketotic hypoglycemia or functional fasting hypoglycemia (Senior & Wolfsdorf, 1979). This condition often is manifest during a lengthy period of fasting, such as sleep subsequent to the child's having missed or refused the evening meal. Alternatively, sleeping later than usual and/or missing breakfast can result in similar changes. The child may become irritable or unarousable, or first may draw attention during a generalized motor seizure. Although typically absent, a history of head trauma, seizures, preceding illness, or possible ingestion of medications or alcohol should be excluded in each case.

Following administration of glucose, the child's symptoms resolve quickly in most cases. The initial blood glucose level is low, and ketones are found in the urine. When measured, levels of hormones and other metabolic parameters are normal.

Children with ketotic hypoglycemia are typically healthy and active. The mainstay of treatment for this disorder is to avoid prolonged fasting. The diet should be well balanced and calorically adequate for the child's chronological age. Often, late evening snacks are given to decrease the duration of fasting during sleep. Parents should be warned to prevent the child from sleeping late into the morning and from skipping meals.

Special concerns arise when children with ketotic hypoglycemia suffer illnesses characterized by anorexia and vomiting or when they voluntarily refuse food intake. The specific case described in the following section involved refusal of food by a young boy diagnosed with ketotic hypoglycemia.

CASE IDENTIFICATION

Ben, a 2½-year-old boy, was diagnosed with ketotic hypoglycemia following his presentation in a semicomatose state at a local emergency room. He was admitted to the hospital with generalized seizures, at which time the second author, a pediatric endocrinologist, was called upon as a consultant by the child's pediatrician.

During hospitalization, Ben responded well to intravenous glucose therapy and was able to rapidly resume oral feeding without problems. His parents, both well educated and in their early 30s, were quite receptive to treatment recommendations, which consisted of frequent feedings and home glucose monitoring.

Within 2 weeks following Ben's discharge from the hospital, his parents indicated that they were experiencing some inconvenience in following the recommended guidelines for treatment. Ben was originally to have been awakened at 11 p.m. for a late evening snack. Not only did this conflict with the parents' schedule but Ben was very uncooperative on being awakened following such a brief interval of sleep. Therefore, it was decided to delay the nocturnal feeding until 2 or 3 a.m. A ready-to-drink liquid nutritional supplement, Ensure Plus (Ross Laboratories), was recommended for use at this feeding because it required no preparation, was palatable, and could be consumed rapidly with minimum disruption of the child's sleep. Ben's parents also were provided with more detailed nutritional information at this time. Approximately 6 weeks later, however, they expressed major concerns regarding Ben's refusal to consume solid foods. It was at this point that the first author also became involved in the case.

PRESENTING COMPLAINTS

In a telephone conversation, Ben's mother indicated that although Ben had gained weight since his release from the hospital, his eating had deteriorated gradually over the past 2 months. She indicated that Ben now was refusing virtually all foods with the exception of the nutritional supplement, Ensure Plus.

During an interview the following day, Ben's mother outlined the difficulties she and her husband were experiencing in feeding this child. Several weeks earlier, Ben had begun to refuse some of his least preferred foods. Owing to the need for him to avoid a fasting state, the parents began to substitute foods Ben preferred for those that he refused, in order to ensure that his total nutritional intake was adequate. However, Ben became increasingly more selective, first refusing all nonpreferred foods and then refusing many of his favorite foods.

At that point, Ben's parents began to offer him Ensure Plus during the daytime also. The child readily accepted this nutritional supplement and requested it frequently. However, with the further use of Ensure Plus, a substance containing approximately 45 calories per ounce, Ben's consumption of solid foods began to decrease even further. During the week prior to the appointment, Ben had refused nearly all of his favorite foods. His diet now consisted of Ensure Plus almost exclusively, since he consumed an estimated 900 to 1,100 calories per day of that substance. In addition to being concerned about his lack of consumption of normal foods, Ben's parents were equally concerned about the possibility that their child would begin to refuse the food supplement, as he had done with other foods, thus increasing the likelihood of recurrent hypoglycemia.

HISTORY

A previously healthy child, Ben was described by his parents as having been a "picky eater" since being weaned from the bottle at 14 months of age. At 26 months of age, he was taken to the emergency room of a local hospital in a semicomatose state with generalized seizures. According to his parents, Ben had appeared healthy on the previous day. He had eaten a scant supper and as usual had eaten nothing else prior to bedtime. Ben reportedly had slept with no apparent difficulty throughout the previous night. His parents left for work the next morning before Ben had awakened.

The child's baby-sitter attempted to wake him at approximately 8:30 a.m. However, Ben was found in a semicomatose state and, while having intermittent seizures, was taken to a local emergency room. Initial examination in the emergency room revealed that Ben was lethargic and unresponsive to pain. He had a normal liver, generalized hypotonia, and rotatory nystagmus. There were no focal neurologic deficits, his heart and lungs were normal, and he did not appear to be dehydrated.

Initial laboratory tests revealed a blood glucose level of 15 mg/dL and the presence of ketones in the child's urine. Additional laboratory procedures, including measurement of corticol, growth hormone, and insulin levels, all were within normal limits. When given concentrated intravenous dextrose, Ben quickly became arousable and recognized his parents.

This child's prior medical history did not appear to contribute to his condition. Although his weight was at the 10th percentile for his age group, Ben's physical growth and attainment of developmental milestones were reportedly within normal limits; his parents reported no history of head trauma or ingestion of medications or alcohol by the child.

Since this child did not appear to have other acute or chronic illness, it was concluded that he suffered from ketotic hypoglycemia. During his hospital stay, Ben was maintained on intravenous glucose, which was gradually tapered and subsequently discontinued when he became able to tolerate oral feeding.

Dietary counseling was initiated during Ben's hospital stay and continued on an outpatient basis. The primary goal of such counseling was avoidance of a fasting state. A combination of frequent feedings high in protein and carbohydrate and a high-protein feeding during the night were recommended. More specifically, Ben was to eat three solid meals and three snacks daily. Two weeks after his discharge from the hospital, Ben's parents requested that a feeding during the night be substituted for, or added to, the other snacks. Due their work schedules, the parents preferred that Ben not be awakended prior to their departure for work in the morning. However, since Ben usually fell asleep by 9 p.m., this would involve a lengthy nighttime fast. In order to reduce the time involved in preparing food and having Ben consume during a nocturnal feeding, Sustacal or Ensure Plus in a premixed liquid form were recommended by the dietician for use at a 3 a.m. feeding.

The etiology of the problem was discussed further with Ben's parents at that time. In addition to nutritional instruction regarding frequency and type of foods to be consumed, the parents were instructed in home blood glucose monitoring and methods for resuscitating Ben from a comatose state in the unlikely event that a hypoglycemic episode did occur.

ASSESSMENT

At the time when the majority of Ben's caloric intake began to consist almost entirely of Ensure Plus, his mother began to keep a diary that contained a narrative account of the parents' efforts to deal with his lack of eating as well as a record of amounts of food consumed each day. The diary was reviewed by the first author during the initial appointment. Records of the previous 4 days indicated that except for Ensure Plus, Ben's intake for that entire period consisted of one bowl of oatmeal, two teaspoonsful each of pancake and mashed potatoes, one taco chip, and less than 1 ounce of milk.

During that time, his parents attempted to get Ben to eat by encouraging him at virtually every opportunity and by making food readily available to him throughout the day. They initially offered him all of his favorite foods, including cereal, pancakes, apples, cheese, and ice cream. Ben's response was always "No, don't want it. Not hungry." At times, he would add, "I'm sick." Not only did Ben refuse soiid foods during this period but he also refused all liquids other than Ensure Plus. In response, Ben's parents only tried harder to get him to eat, leaving attractive foods in areas were Ben would have access to them. Whenever he refused a meal, he would be given 4 ounces or more of the nutritional supplement in order to avoid a fasting state. His consumption of Ensure Plus during the previous 4-day period had been a mean of 20 ounces per day.

When asked about his eating in other settings, Ben's mother indicated that he also would refuse to eat for his grandmother and his baby-sitter. Although he was not a good eater at a preschool he attended 1 to 2 days weekly, Ben *did not* refuse all foods in that setting.

Ben's mother stated that it was clear to her and her husband that they were fighting a losing battle regarding Ben's eating. They readily admitted that they would do anything, including "stand on their heads to get Ben to eat." However, their methods of intervention, including verbal encouragement to eat, free access to food, and use of the nutritional supplement, were providing what appeared to be very potent reinforcers for Ben's refusal of food.

The evening prior to the appointment, Ben's mother reported that she and her husband used what they termed "punishment" when Ben refused to eat. After Ben refused all food and drink during a trip to McDonald's, he was told by his parents that he could go on the restaurant playground only if he ate his food. Once again, Ben refused to eat and, as he had begun to do several days earlier, requested water to drink rather than milk or juice. Ben cried in the restaurant while his older brother was permitted to go onto the playground, but he still refused all food.

Ben's mother reported that she felt as if she had treated Ben in a cruel manner by withholding access to this activity. However, she was praised for her efforts, and it was pointed out that she had not deprived Ben of access to the playground. Rather, Ben had had a choice in the matter and had chosen not to go on the playground.

In order to effect change in this child's food intake, it was determined that the consequences for consumption and refusal of food needed to be altered. For the first time since his hospitalization, Ben's mother had made a desirable activity contingent on eating. Despite her initial reaction of guilt surrounding restriction of Ben's access to the playground at McDonald's, it appeared that she might be willing to make other activities contingent on eating. Because Ben's food intake was at a near-zero level, concern that such an intervention would further reduce his eating was not an issue.

Of greater importance, however, were contingencies involving the use of nutritional supplements. Whenever Ben refused a meal, such refusals would rarely result in increased hunger. Instead, in order to avoid a fasting state, Ben's parents would attempt to cajole him into eating by offering and giving him access to a variety of foods, followed by offers of a substitute for regular food, Ensure Plus. This consequence for refusal of food was actually a substance that Ben had begun to prefer over regular food and drink.

SELECTION OF TREATMENT

A rearrangement of contingencies so that food refusals produced little parental attention as well as a state of hunger—at least temporarily—

appeared in order. Since it was estimated that Ben could likely withstand at least 6 hours of fasting without precipitating a hypoglycemic state, a treatment plan was presented to his parents that involved decreased use or delayed use of nutritional substitutes following refusal of food.

Ben's parents were asked to implement a program that included several major components, each of which was related to consumption or refusal of foods. First, they were instructed to begin offering food to Ben on a regular schedule. This was a dramatic departure from the previous arrangement in which food was available to Ben at virtually all times. They were instructed to refrain from use of the almost continuous verbal prompts that they had been relying on to encourage Ben to eat. Instead, they were told to offer food to this child at specific mealtimes or snack times and to use only one or two verbal prompts at each feeding. Specific guidelines for scheduling of each meal and snack were as follows:

3:00 a.m.	Nighttime snack (Ensure Plus)
8:00 a.m.	Breakfast
10:00 a.m.	Morning snack
12:00 p.m.	Lunch
3:00 p.m.	Afternoon snack
6:00 p.m.	Dinner
8:00 p.m.	Bedtime snack

Ben's parents were further instructed to refrain from discussing food and eating when Ben refused, and to somewhat limit his immediate access to desirable activities following such refusals. Most important, his parents were instructed to refrain from offering more food or Ensure Plus or Sustacal to Ben immediately or shortly after he refused to eat or consumed an inadequate amount of a meal or snack. Rather, Ben would have to wait until the next meal, which was to be offered 1 hour earlier than the above schedule. For the sake of convenience, his parents were to continue to give him Ensure Plus at a 3 a.m. feeding. However, Ensure Plus was to be given to Ben only 1 hour after his refusing breakfast, or 1 hour after refusal or inadequate intake at two successive meals or snacks at other times of the day.

In this way, whenever Ben ate poorly, he would have to wait from 1 to 6 hours before food or nutritional supplements were available to him again. The supplements were only used as a last resort, however, after Ben had fasted for a period of 6 hours. In addition, Ben's parents were instructed to use praise as well as activity and token rewards whenever Ben consumed regular food or drinks.

COURSE OF TREATMENT

According to records kept by the child's mother, Ben's intake during
the 4 days prior to intervention consisted of an average of nearly 900
calories (approximately 20 ounces) per day from Ensure Plus and fewer
than 50 calories per day of other foods and fluids (see Figure 1). On the
first day of the treatment program, Ben refused breakfast. After breakfast,
his mother made "Good Eater" charts for both Ben and his 4-year-old
brother. She explained to both boys that each time one of them was a
"good eater," he could put a star on the chart. The family went about
their normal activities for the remainder of the next hour, and there was
no other mention of eating. One hour after breakfast, Ben was given 4
ounces of Ensure Plus.

At the midmorning snack, Ben again refused all food and observed
his brother receive a star for "good eating." At lunchtime, the family
brought food to a swimming outing, and Ben was told that he and his
brother would get to use newly purchased floating rings only if they were
"good eaters." Ben proceeded to eat a few french fries at that time, was
praised and allowed to use the swimming ring, and continued to eat intermittently throughout the remainder of the outing. Upon arriving home,
Ben initially refused a midafternoon snack until he was reminded that he
would receive a star for eating. He then consumed a small portion of an
apple, for which he received praise and a star.

Ben ate only a few raisins offered him by a baby-sitter at supper and
was given 4 ounces of Ensure Plus after his parents returned home from
a social activity at 11 p.m. and again at his usual 3 a.m. feeding. His total

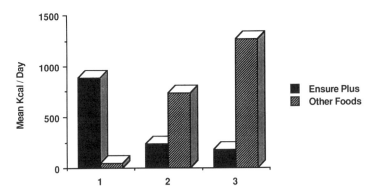

Figure 1.   Mean number of calories of Ensure Plus and other foods consumed per day during
baseline (1), treatment (2), and 9-month follow-up (3).

intake for the 24-hour period was 530 calories from Ensure Plus and 160 calories from other foods.

On Day 2 of treatment, Ben consumed portions of foods offered him at each meal and snack except supper. At supper, he refused all food and drink and cried when his brother received a star for his eating. Before bedtime, Ben initially refused a snack of cereal and milk. Ben again observed his brother being praised for finishing his snack. Ben's brother was then read a book by their mother. Minutes later, Ben said that he wanted "to be a good eater" and consumed what his mother described as "more cereal than he had eaten in a month." After having a book read to him and receiving a star, Ben reportedly kept repeating, "I a good eater." For the day, he had consumed nearly 625 calories from foods eaten at meals and snacks and received an additional 175 calories from Ensure Plus at his usual 3 a.m. feeding.

In a telephone conversation on Day 3 of treatment, Ben's mother reported that she was pleased with his progress over the previous 2 days. She expressed pleasure at having to resort to the use of Ensure Plus on only two occasions other than the 3 a.m. feedings. Although Ben's caloric intake was still well below the 1,200-calorie total recommended for him, his mother expressed confidence that intake would continue to increase.

A return appointment was scheduled for Day 10 of the treatment program to review records of Ben's intake over the previous 2 weeks and to discuss any problems his parents had encountered in implementing the treatment procedures. It appeared that Ben's parents generally had been able to implement the program in the manner outlined. Ben reportedly had refused meals or snacks on only five occasions during the previous 9 days of treatment.

In contrast with Ben's pretreatment average of 20 ounces of Ensure Plus consumed per day, his intake of this supplement had decreased to a mean of 6 ounces per day (237 calories) over the previous 9 days. Of this total amount, a mean of 4 ounces was consumed at the nightly 3 a.m. feeding. More important, Ben's intake of other foods during that time had increased to a mean of 737 calories per day.

TERMINATION

By Day 10 of the treatment program, Ben's parents expressed a great deal of satisfaction with the changes that had been made in Ben's eating. His mother indicated that Ben was now eating as well as he had at any time since he had been weaned from bottle feedings. She further indicated that they expected Ben to continue to be very independent and "a picky eater," but recognized that such behavior was typical of a normal 2-year-old.

As a result of the reported changes in Ben's eating behavior and his parents' expressed satisfaction with the short-term outcome of the intervention, a return appointment was scheduled for 3 months to coincide with his medical recheck. It was suggested to the parents that Ben probably would refuse to eat on an intermittent basis and that they should continue to use the same procedures at those times. In addition, they were cautioned against increasing their use of Ensure Plus over the quantities that had been given Ben the previous 9 days. The parents agreed to continue keeping records of Ben's intake of Ensure Plus and to resume keeping records of Ben's eating, as well, if they detected any change in their use of Ensure Plus or a decrease in Ben's intake. They were further encouraged to contact the therapist at any time concerning questions about Ben's eating.

FOLLOW-UP

Ben's parents reportedly encountered no major difficulties in managing Ben's eating over the next 3 months. At that time, the child's mother noted that they were continuing to adhere to a general eating schedule similar to that which had been outlined at the outset of treatment. She further reported that Ben continued to respond well to the use of social, token, and activity reinforcers contingent on eating. Aside from the 3 a.m. feeding, she and her husband reportedly had resorted to giving Ben the nutritional supplement only on two other occasions during the 3-month period.

Although she described Ben's eating as "still picky," Ben's mother reported that she did not become overly concerned or focus a great deal of attention on his behavior when Ben engaged in selective eating. In general, these parents felt that Ben's overall intake was adequate. Despite the dramatic decrease in his intake of Ensure Plus, Ben's weight had increased slightly (by approximately $\frac{1}{4}$ pound). Therefore, it was suggested to the parents that they might begin to focus more on the various types of foods that Ben was consuming now that they had effectively decreased their previous reliance on the use of nutritional supplements. Use of contingent tangible, token, and social reinforcement procedures similar to those that had already been implemented was discussed with regard to increasing Ben's consumption of foods having higher caloric content and nutritional value. Ben's mother expressed confidence that she could effectively implement such a program if the child did not demonstrate further weight gain in the coming months. She indicated that she would not hesitate to call regarding any additional concerns about Ben's eating before his next appointment scheduled in 6 months (i.e., 9-month follow-up).

When Ben's mother called to schedule the 9-month follow-up appointment, she indicated that Ben's eating had improved considerably. In order to document this, she and her husband were asked to keep records of Ben's intake for the 2-week period prior to the appointment, which indicated that Ben's mean caloric intake for the period had been 1,441 calories per day. Of that total, a mean of 1,266 calories per day came from regular food and fluids and a mean of 175 calories per day from his nocturnal feedings of Ensure Plus. Ben's mother indicated that his eating over the prior 2 weeks was very representative of his pattern throughout the previous 6 months. She reported that parental use of Ensure Plus at times other than the 3 a.m. feeding was quite rare, and that Ben seldom requested the supplement in the interval since the previous follow-up visit.

Moreover, Ben had gained 1.7 kg ($3\frac{3}{4}$ lb.) over the nearly $6\frac{1}{2}$ months since his last appointment, placing his weight at approximately the 42nd percentile for children his age. At this visit, the child demonstrated no symptoms of hypoglycemia, and his mother indicated that blood glucose monitoring at home continued to produce levels of greater than 80 mg/dL. She stated that she felt that Ben was now in better health than at any time since his infancy and again expressed confidence in the parents' ability to deal effectively with any future eating problems that Ben might demonstrate.

OVERALL EVALUATION

This case provides an illustration of how parents may be trained in behavior therapy procedures to effectively deal with selecting eating and food refusal (Palmer, Thompson, & Linscheid, 1975; Riordan, Iwata, Wohl, & Finney, 1980). Furthermore, it provides an example of the use of behavioral treatment methods to avert the potentially devastating effects of a severe metabolic disorder. Had this child's ketotic hypoglycemia been left undiagnosed or nutritional intervention been inadequately implemented, he undoubtedly could have suffered permanent neurological impairment.

Further hypoglycemic states might have been averted—at least temporarily—with continued reliance on nutritional supplements as this child's primary means of caloric intake. However, maintaining Ben's intake by relying exclusively on his continued acceptance of a single nutritional substance is a practice that would likely meet with decreased success and become less practical over time.

Although this case did not involve a controlled single-subject evaluation of the impact of the treatment procedures, it seems unlikely that maturation or other extraneous variables could account for the somewhat dramatic change in this child's intake of Ensure Plus and regular foods. Coinciding with his parents' introduction of treatment procedures, consumption of nutritional supplements rapidly decreased by 70%, and the child's caloric intake from other foods and liquids increased from near-zero levels to what gradually approached nutritionally appropriate levels.

Moreover, a weight increase of 4 pounds was observed during the 9 months following introduction of treatment procedures. The child's weight, which had been at the 10th percentile prior to diagnosis of ketotic hypoglycemia, approached the mean for his age group at 9-month follow-up. Thus, proper medical diagnosis and dietary intervention augmented by methods of managing this child's eating behavior appear to have produced significant change in his overall health status.

REFERENCES

Cornblath, M., & Schwartz, R. (1966). *Disorders of carbohydrate metabolism in children.* Philadelphia: W. B. Saunders.

Palmer, S., Thompson, R. J., & Linscheid, T. R. (1975). Applied behavior analysis in the treatment of childhood feeding problems. *Developmental Medicine and Child Neurology, 17,* 333–339.

Riordan, M. M., Iwata, B. A., Wohl, M. K., & Finney, J. (1980). Behavioral treatment of food refusal and selectivity in developmentally disabled children. *Applied Research in Mental Retardation, 1,* 95–112.

Senior, B., & Wolfsdorf, J. I. (1979). Hypoglycemia in children. *Pediatric Clinics of North America, 26,* 171–185.

Smith, D. W. (1977). *Growth and its disorders.* Philadelphia: W. B. Saunders.

CHAPTER 22

Pica

SUE ANN FULTZ and JOHANNES ROJAHN

DESCRIPTION OF THE DISORDER

Pica is a relatively rare eating disorder that is characterized by the ingestion of nonnutritive items. According to criteria of the *Diagnostic and Statistical Manual of Mental Disorders* (APA, 1980), these behaviors can be diagnosed as pica if they are not a function of another mental or physical disorder. The term stems from the ornithological name of the genus *pica*, which contains the omnivorous bird *magpie*. Pica usually remits in early childhood and is considered pathological only if it persists beyond that age. While the etiology of pica is largely unknown, predisposing factors of pica are mental retardation, mineral deficiencies (i.e., zinc, iron), and neglect. A number of specific forms of pica have been described, such as geophagia (eating of clay) and pagophagia (excessive eating of ice), both of which are associated with iron deficiency anemia. In a recent pilot study involving two mentally retarded adults with chronic pica problems, it was found that the rate of pica was related to the serum zinc blood level (Lofts, 1986). An increase in serum zinc level, which was manipulated by doses of 100 mg and 150 mg of chelated zinc, was associated with a significant decrease in pica attempts.

Pica is frequently conceptualized as a form of self-injurious behavior, owing to the medical complications that can result from the consumption of harmful objects, such as lead paint chips, paper clips, or cigarette butts.

SUE ANN FULTZ • Western Psychiatric Institute and Clinic, University of Pittsburgh School of Medicine, 3811 O'Hara Street, Pittsburgh, Pennsylvania 15213.   JOHANNES ROJAHN • Nisonger Center, The Ohio State University, 1581 Dodd Drive, Columbus, Ohio 43210-1205.

The resulting complications include lead intoxication, intestinal parasites, nutritional anemia, and intestinal obstruction, which often makes surgical intervention necessary.

Among mentally retarded people the prevalence and incidence of pica increases with the severity of retardation, and it is inversely related to chronological age. Estimates of prevalence vary across studies according to definitions of pica, population characteristics, and other criteria. McAlpine and Singh (1986), for instance, reported a prevalence rate of 9.2% among the entire population of a state institution of 607 persons, Danford and Huber (1982) identified 16.7% of pica cases among 991 individuals residing in an institution for mentally retarded persons; and Rojahn (1986) found that pica was observed in 0.3% of a total of 25,872 noninstitutionalized mentally retarded persons.

A variety of treatments have been reported in the literature, ranging from medical interventions and nutritional regimens to long-term mechanical restraints, such as camisoles and helmets with face masks, and behavior modification techniques. The list of employed behavioral procedures covers almost the full range of restrictiveness, depending on the severity of the problem and client characteristics. They reach from benign and indirect reinforcement schedules for the omission of pica to punishment procedures. Reinforcement procedures have not been reported as a unimodal form of pica treatment because they tend to be too slow-acting for such a high-risk behavior. They are usually part of a treatment package that consists of a number of treatment components. Differential reinforcement of other behaviors (DRO), for example, has been successfully combined with time-out, with discrimination training and overcorrection, and with physical restraint and avoidence conditioning. Owing to the self-injurious nature of the behavior, a wide variety of aversive techniques have also been implemented to suppress pica. These techniques include overcorrection, brief physical restraint, (Bucher, Reykdal, & Albin, 1976), and visual screening. Recently, researchers have started to address comparative efficacy issues of punishment programs for pica control. Singh and Bakker (1984) compared the effects of overcorrection versus contingent physical restraint, and Rojahn, McGonigle, Curcio, and Dixon (1987) investigated water mist and aromatic ammonia. Interestingly, no studies have been reported so far that contrasted aversive behavior programs, reinforcement techniques, and their combination.

CASE IDENTIFICATION

The client, Pete, was a 19-year-old profoundly retarded Caucasian male, 170 cm tall and 57.5 kg of weight. His DSM-III Axis I diagnosis

was atypical organic brain syndrome, atypical stereotyped movement disorder, profound mental retardation, and pica; on Axis III a partial complex
seizure disorder was diagnosed. He was ambulating and had no expressive
language, with a Vineland Adaptive Behavior Scale score of less than 20.
It was unclear whether he understood verbal commands. Records indicated that he was allergic to some forms of psychotropic medication,
including haldoperidol, thioridazine, and imipramine. Phenytoin trials for
his seizure disorder were started after the behavioral treatment evaluation
reported below was completed. He remained drug-free throughout the
study. Pete had been institutionalized since the age of 8. Developmental
history was reportedly inconspicuous until he was about 2 years of age,
when he started to regress for unknown reasons.

PRESENTING COMPLAINTS

The treatment evaluations discussed below took place at a psychiatric
hospital inpatient unit for multiply handicapped children and adolescents.
Pete was referred to the psychiatric facility primarily for the treatment
of severe and high-frequency pica and mouthing behavior. His behavior
problems required constant and close supervision by staff to prevent mouthing and ingestion of harmful objects. Reports of earlier pica incidents
included the ingestion of feces, grass, stones, washcloths, a wristband,
and a small toy. Owing to the almost exclusive absence of a gag reflex,
the client could place his entire hand in his mouth, and there was some
risk that objects could become lodged in his throat with no visible signs
that he was choking.

HISTORY

Pete's target behaviors of pica and mouthing had been noted by the
parents prior to his institutionalization at age 8. These behaviors, along
with bruxism, had been persistent and occurring at high rates throughout
his institutionalization. Prior to hospitalization, treatment at the institution involved 24-hour observation and overcorrection procedures, which
consisted of required teeth brushing with a soft-bristle toothbrush dipped
in Listerine after each occurrence of pica. Reportedly, the client was
resistant to the procedure, so that four staff were required to implement
it. This difficulty with implementation resulted in the discontinuation of
overcorrection and Pete's hospitalization. The client also suffered from

recurring nosebleeds, which were closely monitored throughout the study.

ASSESSMENT

Five different observers were trained to participate in the treatment selection and evaluation process. There was one primary observer and four backup and reliability observers. Observations were conducted through a large one-way mirror in the treatment room. A number of behaviors were targeted for observation during all phases of the treatment. The operationalized definitions of the two most important categories are listed below.

Pica was defined as the ingestion of nonnutritive objects of touching of parted lips with nonedible items, such as pieces of paper, Play-Doh, and cloth. *Mouthing* was described as the insertion of hand in mouth, criterion being the fingertips reaching beyond the lips. Occurrences of mouthing with a pica item in his hand were scored as both mouthing and pica.

Frequency recording was conducted for the targeted behaviors and the implementation of the treatment programs. In addition, a 10-second continuous-interval recording system was used to record the above observation categories in order to allow for a more rigorous estimate of observer agreement, as would be possible with frequency data. The kappa coefficient was used to estimate observer agreement, which is based on interval-by-interval comparisons.

SELECTION OF TREATMENT

No diagnostic findings were identified, that would have been suggestive of a medical form of treatment. The items the client chose for ingestion appeared to be nonselective, so that no clue was given as to specific dietary deficiencies. We therefore primarily concentrated on a behavioral analysis of the problem behaviors. Treatment evaluations took place in a 4 m × 4 m treatment room, which was furnished with a small table, a chair, a sink, and a one-way mirror across one wall of the room. Treatment sessions in this environment were considered to be an initial step in order to establish strong control over the behavior. Generalization across other settings on the unit was planned as a next phase in the treatment program.

A first question was whether the client might swallow objects because of relative food deprivation (i.e., hunger before meals). If this were the case, it was hypothesized that Pete would display relatively fewer pica responses after meals than before meals. On each of 3 consecutive days Pete was taken to the treatment room and observed for 50 10-second intervals 30 minutes before and 30 minutes after dinner. He was presented with nonedible items, which were selected on the basis of earlier preference reports. They consisted of small amounts of cotton balls, paper, and pieces of Play-Doh. The resulting data showed that the overall rate of pica was very high, and that the predinner pica attempts were somewhat more frequent (pica attempts occurred on an average of 83.3% of the intervals, with a standard deviation of 17) than the postdinner attempts (mean of 74% and a standard deviation of 22.7), but that there was not a striking difference. This evaluation indicated that the behavior was relatively independent of mealtime schedules and that food deprivation was not a strong contributing factor maintaining pica.

A second hypothesis to be tested was that Pete's pica problem might have been a function of his inability to discriminate between food and nonfood items. If this were the case, a training procedure would be called for that would concentrate on the acquisition of discrimination between edible and nonedible objects. To test the hypothesis, a pilot study was initiated in which the client was systematically presented with pairs of one edible and one nonedible item. Food items consisted of small amounts of pretzels, M&Ms, chewing gum, and marshmallows; nonfood items were the same as listed above. Pairwise comparisons were performed in five sessions, with a total of 79 trials of one edible and one nonedible. Combinations and sequence of combinations within sessions were randomized. In 44% of the trials Pete selected the nonedible item first. This indicated that there was no strong preference of food over nonfood items and that his item selection was not clearly discriminative.

Our findings led us to investigate operant hypotheses of pica as a form of self-injurious behavior. Self-injurious behavior is frequently found to be maintained by either positive reinforcement, such as social attention or sensory stimulation, or by negative reinforcement through escape/avoidance of unpleasant circumstances, such as demands or pain. Frequently, both positive and negative reinforcement mechanisms can be in operation for the same behavior under different setting events. For instance, persons can exhibit head-banging behavior in situations in which they seek social attention or in which they want an ongoing social interaction terminated. In Pete's case, informal observations suggested that the behavior appeared to be primarily maintained by reinforcement involved in the act (presumably sensory reinforcement of some sort). For instance, when left all by himself, Pete continued to mouth and ingest objects, which points to the self-reinforcing property of this class of behaviors. It also indicates that social attention probably had no major main-taining function for pica. Given Pete's high frequency of free operant pica responding, we assumed that there was a strong reinforcing sensory component involved in the act. Owing to the chronicity, frequency, and high risk involved in the behavior, relatively benign forms of treatment, such as shaping of alternative appropriate behaviors, were either not feasible or insufficient at that point. Rapid elimination of the behavior had to be the primary treatment goal.

A first study was initiated to evaluate the aversive properties of two stimuli: aromatic ammonia and water mist. The procedures were compared by means of an alternating treatments design. Eighteen 16.6-minute baseline sessions were conducted first. This was followed by seven sessions for each one of the aversive stimuli in evenly balanced order. Mean frequency of pica during baseline was 31.4 ($SD = 16.8$) as compared with 31.5 ($SD = 28.9$) during the water mist program and 10.0 ($SD = 6.0$) during ammonia conditions. Obviously, water mist had to be discarded since it did not decrease pica below baseline levels. Aromatic ammonia, on the other hand, had a clear suppressive effect.

Punishment alone is generally not considered a feasible treatment program since clients generally do not expand their adaptive behavioral repertoires by passive avoidance of punishment. Punishment is frequently more effective if the individual has alternative behaviors available that can produce reinforcement. Also, the therapist is soon associated with punishment and then becomes avoided by the client. Thus, when the rapid reduction of a behavior is called for, a combination of a punishment program with supportive positive reinforcement procedures is therefore often the treatment of choice. With our client it was decided to first focus on DRO for nonpica intervals in combination with suppression of pica by use of aromatic ammonia. Later, a combination of ammonia with a different reinforcement procedure (DRI) was evaluated. Aromatic ammonia has been demonstrated to be an effective punisher in the treatment of other self-injurious behaviors, and more recently also with pica (Rojahn et al., 1987). However, it has not been explored in contrast to reinforcement techniques, such as DRO. Furthermore, it was decided to investigate whether the addition of a differential reinforcement of a pica-incompatible behavior program (DRI) would enhance the suppressive effects of the ammonia punishment.

COURSE OF TREATMENT

The main purpose of the following evaluation was to identify a small number of potential treatment techniques and to chose the most effective program. Owing to considerable time constraints, treatment decisions had to be made rapidly. For that reason an alternating treatments design was considered useful because it allows for relatively frequent treatment comparisons in a short period of time. The main problem with these designs is multiple treatment interference, a confound in the data, which can occur when more than one treatment is presented to one individual. Multiple treatment interference means that treatments influence each other, and that their true effect is exacerbated or reduced.

In a first attempt, DRO sessions and aromatic ammonia sessions were contrasted against no-treatment conditions. Scattered in the treatment room were small pieces of tissue paper, Play-Doh, and cloth. The no-treatment condition was continued after baseline in order to control for multiple treatment interference. After the first comparison was completed, a second one involving aromatic ammonia and a DRI schedule against ammonia conditions alone was started. In addition to these two sequential alternating treatments designs, an atypical multiple baseline design across two behaviors (pica and mouthing nonedible objects) was added in order to provide additional experimental control. Each condition lasted 7.5 minutes, with short breaks between conditions.

During the first phase of the study, baseline conditions were scheduled that established rates of pica under baiting conditions. These sessions consisted of three 7.5-minute time blocks, with 2-minute breaks in between in which no active treatment program was provided. The therapist sat in a chair and did not interact with the client. The client was permitted to wander throughout the room and was not restrictred from engaging in any activities. Four nonfood items (a selection of those described above) were constantly available. They were placed at four different areas in the treatment room (on the sink, the table, the windowsill, and the floor). Each time the client attempted to swallow an item, the therapist tried to remove it from his mouth and replaced the item at its respective location in the room. The therapist completed this with no further interaction and the client never resisted the removal of the items. Between the time blocks the client had to leave the room.

The second phase of the study was designed to compare DRO and aromatic ammonia conditions. It consisted of three component sessions daily, one of which was a no-treatment component, one a DRO component, and one an ammonia component presented in randomized order. The no-treatment condition was conducted in a manner identical to the baseline described above. During the aromatic ammonia condition, occurrence of pica produced a verbal reprimand (a loud "No!"); simultaneously, the therapist quickly removed the lid of a test tube containing two crushed ammonia capsules and held it directly under the client's nose for 10 seconds. The capsules (Burroughs Wellcome Co.) contained 0.33 cc alcohol (36%). After approximately 10 openings of the tube the capsules were replaced by new ones. Also, the pica item was removed from the client at this time. Under DRO conditions, the client was reinforced with edibles (e.g., raisins, potato chips) and social praise (e.g., "Good job, keeping your hands down") for each 5 seconds of nonoccurrence of pica. All other behaviors were ignored. The therapist provided the client with discriminative stimuli (SD) at the beginning of each condition, in an effort to facilitate differentiation of the experimental conditions. The SDs were either the test tube with the ammonia capsules (ammonia condition) or edible reinforcers (DRO condition). In addition, the therapist wore a light blue smock during DRO conditions and a yellow smock during ammonia.

Unfortunately, the data gathered in phase 2 indicated multiple treatment interference among the treatment components. Therefore, during phase 3 of the study, an attempt was made to reduce multiple treatment interference by expanding the intervals between different treatment conditions from 2 minutes to 24 hours; i.e., instead of treatment conditions being alternated back to back within a short period of time, they were alternated between days. The no-treatment condition was dropped to save time. Each session consisted of three 7.5-minute components under either ammonia or DRO conditions.

After the comparison between DRO and ammonia was completed, it was decided to replace DRO with another reinforcement schedule. The main reason was that the edibles produced substantial increases in mouthing behavior (see Figure 1). Mouthing usually occurred immediately after a reinforcer was delivered, before the edible had been completely chewed and swallowed. This was an unsightly event that was aversive to staff interacting with him (saliva and pieces of partially chewed food covering the client's hand). A reinforcement schedule was needed that would reduce pica and mouthing. Therefore, a differential reinforcement of incompatible behavior (DRI) was chosen. The new evaluation phase was initiated by a return to baseline conditions in phase 4. Baseline conditions were identical to the ones described above. In phase 5, ammonia, in combination with a DRI component, was compared to ammonia alone. It had to be determined whether an addition of a DRI schedule would enhance the suppressive effects of ammonia on pica and at the same time reduce the rate of mouthing behavior. The no-treatment blocks were a continuation of baseline conditions. The aromatic ammonia with DRI procedure prescribed that after each 10 seconds during which pica was not observed, the client was prompted to engage in an appropriate activity (e.g., stacking rings, putting pieces into a puzzle). The completion of one appropriate

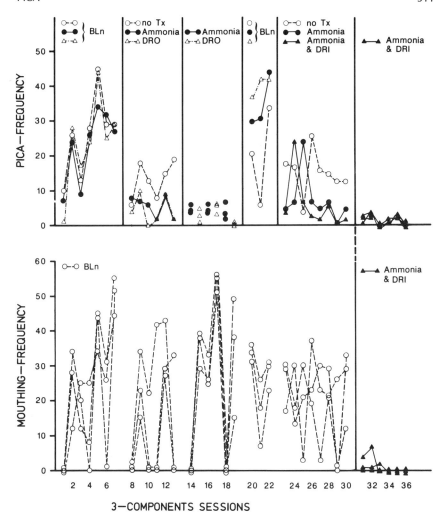

Figure 1.   Frequency of pica and mouthing behaviors during three 7.5-minute time blocks per session.

response was reinforced with edibles and praise. Application of ammonia for occurrences of the targeted behavior(s) proceeded as described above.

In the final phase of the study both pica and mouthing were treated with the combination of ammonia and DRI. At the same time the treatment was implemented throughout the whole day, on the whole unit, and by every direct care staff on site.

Treatment Results

Observer agreement was completed in 25% of the three component sessions. Kappa computations for pica behavior resulted in a mean observer agreement of 0.88, with a range from 0.54 to 1.0; mean Kappa for mouthing was 0.91 with a range from 0.74 to 1.0.

The frequency of pica and mouthing for the three components in each daily session is shown in Figure 1. High but variable rates were observed during baseline for both targeted behaviors; however, intersession variability occurred for pica, whereas both inter- and intrasession variability occurred for the longer mouthing baseline. The mean baseline rate of pica was 72.0; mean baseline rate of mouthing was 64.9.

In the second phase of the study, both ammonia and DRO treatments resulted in similar reductions of the targeted behavior (an average of 5.6 and 4.5, respectively). The no-treatment condition also resulted in a slight reduction of pica, although it continued to occur at a somewhat higher rate than the two treatments (mean of 13.0). The deceleration of pica during the no-treatment condition indicates that multiple treatment interference had occurred. To control for such error, discontinuation of the no-treatment conditions and alternating treatments across days rather than across treatment components within sessions was initiated in phase 3. Again, ammonia and DRO conditions both produced reduction in the behavior. Interestingly, lower rates of pica were observed during the DRO condition (the mean pica rate during ammonia condition was 13.3 during DRO of 8.6). Inspection of Figure 1 suggests a concurrent increase in mouthing behavior during the DRO condition of treatment of pica.

A return to baseline in phase 4 resulted in recovery of pica to levels exceeding the original baseline (average of 95.6 per session), which can be expected after the withdrawal of punishment contingencies. During phase 5, ammonia and no-treatment conditions were reinstated, with results similar to those achieved in previous phases (a mean of 7.6 and 15.25, respectively). Implementation of combined ammonia and DRI treatments, however, produced the greatest suppression of pica achieved thus far (a mean of 6.0). Therefore, introduction of the combination treatment across all three components in each session for both pica and mouthing was indicated for phase 6. The best reduction of both behaviors was achieved during this phase, with the mean rate of pica being 5.3 and the mean rate of mouthing being 2.5.

TERMINATION

At the end of the treatment evaluation study in the laboratory setting, the DRI and ammonia procedure was implemented first in the learning center of the inpatient unit for 3 hours/day and then unitwide during all waking hours. The client was soon to be discharged and the swift generalization of the procedure was necessary. Since it was impossible to continue with the previously described data-collection system for such extended periods of time, a simple frequency count by direct care staff served as the data-collection system during this generalization period. A decrease in both pica and mouthing behaviors were reported on the unit.

FOLLOW-UP

Following discharge from the hospital, Pete returned to the facility where he had previously been institutionalized. In anticipation of this move, staff from that institution were invited for training on our inpatient unit. Here they were observed and trained in the implementation of the combination treatment (aromatic ammonia and DRI) since this proved to be the most effective strategy for reducing the client's pica and mouthing behaviors. However, despite the initial agreement to continue implementation of our recommended procedures, institutional administrators then recanted. They were concerned with the client's history of nosebleeds and aromatic ammonia as a potential irritant.

Follow-up data in form of institutionalized records indicated that the behaviors returned to baseline levels following discontinuation of aromatic ammonia and DRI: 1,514 episodes of pica in the first 13 days, 6,228 episides of mouthing in the same period. Institution staff reported that after 5 days, an overcorrection procedure, similar to the one that had been previously implemented (and which had not prevented Pete's hospitalization), was reinstituted. Subsequently, the behaviors were reported to have "dropped dramatically." However, soon after the implementation of overcorrection, the client experienced severe nosebleeding and all programming was discontinued. Mechanical wrist restraints were applied, although these were not totally effective in preventing the behaviors. At 5-month follow-up, restraints were still being implemented, and the rates of the target behaviors were reported to be as high as 624 pica and 616 mouthing incidences per month.

OVERALL EVALUATION

The results of the present study demonstrate the effective control of longtime and high-rate behavior problems with behavior therapy procedures. Both the application of the aversive aromatic ammonia and the implementation of a dense reinforcement schedule resulted in dramatic decreases of pica in the first part of the study. It should be emphasized again that DRO conditions resulted in even lower rates of the behavior than aromatic ammonia, which is an unexpected finding. However, DRO also produced substantial increases in the untreated mouthing, as was made evident during phase 3 (see Figure 1) (a surprising finding that does not typify reinforcement techniques). It can be assumed, however, that this negative concurrent effect of DRO was idiosyncratic for our client and the specific behaviors involved. Mouthing appeared to increase with the ingestion of objects, owing to the client's difficulties swallowing.

We do not wish to suggest that negative side effects are a general feature of DRO procedures. The application of the aromatic ammonia resulted in low rates of pica and near suppression of the untreated mouthing, as demonstrated during phase 3. However, our results comparing DRO and ammonia programs have to be viewed with some caution since they were presumably flawed by multiple treatment interference. Nevertheless, passive avoidance of aromatic ammonia fumes was found to be an effective treatment component with positive behavioral side effects on mouthing behavior, while water mist did not suppress pica. However, complete suppression of pica was never lastingly achieved with ammonia alone. Therefore, a second evaluation was required to investigate whether ammonia effects could be enhanced by a combination with DRI. Such combination treatment was eventually found to be the most effective and most desirable for both pica and mouthing. Whether DRI was a better treatment addition to ammonia than DRO was not tested.

Unfortunately, the treatment package was discontinued by the institution staff after discharge of the client from our hospital. Such discontinuation produced unfortunate results for Pete, as was discussed earlier. Concerns by institution staff that the inhalation of ammonia would irritate his nasal cavity and produce nosebleeds appeared to be unfounded since Pete did not experience any nosebleeds or other medical complications during hospitalization. Proper precautions were taken at the hospital, which included periodic examinations of the client's nasal cavity throughout the study by a physician and a nurse practitioner. The client did experience an incident of nosebleeding *after* he returned to the original institutional setting after implementation of the overcorrection procedure (contingent toothbrushing with a tootbrush dipped in Listerine). There was no indication that this incident was related to the ammonia program. Neither a review of the literature nor consultation at an ear-nose-throat clinic obtained prior to the initiation of ammonia treatment produced any data associating inhalation of aromatic ammonia with nosebleeds. Yet it is still strongly recommended, of course, that medical precautions be taken to ensure the client's safety during the use of aromatic ammonia.[1]

A few words should be added concerning the evaluation design. As was mentioned several times earlier, this study was partly troubled by multiple treatment interference, which may be a general problem with alternating treatments designs. In phases 2 and 5, pica was decreased under all three conditions, including the no-treatment condition. One way to test for multiple treatment interference is to include a no-treatment condition during the alternating treatments phase, as demonstrated in this study. A change in the behavior during the no-treatment component relative to baseline should alert the researcher. It suggests that multiple treatment interference might affect the treatment conditions too. In this particular case it is unclear which of the treatments, if not both, had caused multiple treatment interference. The attempt to control for multiple treatment interference was not successful. Daily alternation of treatments during phase 3 still showed low rates of pica behavior for both treatments, which still did not answer our questions. Owing to the discontinuation of the no-treatment condition during the third phase, it remains ambiguous as to which treatment (or if indeed both treatments) caused multiple treatment interference. The lack of the client's ability to discriminate between the contingencies operating during each condition appears to be partially responsible for the multiple treatment interference in this study. There was not enough time to test this any further, however, because clinically more important questions had to be addressed. Clarification of the contingencies was attempted through the use of cues, as described in the section on course of treatment. However, Pete's low level of functioning may have been responsible for the lack of discrimination.

REFERENCES

American Psychiatric Association. (1980). *Diagnostic and statistical manual of mental disorders* (3rd ed.). Washington, DC: Author.

Bucher, B., Reykdal, B., & Albin, J. (1976). Brief restraint to control pica in retarded children. *Journal of Behavior Therapy and Experimental Psychiatry, 7,* 137–140.

Danford, D. E., & Huber, A. M. (1982). Pica among mentally retarded adults. *American Journal of Mental Deficiency, 87,* 141–146.

---

[1] In a treatment of a different case with ammonia capsules, first-degree skin burns were observed under the client's nose, which led to the termination of the ammonia program. It has to be noted, however, that with this latter client, ammonia had to be administered at very high rates, that *new* capsules were crushed each time, that the capsules were not kept in a test tube, and—most important—that the irritation was caused by incidental contact of the crushed capsule with the client's skin.

Lofts, R. (1986). The effect of zinc on pica in a mentally retarded female [Summary]. *Proceedings of the 19th Annual Gatlinburg Conference on Research and Theory in Mental Retardation and Developmental Disabilities*, p. 32.

McAlpine, C., & Singh, N. N. (1986). Pica in institutionalized mentally retarded persons. *Journal of Mental Deficiency Research, 30*, 171–178.

Rojahn, J. (1986). Self-injurious and stereotypic behavior of noninstitutionalized mentally retarded people: Prevalence and classification. *American Journal of Mental Deficiency, 91*, 268–276.

Rojahn, J., McGonigle, J. J., Curcio, C., & Dixon, J. (1987). Suppression of pica by water mist and aromatic ammonia. A comparative analysis. *Behavior Modification, 11*, 65–74.

Singh, N. N., & Bakker, L. W. (1984). Suppression of pica by overcorrection and physical restraint: A comparative analysis. *Journal of Autism and Developmental Disorders, 14*, 331–341.

CHAPTER 23

Rumination

LORI A. SISSON, BRENDA S. EGAN, and
VINCENT B. VAN HASSELT

DESCRIPTION OF THE DISORDER

Rumination is a behavior consisting of the regurgitation of previously consumed food without nausea or retching. This food is then reswallowed or ejected from the mouth. The incidence of this disorder in the general population is unknown since it often is confused with food allergies. Although rumination is thought to be relatively rare in normal developing children, it is not uncommon among severely mentally retarded persons (Rast, Johnston, Drum, & Conrin, 1981).

Serious medical problems may ensue if this behavior is not controlled. Major difficulties are malnutrition, electrolytic imbalance, dehydration, aspiration, pneumonia, and lowered resistance to disease. These consequences are sometimes life-threatening. Indeed, the mortality rate attributed to chronic rumination ranges from 12 to 20% (Rast *et al.*, 1981). Ruminative vomiting may have an additional negative social impact since it detracts from the individual's appearance and approachability. Hence, opportunities for positive social interaction and learning may be decreased.

The etiology of rumination has yet to be clearly ascertained. Thus,

LORI A. SISSON • Department of Psychiatry, Western Pennsylvania Institute and Clinic, University of Pittsburgh School of Medicine, 3811 O'Hara Street, Pittsburgh, Pennsylvania 15213.   BRENDA S. EGAN • Western Pennsylvania School for Blind Children, Bayard Street at Bellefield Avenue, Pittsburgh, Pennsylvania 15213.   VINCENT B. VAN HASSELT • Department of Psychiatry and Human Behavior, University of California Irvine Medical Center, 101 City Drive South, Orange, California 92268.

treatment procedures applied to remediate the disorder are diverse. Early interventions frequently were based on medical or psychodynamic models. These included surgery, drugs, mechanical devices (e.g., chin straps, esophagus blocks), thickened feedings, and very high levels of maternal attention. The primary shortcoming of these strategies was that even when they were successful, cessation of rumination generally was slow (Sajwaj, Libet, & Agras, 1974).

More recent treatment programs are based on two observations that suggest that this condition may be under environmental control. First, there is an apparent lack of organic pathology. Individuals referred for psychological remediation of rumination usually have undergone an extensive medical workup to rule out physical causation. Typically, no physical bases for the disorder are found. Second, children and adults who exhibit chronic rumination have been found to engage in a sequence of intentional behaviors that induce the response. For example, these persons may strain vigorously to bring food back into their mouths. Several behavioral strategies for eliminating rumination have been reported to be both effective and fast-acting. One intervention involves controlling antecedent stimulus conditions, as in altering food texture and quantity (Rast *et al.*, 1981). Alternatively, differential reinforcement of other behavior combined with ignoring ruminative responding has been investigated (Mulick, Schroeder, & Rojahn, 1980). Finally, punishment with overcorrection (Duker & Seys, 1977), a bitter-tasting substance (Sajwaj *et al.*, 1974), or electric shock (Toister, Condron, Worley, & Arthur, 1975) has produced positive results.

CASE IDENTIFICATION

Amanda was a 10-year-old black female who suffered from multiple severe handicaps as a result of subarachnoid hemorrhage incurred at 7 weeks of age. She was the product of a full-term pregnancy and an uncomplicated delivery. Amanda showed no evidence of mental retardation or physical disorder following birth or during the first 7 weeks of life. However, at 7 weeks she was admitted to the hospital unconscious and with multiple bruises. Child abuse was suspected. Subsequent to this event, Amanda failed to develop normally in all areas (e.g., motor control, social responsiveness, language acquisition).

Amanda attended a residential school for blind children for 6 years prior to initiation of this intervention. She resided at the school during the week and visited her home on weekends and holidays. Her classroom included five additional multihandicapped peers ages 8 to 13 ($\overline{X} = 11.0$).

One teacher (the second author) and two classroom aides carried out individual and group instruction in self-help, communication/social, and preacademic areas.

At the time of referral, Amanda was diagnosed as profoundly mentally retarded on the basis of performance on educational and psychological tests and observation of adaptive behavior. She also was visually impaired, secondary to optic atrophy. Further, Amanda had cerebral palsy and a seizure disorder. Major motor seizures were controlled by Phenobarbital, although she continued to exhibit brief periods of staring and to drop objects, both of which were thought to be seizure-related.

Anecdotal observations revealed that Amanda was completely dependent on others for care. She did not feed, dress, or toilet herself independently and showed no expressive or receptive communication. Her response to visual stimuli, such as light, was inconsistent. Mobility was impaired, although Amanda recently had learned to walk with minimal adult assistance (i.e., light physical prompts). In addition to self-care and learning deficits, Amanda exhibited numerous maladaptive behaviors, including self-stimulation (head weaving, tooth tapping), self-abuse (self-biting, self-scratching, hair pulling), and aggression (scratching, pinching). However, the problem of greatest concern was chronic rumination.

PRESENTING COMPLAINTS

Amanda's classroom teacher requested consultation in behavioral assessment, treatment planning, and staff training to eliminate the child's chronic rumination. Rumination occurred almost continuously, and vomitus frequently was expelled onto clothing, objects in the classroom, and the floor, causing staff and peers to avoid interaction with Amanda. The high rate of this behavior was the impetus for increased concern by the mother, teacher, and school medical staff regarding the health of the child. In addition, Amanda's rumination was a health hazard to the staff members and children with whom she came into contact. Despite consistent efforts on the part of classroom staff to monitor and clean up after rumination, vomitus was sometimes found on classroom materials and furniture used by others. In particular, there was heightened concern about the spread of communicable diseases, such as colds and flu, from contact with regurgitated material.

HISTORY

Rumination had been a problem for approximately 3 years. Amanda was significantly below height and weight norms for children her age. She was 48 inches tall and weighed 46 pounds, which placed her below the fifth percentile for both height and weight, according to the National Center for Health Statistics norms. However, this must be attributed in part to the fact that numerous other medical, physical, and behavior problems interfered with normal eating patterns and growth. Previous attempts on the part of classroom teachers and aides to reduce rumination had met with minimal success. These efforts included differential reinforcement of other behavior (DRO) and restitutional overcorrection.

DRO procedures involved the presentation of social attention (verbal praise and light stroking of arms and face) when rumination was not occurring. Also, staff members turned and/or walked away whenever rumination was observed. Necessary clean-up of rugurgitated material was carried out as matter-of-factly as possible. However, DRO alone failed to have a significant impact on the duration or rate of rumination. In fact, rumination was so frequent, particularly during postmealtime periods, that there were few opportunities to apply positive consequences. Further, Amanda showed little interest in the presence or absence of the adult who administered positive reinforcement. She generally appeared content to sit alone and engage in ruminative and/or stereotypic self-stimulatory behaviors.

Next, DRO was paired with restitutional overcorrection. In this procedure, whenever food and/or saliva was ejected from Amanda's mouth, a staff member provided her with a bucket and a scrub brush, placed her on her hands and knees, and manually guided her through scrubbing motions for 20 minutes. This was an extremely laborious procedure since Amanda was unable to complete the motions independently. She also struggled with the adult continuously throughout the 20-minute clean-up period. Further, although this treatment had been applied for approximately 1 year, ruminative vomiting continued to occur at significantly high rates. Initial assessment indicated that overcorrection was applied as frequently as six times per day. That is, Amanda was manually guided through scrubbing exercises for as long as 2 hours. Staff members were vocal about their dislike of this treatment approach and would sometimes ignore the targeted behavior to avoid carrying out the time-consuming overcorrection procedure. On other occasions, they were involved in the treatment or care of remaining students in the classroom and were unable to interrupt these activities to engage in the lengthy clean-up procedure with Amanda.

Another problem was that Amanda's mother failed to carry out overcorrection when the child was at home. Therefore, ruminative vomiting recurred at pretreatment levels following weekends, illnesses, or vacations. Further, treatment was administered only as the consequence of expulsion of regurgitated food from the mouth. Other ruminative responses, such as chewing regurgitated food and swishing it around in the mouth were not targeted. Thus, decreases in rumination *per se* were modest at best.

ASSESSMENT

The first step in the assessment of ruminative responding was to determine baseline (pretreatment) levels of occurrence. This allowed comparison with rates achieved under subsequent intervention conditions so that treatment efficacy could be determined empirically. Baseline assessment of the target response involved three steps: (a) defining the behavior, (b) developing and employing observation procedures, and (c) evaluating the data obtained.

Response Definition

Rumination was defined as any regurgitation, chewing, swishing, reswallowing, or expelling previously consumed food. Each aspect of the rumination response was easily detected since it was accompanied by characteristic throat, tongue, and/or mouth movements. For example, regurgitation involved a sequence of behaviors that began with tongue thrusting and jaw protrusion, often proceeded to choking, and terminated with lip smacking as food was brought into the mouth. Chewing and swishing were up-and-down and side-to-side jaw movements. Reswallowing could be identified by expansion of the throat and neck. Finally, expelling food included any food or liquid dripping from Amanda's mouth or forcefully projected from her mouth as in spitting.

Observation Procedures

Three 32-minute samples of Amanda's behavior were obtained each day. These samples directly followed meals and snacks and began at 9:00 a.m., 10:00 a.m., and 12:30 p.m. These periods were selected in light of staff reports that rumination was most frequent at these times. During these periods, Amanda was involved in self-care activities, including toileting, teeth brushing, and hand and face washing.

Direct behavioral observations were carried out by trained raters stationed within the classroom. Experimental assistants served as raters.

Use of independent observers offered several advantages: (a) the teacher and aides were freed of time-consuming data-collection activities and were able to attend to the needs of other students; (b) raters were able to objectively record the target behavior since they had little investment in treatment outcome (i.e., therapist bias was eliminated); and (c) a sensitive and reliable measure of rumination was obtained via interval recording techniques (described below). Rater training consisted of instructions in use of recording procedures and several hours of direct observations. Obtrusiveness of raters in the classroom was minimized by a number of adaptation sessions prior to formal baseline assessment. These adaptation sessions also were used for rater training.

A 10-second noncontinuous partial-interval recording system was employed to monitor rumination. To facilitate recording, raters wore earphones connected to a cassette tape player. An audiotape had been prepared to assist in behavioral observations. Observation intervals had been timed and recorded onto the audiotape by voice. A verbal cue signaled raters to observe the child for 10 seconds. During this observation interval, raters watched the child for occurrences of rumination. Following this observation interval, a second cue signaled a recording interval of 5 seconds' duration. At this time, raters recorded whether rumination had occurred onto specially prepared data sheets. Rumination was scored as occurring if it was seen during any part of the 10-second observation interval. This sequence of observation and recording intervals was repeated for the entire 32-minute period. Thus, for each session, there were 128 opportunities to record the target behavior. Data were expressed in terms of percentage of intervals in which rumination was scored.

Generally, one rater observed Amanda. A second rater independently recorded behaviors periodically across baseline and treatment sessions. The extent to which the two raters agreed on the occurrence of the target behavior was calculated by dividing the number of behaviors recorded in agreement by that number plus the number recorded in disagreement, then multiplying by 100. Only intervals in which at least one rater recorded the behavior were used in the analysis. Agreement was reached when both observers marked the child as emitting the target behavior within the same interval. This measure of *percentage occurrence agreement* provides an index of the reliability of the observation system. Percentage occurrence agreement in this case always exceeded 80%.

Evaluating Baseline Data

Baseline data were collected during 9:00 a.m., 10:00 a.m., and 12:30 p.m. periods for 10 days. As illustrated in Figure 1, these data indicated

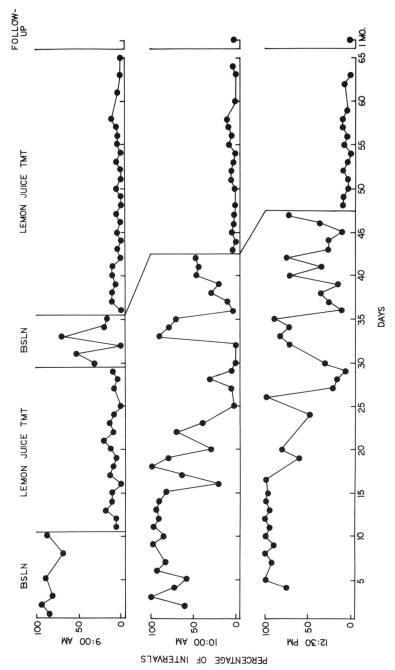

Figure 1. Percentage of intervals in which rumination was observed across baseline and lemon juice treatment phases, during three 32-minute time periods beginning at 9:00 a.m., 10:00 a.m., and 12:30 p.m.

that Amanda engaged in a very high and stable level of ruminative responding during baseline. Mean percentage of intervals in which rumination occurred was 93% during the 9:00 a.m. observation period, 82% during the 10:00 a.m. period, and 96% during the 12:30 p.m. period. These findings underscored the need for immediate intervention.

SELECTION OF TREATMENT

There were several considerations that guided the selection of a treatment program to reduce rumination in this case. These included ethical issues, potential treatment efficacy, and the acceptability of the intervention to care providers.

Ethical Issues

Ethical guidelines dictate that the *least restrictive* but effective intervention must be utilized in the treatment of maladaptive behavior. This is usually interpreted to mean that positive approaches to behavior change are attempted first. Only when these strategies have proven ineffective should punitive procedures be employed. When aversive methods are considered, there must be clear substantiation of their utility with similar problems. Further, those techniques that are least aversive should be attempted first. In Amanda's case, a positive approach (DRO) alone already was shown to have little impact on rumination. Overcorrection, generally considered a less aversive method than other punitive interventions (e.g., contingently administered bitter-tasting substances, electric shock), also was found to have limited effect on the target behavior. Consequently, a more aversive treatment approach was indicated.

Contingent presentation of a bitter-tasting substance (lemon juice) was chosen for treatment of ruminative behaviors. This approach seemed particularly applicable since it involved applying an aversive gustatory stimulus for a gustatory response. Lemon juice has been employed with infants who ruminated (Sajwaj *et al.*, 1974) and was considered to be milder than other bitter substances, such as tabasco sauce or a commercially available substance used to control nail biting. Prior to initiation of treatment, approval for use of an aversive treatment technique was obtained. This involved meetings of a Human Rights Committee, including the child's mother, her teacher, the school physician, a psychologist, school administration personnel, and members of the community, to discuss the program and its possible contraindications. Lemon juice treatment was begun only when all members of this committee agreed to its implementation. Approval of this program was conditional upon close monitoring of the target response so that treatment effectiveness could be ascertained on a continual basis. This would guard against the unnecessary extended use of an aversive treatment in the event that it was ineffective in reducing rumination.

Treatment Efficacy

As described above, the selection of lemon juice treatment was based on ethical guidelines to use the least restrictive procedure as well as reports of successful application of this intervention with other children exhibiting rumination. There is a consensus that when punishment techniques are used to reduce maladaptive behaviors, positive reinforcement programs promoting adaptive, alternative responding should be utilized concurrently. Thus, previously employed DRO procedures were combined with lemon juice treatment in the present intervention.

Since reinforcement of appropriate behavior was considered requisite to behavior change, identification of effective positive reinforcers was of considerable import. Casual observation indicated that Amanda was uninterested in the adult attention used in prior DRO administrations. Potential reinforcers are identified quite readily for some individuals by simply asking them what they prefer, or by exposing them to an array of stimuli and recording the duration or frequency of interaction with each stimulus item. In contrast, for many severely impaired individuals, such as Amanda, who are nonverbal, do not engage in spontaneous play, and have limited sensory and motor capabilities, identification of reinforcing stimuli is problematic.

To identify stimuli with potential reinforcement value for Amanda, a variety of items and events were presented and her response to them was monitored. These were edible (e.g., cracker, M&M, juice), tactual (e.g., vibrator, fan), visual (e.g., light), auditory (e.g., music), and social (e.g., tickle, hug) stimuli. Items and events to which Amanda responded with smiles or vocalizations, or by orientating or reaching, were noted and later used in DRO contingencies. These stimuli included gentle touch to her face and neck, the breeze from a fan, and a basin of water in which she could play.

Treatment Acceptability

In addition to requesting an effective treatment for rumination, Amanda's teacher desired an intervention that could be carried out within the constraints of the classroom situation. Although the staff-to-student ratio was adequate (minimum: 2:5) and staff were enthusiastic about educational and behavioral programming for class members, the nature of the (multiple) disabilities of the students required that each child receive frequent and intensive attention from the teacher and aides. Thus, it was unrealistic to expect the target child to receive consistent and continuous one-to-one attention over long periods of the day on an extended basis.

Further, the child care, teaching, and behavior management responsibilities of classroom staff were quite demanding. These individuals spent much of their day concentrating on self-care activities, conducting individualized instruction, and maintaining control of aggressive and disruptive behaviors exhibited by children in the class. The slow progress and severe behavioral disturbances of multihandicapped students taxed staff members' patience and physical endurance. In designing a treatment program for Amanda's rumination, it was important to avoid unnecessary physical and emotional demands on classroom personnel.

It was felt that the acceptability of the intervention by staff would be important to ensure its consistent administration. In this case, treatment acceptability was predicted to be directly related to time required by the program and its ease of application. These two factors would be even more important during late afternoon and evening hours when lower staff-to-student ratios and fewer structured activities would make systematic implementation of treatment even more difficult. The failure of overcorrection to satisfy these requirements might have contributed to its inconsistent use and, therefore, to its poor results. Contingent lemon juice treatment was considered to be relatively quick and easy to administer.

COURSE OF TREATMENT

Since lemon juice treatment is viewed as an intrusive procedure, it was felt that treatment should be carefully applied and evaluated in as controlled a situation as possible. Once the utility of the strategy was ascertained, recommendations regarding application of treatment throughout the day could be made. Thus, rumination initially was treated during one 32-minute period each day (beginning at 9:00 a.m.). This period was chosen to correspond to one of the times data were obtained by behavioral raters. During this session, Amanda received one-to-one attention from a staff member so that the intervention could be carried out consistently. Whenever Amanda engaged in rumination, she was told "No!", her hands were held at her sides to avoid interference with treatment, and 5 cc of lemon juice (Realemon brand reconstituted lemon juice) were injected into her mouth using a plastic syringe. This procedure was carried out without additional comments or conversation. When Amanda was not ruminating, she was provided with one of the previously identified positive reinforcers (stroking, fan, or water basin). Assessment procedures, described previously, continued in this period as well as at 10:00 a.m. and 12:30 p.m.

Figure 1 shows the effects of lemon juice treatment on the percentage of intervals in which rumination was observed across baseline and treatment phases during the three daily assessment sessions. It is clear from this figure that lemon juice treatment had a marked effect on rumination when it was applied during the 9:00 a.m. period. At this time, rumination was immediately reduced to near-zero levels ($\overline{X}$ = 6%). Interestingly, treatment effects appeared to generalize to the other periods, with gradual but variable declines noticed during 10:00 a.m. and 12:30 p.m. sessions, even though treatment was not applied at these times.

In order to rule out the possibility that some other uncontrolled variable could account for the change in level of rumination, treatment was briefly withdrawn (days 30–35). This was particularly important given that small but positive changes were seen in the level of the target response during periods in which no treatment was carried out. Levels of rumination increased to a mean of 23% upon return to baseline. Reinstitution of treatment decreased rumination again, thus replicating earlier effects. The controlling effects of lemon juice treatment were demonstrated using the withdrawal single-case design during the 9:00 a.m. session.

Once level of rumination was reduced during the 9:00 a.m. period, lemon juice treatment was introduced in the 10:00 a.m. period (day 43). Percentage of intervals of rumination was quickly reduced during that session. Next, lemon juice treatment was initiated in the 12:30 p.m. period (day 47). Again, lemon juice treatment suppressed ruminative responding. Sequential application of treatment across these three sessions showed that significant behavior change occurred when, and only when, lemon juice treatment was implemented. This documented the controlling effects of treatment within a multiple-baseline design across time periods.

At this point, it was clear that lemon juice treatment was responsible for clinically significant reductions in the amount of time Amanda spent ruminating. Anecdotal observations indicated that treatment was easily applied and accepted by staff. Although Amanda struggled to avoid the injection of lemon juice into her mouth, holding her arms to her sides was sufficient to allow this brief treatment to be carried out. Also, as rumination decreased, staff interacted with Amanda and delivered reinforcing activities more frequently. Since few injections of lemon juice were required, staff were able to direct increased attention to the needs of other children in the classroom, rather than to Amanda exclusively.

TERMINATION

Following evaluation of treatment effectiveness in these three periods, lemon juice treatment was applied throughout the day. Anecdotal reports from classroom staff revealed that gains were noted during all other class periods. Amanda's program was continued successfully for 1 month under the direct supervision of the classroom teacher, with periodic consultation from the behavior therapist.

FOLLOW-UP

One month following termination of data-collection procedures, behavioral raters returned to Amanda's classroom to obtain a follow-up probe. Data-collection procedures were carried out as before. Data were obtained in two of the three daily sessions (10:00 a.m. and 12:30 p.m.). During this follow-up probe, Amanda showed no rumination responses at all. Staff commented that although materials required by treatment were continually available in the classroom, lemon juice treatment was rarely required.

OVERALL EVALUATION

Amanda's rumination dropped from nearly 100% of the time to near-zero levels as a function of the lemon juice treatment. Feedback from classroom staff indicated that they were quite pleased with the results of the treatment program. In particular, they were less frustrated with Amanda once rumination was suppressed with a treatment that was not only effective but also easy to apply. However, rumination was only one of many maladaptive responses exhibited by this child. Amanda continued to display other self-stimulatory, self-abusive, and aggressive behaviors that were not specifically targeted with the current intervention. Because of these problems, she was referred for inpatient psychiatric hospitalization for evaluation and treatment. During this 3-month hospitalization and in subsequent months at the school, Amanda continued to show low levels of rumination. Such was the case despite the fact that lemon juice treatment was suspended during hospitalization and was not resumed following Amanda's return to the school.

ACKNOWLEDGMENTS

Preparation of this manuscript was facilitated by a grant from The Buhl Foundation. The authors wish to thank Judith A. Lorenzetty, Carole McCracken, Louise E. Moore, and staff of the Western Pennsylvania School for Blind Children for their varied contributions.

REFERENCES

Duker, P. C., & Seys, D. M. (1977). Elimination of vomiting in a retarded female using restitutional overcorrection. *Behavior Therapy, 8,* 255–257.

Mulick, J. A., Schroeder, S. R., & Rojahn, J. (1980). Chronic ruminative vomiting: A comparison of four treatment procedures. *Journal of Autism and Developmental Disorders, 10,* 203–213.

Rast, J., Johnston, J. M., Drum, C., & Conrin, J. (1981). The relation of food quantity to rumination behavior. *Journal of Applied Behavior Analysis, 14,* 121–130.

Sajwaj, T., Libet, J., & Agras, S. (1974). Lemon juice therapy: The control of life threatening rumination in a six month old infant. *Journal of Applied Behavior Analysis, 7,* 557–563.

Toister, R. P., Condron, C. J., Worley, L., & Arthur, D. (1975). Faradic therapy of chronic vomiting in infancy: A case study. *Journal of Behavior Therapy and Experimental Psychiatry, 6,* 55–59.

CHAPTER 24

Obesity

ALLEN C. ISRAEL and LAUREN C. SOLOTAR

DESCRIPTION OF THE DISORDER

The problem of overweight in the adult population is one of longstanding and serious professional concern and has become a national obsession. In contrast, the problem of obesity in children has, until recently, received relatively little attention. Difficulty in treating adults and the persistence of the problem, recognition of family patterns of obesity, alarm over an increasing percentage of overweight and a decreasing percentage of physically fit youngsters, and greater attention to problems of children in general have contributed to increased awareness of childhood obesity as a problem.

Childhood obesity is most frequently defined as a weight above the 20th percentile for height, age, and gender. This is, of course, a measure of relative weight and not body fat, which would need to be assessed by other means. However, weight for height represents, except in rare cases, a reasonable index of obesity in children. Childhood obesity not only is associated with immediate medical concerns such as hypertension and diabetes but also, because of the likely persistence of obesity into adulthood, offers an arena for the potential prevention of medical disorders associated with adult obesity. The clinician working with the obese child needs also to be sensitive to the potential social and psychological difficulties that these children are likely to experience. Stigmatization associated with obesity, as well as restrictions in physical activities, puts

ALLEN C. ISRAEL and LAUREN C. SOLOTAR • Department of Psychology, State University of New York, 1400 Washington Avenue, Albany, New York 12222.

the child at risk for peer-related difficulties. These and other factors also increase the risk of other psychological problems (Israel & Shapiro, 1985).

This suggests that in working with the obese child the clinician is faced with a complex task. Clearly, attention must be given to the modification of energy intake and expenditure behaviors. However, with the clear indication that the problem is multifaceted in its etiological and maintaining variables and varied in its consequences to the child, it is likely that the clinician will need to attend to a variety of familial and social variables. The recognition that, for example, parental control of food intake was central resulted in early attention to viewing the problem as broader than the child's behavior and weight. Thus, this area of behavior change has from the start been sensitive to variables beyond the individual. The challenge remains for the clinician, however, to design interventions appropriate to the individual child.

CASE IDENTIFICATION

The hypothetical, yet representative, case that will be discussed in this chapter involves Sean C., a 10-year-old white male who resides with his parents and two siblings. Sean is in the fifth grade and is of average intelligence. He is from a middle-class family; his father is a state employee and his mother is a secretary.

At our first contact with Sean, he was 57.25 inches tall, weighed 127.75 pounds, and was 50.19% overweight. Although only one parent is required to attend treatment, we request that both parents of two-parent families attend the initial evaluation. Sean's father was of normal weight status (6.58% overweight), whereas Sean's mother was overweight (40.53% overweight). Neither of Sean's siblings was overweight, thus making Sean the only overweight child in his family. This was immediately noted since prior research (Israel, Silverman, & Solotar, 1986) has revealed that in comparison with only children and children with one or more overweight siblings, children whose siblings are not overweight are least successful in their weight-loss efforts. Difficulties in being the only overweight child were addressed in treatment.

PRESENTING COMPLAINTS

Overweight is almost always identified by families as the presenting complaint. However, a comprehensive evaluation usually reveals that this is a multifaceted problem. During the initial evaluation, families are first seen together as a unit and then the parents and the target child are seen individually. In the present case, both Sean and his parents identified Sean's overweight status as the primary problem, reporting that Sean snacked frequently and ate an unusually large amount of high-calorie food. Mr. and Mrs. C. reported that Sean frequently "sneaked" food out of the kitchen and spent most of his weekly allowance on snack foods. Mrs. C. reported that she often found candy wrappers in Sean's room and stuffed into his clothes pockets. She believed that the majority of Sean's eating occurred after school when both she and her husband were at work. Sean's restricted physical activity was also noted. Both parents reported that as Sean gained weight, his physical activity had substantially decreased. Currently, Sean's physical activity was limited to gym class at school, and most of Sean's leisure time was spent watching television. Both also voiced concerns about Sean's medical condition, stating that they noticed Sean would lose his breath after walking up a flight of stairs. Sean's mother was also concerned about the possibility of future health problems. Mr. and Mrs. C. further stated that they were having more and more difficulty finding clothes for Sean and were disturbed about Sean's appearance.

Sean's parents were concerned about damage to his self-esteem caused by his weight and the teasing to which he was subjected. They reported that Sean had no close friends and was somewhat of a loner. Sean reported that he frequently was teased about his weight both at school and at home. He reported that his siblings often called him such names as "fatso" and "pig." Sean stated that he was content with his peer relationships, although he occasionally felt left out of games and activities at school.

An important concern raised by Sean's parents was his ambivalence about losing weight. They reported that although he agreed to attend the program, he seemed to care little about his appearance and weight problem. Sean's ambivalence was obvious during our initial meeting. Sean reported that his family constantly "nagged" him about his weight, especially his father, who frequently yelled when Sean was caught snacking.

A final problem, not presented by the family, but noted by the interviewer, was the likelihood of some familial sabotage. Mr. C. stated at the onset of the interview that he was a gourmet cook and that it would be very difficult to make any changes in his food preparations. In addition, Sean frequently visited his grandmother, who lived near the family. The grandmother took great pleasure in providing food and snacks for Sean.

HISTORY

Sean's medical records, obtained from his pediatrician along with approval for program participation, revealed consistent greater-than-expected weight gains over the past 7 years, with extreme increases in the past 3 years. Questioning regarding previous weight-loss attempts revealed two unsuccessful attempts for Sean that were initiated by his parents. Mr. and Mrs. C. reported that on both occasions they promised Sean a new bicycle if he lost 25 pounds. They stated that on both occasions Sean was able to control his intake for approximately 1 week and then seemed to lose interest. Mr. C. reported that he became very angry with Sean when he "gave up" and began punishing Sean whenever he caught him snacking.

Mrs. C.'s weight history revealed that she was always slightly overweight but had gained a significant amount of weight over the last 10 to 15 years. She reported frequent, but unsuccessful, weight-loss attempts, including "fad" and "starvation" diets and enrolling in a commercial weight-loss program. Mr. C., in contrast, reported never having a weight problem and always being physically fit.

In addition to the above information, the role of food and eating in the family was also assessed. If this issue were not addressed, it might impede the child's progress in the program. Much of this family's life and daily activities revolved around food. Food was used as a reward, and of even greater significance was the fact that Mr. C was a gourmet cook. Consequently, the family often ate high-calorie, high-fat meals, and such meals were "family times." Initially this proved difficult to modify, although by the end of treatment Mr. C. initiated many changes in his food preparations.

ASSESSMENT

Like the problem of childhood obesity itself, the task of assessment faced by the clinician is a multifaceted one. Weight/obesity itself must, of course, be assessed. In addition, the problematic behaviors that are assumed to contribute to the maintenance of the weight problem must be measured and evaluated. Such an assessment needs to include not only the child but other family members as well. The approach to treatment also requires that the child's environment be assessed regarding cues associated with food intake and/or energy expenditure. Finally, since it is assumed that the problem of childhood obesity may bring with it difficulties in the social/psychological realm, these too need to be evaluated.

Weight-Related Measures

Since children are in a period of expected growth, the standard against which degree of overweight is judged is a changing one. Thus, a relative measure, such as percent overweight, rather than an absolute one is required. From available norms the percentile of the child's height for gender and age is determined. The child's ideal weight is then presumed to be at this same percentile, and percent overweight equals (actual weight − ideal weight)/ideal weight. While this is the principal measure that will be employed, it would be advantageous for the clinician to obtain a number of other measures. Most investigators in the field obtain measures of skinfold thickness employing special calipers. Measurements are often taken at multiple sites (triceps, biceps, subscapular). If such calipers and the necessary training are available, such measurement may be helpful. More readily available is the measurement of body circumferance at a variety of sites (chest, waist, hips, thighs). These provide an additional index beyond weight change or weight-related change. Finally, it should not be ignored that the *perception* of degree of obesity is often central in the initial decision to seek treatment. Many of the potential psychological and social difficulties experienced by the obese child are related to these perceptions. Thus, the child's perception, and that of others, of the degree of overweight should be obtained.

Weight-Related Behaviors and Cues

Assessment of weight-related behaviors and of environmental cues that may effect food intake and/or energy expenditure are central to behavioral interventions for childhood obesity. Much of this assessment is based upon monitoring required of the child and family. Such monitoring provides an ongoing assessment to guide the therapist in shaping the intervention, but it also provides the family with a mechanism for organizing and observing treatment-related behavior. This dual function of these tasks and their importance should be stressed with the families.

Central to the treatment effort is monitoring of food intake and energy expenditure. The former has been more fully recognized and developed. Prior to beginning treatment, families are required to keep structured food-intake diaries of all food intake for a 2-week period. The kind of food, the amount, and the number of calories for each meal or snack is recorded. Activity is recorded in a similar fashion in an activity book. Daily activity records are broken down into four time periods during weekdays (before school, during school, after school, and after dinner) and three time periods on weekends (morning, afternoon, and evening). Any active behavior is recorded by indicating the behavior (e.g., biking, walking) and the number of minutes of this activity. In a similar fashion all TV watching is recorded.

Regular monitoring of intake and activity continue throughout treatment. In addition to guiding calorie limits, these intake records are used to conduct nutritional analyses aimed at educating families and ensuring adequate nutritional practices. Intake records are also employed at various stages to assess cues that may be associated with food intake. At various times, families are asked to record, along with actual food intake, information concerning a variety of related cues (e.g., place where eating occurs; associated activities, such as TV watching, degree of hunger, and mood). These can then be employed to help the families assess eating patterns and also provide evaluations of interventions aimed at changing such patterns.

Families also keep daily habit records on which they record whether or not they completed prescribed program assignments for the child (e.g., completing food intake record, staying below calorie limit, following activity program, doing nothing else while eating). Parallel habit records are completed by the parents. These include behavior change prescriptions required of the parents (e.g., helping child fill out intake record, praising child's appropriate behavior, keeping high-calorie foods out of sight). These records allow evaluation of the family's adherence to prescribed assignments and also serve as the basis for reward contracts negotiated by the family.

Social/Psychological Functioning

While the major thrust of this section is, by necessity, descriptive of the assessment of weight and weight-related behavior and cues, it is also important to assess social/psychological functioning. As indicated above, this often contributes to the family's decision to seek treatment. Use of standard assessment instruments for evaluating the child's psychological adjustment, such as Achenbach's Child Behavior Checklist (CBCL), are recommended. Comparisons with available norms and findings in the childhood obesity literature are thereby available. Assessment of peer functioning is another important domain. Here, standardized instruments are less available and some combination of interview and written input needs to be employed. Other constructs that are likely to be of interest are self-control (e.g., Kendall's Behavior Rating Scale for Children), self-concept (e.g., Harter's "What Am I Like" or the Piers-Harris), and knowledge of parenting skills (e.g., the O'Dell *et al.* "Knowledge of Behavioral Principles Applied to Children"). Evaluations of these and other dimensions can provide the clinician with important information in individualizing treatment plans and anticipating associated concerns. For example, Sean's CBCL profile indicated behavior problems exceeding norms, particularly on the Social Withdrawal subscale. This pattern is consistent with concerns expressed at intake and indicative of a pattern that may be characteristic of young overweight boys presenting for treatment. Whenever possible, multiple sources of input on any of the above areas of functioning (child, mother, father, siblings, teacher) should be sought.

SELECTION OF TREATMENT

Treatment of childhood obesity has usually been conducted in a group format. While this may have been, in part, a clinical and research convenience, our clinical impressions suggest that both parents and child benefit from such a strategy. Information and examples are then provided in a standardized format, with discussion and assignments allowing for individualization. Involvement, at some level, of all family members seems desirable. However, it is most frequently the case that one parent regularly attends. It seems important from the start to relay the information that change is not focused on the target child alone but rather on the family's intake/activity system. In the case of the attending parent, this is addressed as recognition that the parent will be asked to make changes in her/his behavior. To ensure such involvement in change, the parent is asked to select one of two roles—weight loss or helper—both of which have been shown to be successful (Israel, Stolmaker, Sharp, Silverman, & Simon, 1984). These then become the focus of the parent's behavior change effort. Weekly behavior change assignments and programming are built around either the parent's own weight-loss effort or systematic attention to that parent's role as a helper for the child. Thus, habit records, reward contracts, and similar aids, as described below for the child, are provided for the parent. The parent, along with the therapist, needs to give careful consideration to choice of role. Mrs. C. chose the helper role. Concern over her own inability to sustain a successful weight loss and the decision to make this something special—"just for Sean"—guided this decision.

With young children much of the responsibility for changing the child's behavior rests with the parent. Thus, an integral part of the treatment is assuring parenting skills that are sufficient to implement and sustain such a change effort (Israel, Stolmaker, & Andrian, 1985).

COURSE OF TREATMENT

Treatment consists of three phases—intensive, extended, and followup—spanning a 1½-year period. Families are seen in separate child and parent groups. The content of these sessions is similar, although the last half hour of each children's group is spent doing some physical activity.

Intensive Treatment

The first phase of treatment consists of a 2½-session general parent training module, an orientation session, and eight weekly 90-minute sessions. Phone calls are made between sessions to assist with the weekly homework assignments and with individual problems. It is during this phase of treatment that most of the program information is disseminated.

The parent training module is intended to give parents some brief training in parenting skills from a social learning perspective. In addition to some didactic material, parents practice several of the skills that will be employed later. At this point they focus on non-weight-related behaviors and need not focus on the target child. Parents are told that these presessions are to provide exposure to general parenting skills they will use in the program, but that they may indeed be helpful with other problems and other children. These sessions also begin to acquaint them with some of the terminology we will employ. This parenting information/orientation is also continued in all succeeding treatment sessions.

Initially, when weight-loss-related sessions begin, the philosophy of the program is reviewed. Families are informed that habit change, not dieting, is our primary focus and that children are expected to lose weight gradually. They are told that poor eating and exercise habits are a primary cause of obesity and that their children can gradually learn new habits that will enable them not only to lose weight but, more importantly, to maintain their weight loss. This philosophy is reinforced by the reward program. Rewards are based on following prescribed behavior changes. Reward contracts are reviewed each week to ensure that parents are focusing on habit change.

In the explanation of the philosophy to children, children are informed that they need not entirely give up their favorite foods and snacks (which usually provides some relief to them!). Rather, they are told that they will learn new ways of eating and being active so that they can continue to enjoy some of their favorite foods and still lose weight. For children who are ambivalent about the program, this is usually very helpful.

During the first eight sessions, families receive systematic training in behavioral skills for weight control. The material presented follows the CAIR approach (cues, activity, intake, and rewards). Each week families receive information and homework from the four categories, usually presented in the following order.

Intake. Although decreasing intake and increasing physical activity are equally emphasized in our program, intake is initially addressed so as not to overwhelm the children with too many changes. Calories are defined for both parents and children, using the metaphor of a car and gas to provide energy. Individualized calorie limits (not below recommended minimums) based on the intake records and weight change are set for each child to lose approximately 1 pound per week. These limits are frequently reviewed and adjustments are made when necessary. Nutritional information is presented each week and guidelines are reviewed. In addition, families are taught our color-coding system, which tells families which foods are high and low in calories. This system corresponds to a modified traffic light. Green-coded foods are lowest in calories and children can eat unlimited quantities of them (GO foods), then yellow- (SLOW DOWN), then orange- (WATCH OUT), and red-coded foods, which are highest in calories (STOP). Weekly red-food limits and green-food goals are set for each child.

Activity. The beneficial effects of increased physical activity and the differential effects of various activities are discussed. Families are asked to monitor their activity and to increase their activity level above baseline rates. Individualized activity goals are established at the third week of treatment (minimum goal is 20 minutes/day) and families are instructed in activity planning. The inverse relationship between activity and television viewing is also discussed.

Two types of activity are addressed in the groups. First, children are encouraged to increase the amount of effort they expend in accomplishing their regular daily activities, such as taking the stairs instead of the elevator, taking a longer route to get somewhere, and walking whenever possible. We call this ''taking the long road,'' and children are required to ''take the long road'' twice a day. Second, children are encouraged to select enjoyable physical activities that are likely to be done on a regular basis.

Rewards.   Reinforcement principles are introduced and discussed. Social and nonsocial reinforcements are emphasized and parents are encouraged to "catch their children being good." Parents and children are asked to make contingency contracts with one another. Children's reward contracts are based on compliance with behavior change assignments listed on the weekly habit record. Staying below calorie limits and activity homework are regular items on all children's habit records. Parallel behavior change contracts and rewards are negotiated for parents.

Cue Management.   Families are made aware of the effects of external cues and strategies, and assignments for the elimination of cues are presented to parents and children.

During this phase of treatment, with all of the changes we ask families to make, it is not uncommon for difficulties to arise. The following are scenarios depicting some of the difficulties experienced by Sean and his family. The first scenario illustrates how a therapist might handle the problem of inaccurate recording.

MRS. C.:   I believe Sean isn't being honest in reporting what he eats when we aren't home, and I don't know what to do.

GROUP LEADER: I will talk to the children's group leader, who will address this issue in the children's group. In addition, you can tell Sean that this is his program. It is important that he understands that neither you nor I can help him if we don't know what he is doing.

CHILDREN'S GROUP LEADER: I want to talk to the group today about completing your intake sheets honestly. It is very important that you write down everything you eat. Does anyone know why?

CHILD: Because then you won't know what we are eating and we might go over our calorie limit.

CHILDREN'S GROUP LEADER: You're right. If you don't write down everything you eat, we will think you are eating less than you really are. Then, if you don't lose weight, your calorie limit will be lowered even further. Does anyone know what will happen then?

CHILD: It will be real hard to stay under our calorie limit.

CHILDREN'S GROUP LEADER: That's right. It will become even more difficult for you to meet this even lower goal and you will lose out. So it is very important to write down everything that goes in your mouth.

The next scenario describes how to handle the problem of family sabotage.

MRS. C.:   Whenever Sean's father cooks, Sean exceeds his calorie limit. I don't know what to do because my husband, as you know, is a gourmet cook.

GROUP LEADER: Have you spoken to your husband about this?

MRS. C.:   Not exactly. I was hoping that Sean would just eat smaller portions and that would solve the problem. However, that doesn't seem to be working.

GROUP LEADER: Can anyone think of any suggestions?

PARENT 1:   What about preparing a separate low-calorie meal for Sean?

GROUP LEADER: That's a good idea, although it might make Sean feel excluded from the family. I wonder if Mrs. C.'s husband would consider making some small changes in his cooking. What are some ways to cut calories?

PARENT 2:   What about using low-calorie margarine instead of butter, or baking instead of frying foods?

GROUP LEADER: Those are very good ideas. Anyone else?

PARENT 1:   Preparing poultry dishes instead of meat dishes, and using low-fat ingredients such as using part-skim cheeses instead of whole-milk cheeses.

PARENT 3:   Preparing foods with lighter sauces.

GROUP LEADER: Those are all excellent ideas, which would significantly decrease the caloric and fat content of a meal. It would also make it easier for Sean to stay under his calorie limit. In addition, since your husband enjoys cooking so much, he might enjoy experimenting with low-calorie recipes.

MRS. C.:   All those suggestions sound good and I will try them. However, I'm not sure my husband will agree to any of them. I don't think he really knows much about weight loss or understands what goes on here.

GROUP LEADER: Maybe it would be helpful if your husband came to some of our sessions with you. This might give him a greater appreciation for what it takes to lose weight. The other group members could share cooking tips with him. He might be more willing to make some changes if he were actively included in Sean's weight-loss efforts.

The last scenario addresses the problem of being the only overweight child in a family.

MRS. C.:   I'm having a problem following cue control rule number three—Keeping high-calorie foods out of the house. My two other children are thin and I don't want to deprive them. Yet I don't want to make it more difficult for Sean.'

GROUP LEADER: This is a common problem. It is important to discuss this with your children and try to make them see this as a family's change. Also, one possible compromise is to not have Sean's favorite high-caloire foods in the house, things he just can't resist.

MRS. C.:   I already do that. However, Sean really likes almost everything.

GROUP LEADER: If high-calorie foods are in the house, keep them out of sight. Put them away, wrap them up in foil, or put them in opaque containers. Freeze things, if that works. Above all, don't leave out dishes of candy or cookie jars. They're just booby traps and we don't want to set the children up to fail.

MRS. C.:   That sounds good. Maybe if we keep a lot of low-calorie snacks around the house and all eat more of them it would help.

GROUP LEADER: That's an excellent idea. It is very important to have many low-calorie snacks easily accessible, especially some special foods just for Sean. Unfortunately, higher-calorie snacks, such as cookies or candy, are much easier to quickly grab and snack on. They usually don't need to be washed, peeled, or cut up. What are some of the low-calorie snacks other parents have given their children?

Extended Treatment

During the extended phase of the program, meetings are held every other week. During this phase, daily monitoring is no longer required. Families are encouraged to gradually decrease intake and activity monitoring to 2 days per week by week 26. Families are told to monitor their children's weight while decreasing their monitoring and to return to daily monitoring if an increase in weight is noted.

Between sessions, families are encouraged to weigh themselves in their home once a week, preferably the same day they come for treatments. Parents and children are asked to set aside some time after their weigh-in to discuss their weight change. This provides an opportunity for parents to give children positive feedback or to discuss any difficulties during the previous week.

During the early part of the extended treatment, the family's experience with the greater time between sessions is discussed. Many times parents report that their children take "a week off" from the program. The following scenario is not uncommon:

PARENT: Since we have been coming to treatment every two weeks, I find that Sean isn't doing as well as he had been.

GROUP LEADER: What are some of the differences you noticed?

PARENT: Well, Sean is still following his activity program, but it seems that he snacks more often during the week that we don't come to group. He not only snacks more but snacks on very high-calorie foods—snacks he didn't eat at all during the first eight weeks.

GROUP LEADER: Are you and Sean weighing in and discussing weight-related issues on the weeks we don't have group?

PARENT: Well, every now and then. We don't have anything regular set up.

GROUP LEADER: As I remember, snacking seemed to be one of Sean's most difficult problems, and therefore it is probably most resistant to change. Sean probably still needs some external support to control the behavior. He received this support in the past by coming to group each week. I think that Sean still needs that additional structure. Weighing in and spending some time together on a consistent basis during the weeks we don't meet would also be helpful for Sean. This would let Sean know you were still interested in his treatment. It would also provide a forum for reinforcement and give Sean the opportunity to see the effects of frequent high-calorie snacking. In addition, I wonder if structuring a specific behavior contract based solely on Sean's snacking might be helpful.

PARENT: Those suggestions sound good and I will try to set aside time for Sean on a weekly basis. I'm also concerned about Sean snacking on foods he shouldn't have.

GROUP LEADER: Sean might be feeling deprived and "sick" of watching his weight. Eating high-calorie snacks might be his way of letting you know that. Allowing Sean two snacks of his choice, provided that he stays under his calorie limit, may help with this problem. Since these snacks will "always" be around, it might prove beneficial for Sean to learn to eat them in limited quantities. Providing a variety of low-calorie snacks might also be helpful.

As indicated in the above scenario, consistent family meetings were stressed. Families need to be told that continued success depends on both the parents' and children's efforts over the long run. For especially problematic behaviors, additional reward programs negotiated between parents and children usually have beneficial results.

In general, session time during all extended treatment meetings is spent on problem solving. Parents are taught general problem-solving skills. An example is provided for the group and then parents receive problem-solving work sheets with the problem-solving steps outlined. The group leader talks with each parent during the session to determine what behavior needs to be focused on with their child.

Child-management issues frequently are raised, either implicitly or explicitly, by parents. The parents' group leader should be alert to signs of lowered cooperation between parents and children, and this should be addressed. Both the parents and the children need encouragement, acknowledging the difficulty of the task they are engaged in. It is stressed that this treatment phase is as important as the first phase of treatment and that families are still expected to exert a great amount of effort. Since the groups meet less frequently, families need to be told that more of the responsibility of the program now lies with them.

TERMINATION AND FOLLOW-UP

Group meetings are held every month after week 26 for a 1-year period during the follow-up phase. Between group meetings, families are given a packet of postcards (one for each month) to send to us with their weekly weights. Program-initiated phone calls are also made once a month to determine how families are doing and to help with any difficulties. Families are told that they may call us if they want to discuss a difficulty or to share a success. No new material is presented in the follow-up meetings. Thus, the primary purpose is to assess progress and to do some problem solving for those families having difficulties.

No meetings are routinely scheduled after the 12-month follow-up period. However, families are informed that program personnel are always available to them. These contacts are family-initiated until yearly follow-ups intended to assess continued maintenance/progress. Thus, termination has been an arbitrary, time-defined procedure. Clearly, not all children reach nonobese status by this 1-year follow-up time. The issue of continued extended treatment is clearly worthy of clinical/research attention.

OVERALL EVALUATION

At the start of treatment Sean was 57.25 inches tall, weighed 127.75 pounds, and was 50.19% overweight. By the end of intensive treatment Sean was 57.75 inches, 120.29 pounds, and 30.39% overweight. At week 26, the end of extended treatment, the comparable figures were 58.25 inches, 118.50 pounds, and 18.17%. One year later Sean was 61.00 inches tall, weighted 125.00 pounds, and was 13.64% overweight. This pattern of weight change is representative of our successful cases. In-treatment weight losses are followed by weight stabilization or rates of gain that are appreciably lower than those that existed prior to treatment. In a period of expected growth this results in decreases in percentage overweight. Sean's family was clearly an example of a successful outcome. Sean was no longer obese, and improvements were noted in other areas as well. The family came to view this problem as one that they all were involved in. Changes were made in calorie intake and energy expenditure behaviors, and these appear to have been maintained. Food preparations and eating had been central to family activities and some shift in such emphasis occurred. This still remained an important part of family life. However, changes to more healthful and less caloric eating became part of the family's shared activity. The parents improved their parenting skills and the consistency with which they applied them.

Clearly, not all families will be as successful as Sean's. However, defining success with these children and their families is a difficult issue. Many of the children who do not become nonobese, or perhaps do not show appreciable reductions in percentage overweight, must be judged against a prior weight history. In many of these cases the record was one of increasing *percentage overweight* in the years prior to treatment. Perhaps in this context even stabilization of percent overweight is a measure of success. Nonetheless, treatments that result in greater long-term decreases in relative weight are still needed for many of these families.

REFERENCES

Israel, A. C., & Shapiro, L. S. (1985). Behavior problems of obese children enrolling in a weight reduction program. *Journal of Pediatric Psychology, 10*, 449–460.

Israel, A. C., Silverman, W. K., & Solotar, L. C. (1986). An investigation of family influences on initial weight status, attrition, and treatment outcome in a childhood obesity program. *Behavior Therapy, 17*, 131–143.

Israel, A. C., Stolmaker, L., & Andrian, C. A. G. (1985). The effects of training parents in general child management skills on a behavioral weight loss program for children. *Behavior Therapy, 16*, 169–180.

Israel, A. C., Stolmaker, L., Sharp, J. P., Silverman, W. K., & Simon, L. (1984). An evaluation of two methods of parental involvement in treating obese children. *Behavior Therapy, 15*, 226–272.

CHAPTER 25

Enuresis

GLENN R. CADDY and JEFFREY BOLLARD

DESCRIPTION OF THE DISORDER

Nocturnal enuresis is conventionally defined as the persistent and involuntary passing of urine during sleep beyond about 4 years of age and in the absence of demonstrable urologic or neurologic pathology. In establishing the diagnosis of functional enuresis it is crucial to distinguish between nocturnal enuresis in the absence of other micturitional difficulties and nocturnal enuresis accompanied by diurnal frequency and urgency. Also noteworthy is the distinction between primary (never continent) and secondary (return to bedwetting after a period of continence) enuresis.

Patterns of bedwetting vary markedly, with some children wetting more than once per night while others wet regularly once or twice per week and still others wet more sporadically. Enuresis is a very common and apparently worldwide phenomenon, though survey data are generally available only from the technologically more advanced countries. These surveys indicate that approximately 15% of 5-year-olds, 5% of 10-year-olds, and approximately 2% of teenagers are bedwetters, the remainder becoming continent without specific treatment. Throughout the age span the incidence of enuresis is somewhat higher among males than among females, the ratio being approximately 3:2.

Several different and sometimes contradictory theories about the nature and etiology of bedwetting have been advanced over the years. Similarly, a wide array of remedies have been proposed, since the form of

GLENN R. CADDY • Department of Psychology, Nova University, 3301 College Avenue, Fort Lauderdale, Florida 33314. JEFFREY BOLLARD • The Adelaide Children's Hospital, North Adelaide, South Australia 5006.

treatment recommended usually reflects the therapists' theoretical orientation. Nonetheless, in broad terms, etiological explanations of bedwetting fall into three main categories—psychodynamic theories, physiological theories, and behavioral theories.

The essence of the psychodynamic approach is that bedwetting is the surface indicator of some underlying emotional disturbance. Yet comparative studies of enuretics and nonenuretics show that the vast majority of bedwetters do not exhibit a greater degree of emotional maladjustment than nonenuretics (Cullen, 1966). Of course, if the enuresis persists into adulthood, it is likely that at least some psychological pathology will coexist along with the bedwetting. Second, the psychoanalytic approach recommends that the treatment of choice must be psychoanalytically oriented psychotherapy since such therapy addresses the underlying disturbance. This form of therapy, however, has not been shown to be effective in the treatment of bedwetting.

The physiological theories attribute bedwetting either to an immaturity of the central nervous system connections governing bladder control, an immaturity of the bladder resulting in reduced functional capacity, or a defect in the sleep-arousal mechanisms. Failure of appropriate maturation of either the central nervous system or the bladder is considered important in the bedwetting of younger children, but this view is difficult to sustain for older children. Furthermore, treatment strategies that follow from this perspective, such as the use of bladder-training exercises (retention control training) and the use of medications, like imipramine (Tofranil), have met with only moderate success in the long-term arrest of bedwetting. There is a growing body of evidence that bedwetting is closely associated with faulty sleep arousal mechanisms, but the exact nature of this association is unclear.

We consider the most parsimonious explanation of the nature and etiology of bedwetting to be that proposed by the behavioral theorists, perhaps also implicating elements of the physiological approach. According to the behavioral viewpoint, bedwetting results from the child's failure to learn the response of sphincter contraction during sleep in order to prevent reflex voiding. The bladder collects urine during sleep, and when it reaches a certain volume the limits of tonal compensation of the smooth detrusor muscle in the bladder wall are exceeded and a complex chain of reflexes is triggered, culminating in the voiding response. Most children above the age of 4 years have learned to inhibit this response, thereby retaining urine throughout the hours of sleep and then voiding appropriately the next morning. The behavioral/learning theory proposes that the majority of bedwetters fail to learn the response of sphincter contraction during sleep. Actually, bedwetters fail to transfer the inhibitory control of detrusor activity learned during the day to the sleeping state, and/or, when the limits of compensatory adjustment of the detrusor muscle are exceeded during sleep, they fail to respond to the feedback stimuli from the distended bladder and do not wake prior to voiding. The main reasons for these learning failures are the absence of environmental conditions ordinarily necessary for the learning to take place and/or low levels of conditionability. In a minority of cases, failure to develop control may be due to high levels of anxiety, nervous tension that produces inefficient learning, or the breakdown of previously established linkages.

The treatment that follows from the behavioral viewpoint is aimed at conditioning the sphincter to contract in response to the stimuli arising from a filling bladder during sleep. The most common form of behavioral therapy for bedwetting has been the standard conditioning procedure employing the Mowrer-type urine-alarm instrument (Mowrer & Mowrer, 1938). This general approach has been demonstrated in many studies to be highly effective in arresting bedwetting (see Lovibond & Coote, 1970).

A major development in the behavioral treatment of bedwetting since Mowrer's original work has been the introduction of dry-bed training by Azrin, Sneed, and Foxx (1974). The dry-bed training program utilizes the urine-alarm device but adds to it an intense training schedule that includes practice in correct toileting, practice in waking quickly, retention control training, and increased social motivation to become dry. This procedure has been modified and simplified over the ensuing years, and Bollard and Nettlebeck (1982) have argued, on a cost-effectiveness basis, that the standard conditioning procedure combined with the waking schedule from dry-bed training offers the most efficient large-scale treatment for bedwetting currently available. The standard conditioning plus waking schedule regimen formed the basis for the case treatment presented herein.

CASE IDENTIFICATION AND PRESENTING COMPLAINTS

The patient, Sophie, was a 9-year-old female, the youngest of three children. The father was a self-employed accountant. The mother was primarily engaged in home duties but did casual work to assist the father in his business. The family enjoyed a comfortable middle-class life-style.

Sophie initially was referred because of concerns for her learning progress. She was in the fourth grade at school but was stated to be below the class average in basic literacy and numeracy. More to the point for the present purposes, in the course of the comprehensive assessment to be reported it also was revealed that Sophie was still bedwetting.

HISTORY AND ASSESSMENT

The case history was developed during the assessment phase. The assessment of Sophie involved an initial appointment with her parents, during which time a detailed developmental, psychosocial, educational, and clinical history of the child was undertaken. (As a general rule, we recommend that the child(ren) not attend during this initial visit with the parents. We prefer to see the parents first for initial data collection because we do not wish to have the child(ren) spend their first visit largely in the waiting room.)

The history in this case proved developmentally unremarkable in that Sophie reached all her various developmental milestones age-appropriately, save for her control on nocturnal voiding. A focus on the history of this problem was then undertaken. This history revealed that Sophie was toilet-trained for diurnal bladder and bowel control without fuss by about 2 years of age. However, she had never mastered nocturnal bladder control and had wet the bed almost every night of her life. As a preschooler Sophie had exhibited urinary frequency and urgency during the day and even an occasional wetting accident. These symptoms, however, had not been evident since she started school.

Sophie had been examined medically in the past, but no evidence of underlying organic disease had been found. Specific investigations, including microurine analysis, intravenous pyelogram, complete blood picture, and blood pressure check, all had proven to be normal.

The parents had tried a variety of strategies in the past to arrest Sophie's bedwetting. These included fluid restriction after the evening meal, waking during the night for toileting, reward systems for dry nights, and a trial on medication (imipramine). They had never punished her for wetting accidents and had not overreacted to the problem, though both parents were keen to arrest Sophie's symptoms as soon as possible.

All of the above strategies had been unsuccessful. In addition, Sophie had had a trial on a bed buzzer device, which also had proven to be ineffective. This device was hired from a local pharmacy and was reported to have been unreliable and ineffective in waking Sophie in response to bedwetting events. Furthermore, there was no supervision of the program—the parents were simply given an alarm and a set of very basic instructions and left to their own resources. They were charged a weekly rental fee and were instructed to return the alarm when the child had stopped wetting the bed.

In terms of Sophie's psychosocial development, the parents described what appeared to be a socially well-adjusted child with significant friendships and no indices of psychopathology or behavior disorders. The parents did note that Sophie was a particularly deep sleeper. With the exception of the bedwetting, however, the parents' concerns focused on what they regarded as Sophie's probable scholastic difficulties.

During the course of this initial, rather structured interview with the parents, questions also were directed at evaluating the parents child-rearing/management skills and the relationships among the various family members. In Sophie's case, the qality of both the parenting and the familial interrelationships appeared very favorable to her competent development. Finally, in this interview, an extended family history for developmental or clinical pathology was investigated. During this process it was revealed that Sophie's mother had been a bedwetter until age 14 years, whereupon the problem remitted spontaneously.

The comprehensive assessment of Sophie was completed over the next two sessions. Intellectual and psychoeducational testing revealed that Sophie was functioning within quite normal limits intellectually, and that there appeared no specific deficits on her Wechsler Intelligence Scale for Children-Revised subtest profile scores. Her scholastic attainment scores showed Sophie's reading, spelling, and arithmetic skills to be only marginally below her grade level, and it was understood that these indices of achievement were age-appropriate—Sophie was substantially younger than most of the children in her class. Further inquiry revealed that Sophie was attending a school where the standards of achievement were higher than average, and no doubt this finding also contributed to the parental focus on their child's learning limitations. These "limitations" notwithstanding, Sophie indicated that she enjoyed her school life and got along well with both her teachers and her peers.

Additional assessment with sentence completion, family drawing procedures, and continued clinical interviewing indicated a cheerful and confident child capable of talking openly about her difficulties. She related that she was wetting the bed virtually very night, sometimes more than once. She knew this because sometimes her mother would wake her for toileting and they would discover a wet bed. Then she would wet again before the morning. Sophie did not feel that she had to use the toilet during the daytime more often than most children, nor was she having any wetting accidents during the day. She was annoyed and embarrassed by her bedwetting, particularly since it prevented her from having friends stay overnight or going to school camps. She did not get into trouble from her parents when she wet, but she worried that it was an inconvenience for her mother, who had to do extra washing and cleaning. She was very highly motivated to be rid of the problem.

Given the quality of the data collected during the course of this assessment, it was not considered necessary to interview other family members, teachers, and the like. Moreover, we were satisfied that the quality of the pediatric urological consultation that the parents had sought was adequate to rule out organic pathology as a basis for Sophie's bedwetting. (Sometimes this is not the case, and further specialist medical consultation is recommended to the parents prior to undertaking the comprehensive psychological assessment of the child.) Nevertheless, Sophie had not had a medical examination in nearly 2 years, and so, being somewhat conservative, we decided to arrange yet one more medical examination for Sophie. Again no physical impairment was noted.

The next visit involved both the parents and Sophie. The trio were debriefed regarding the findings of the assessment and a series of treatment recommendations were offered. Regarding the initial primary concern of possible learning impairment, the parents and Sophie were assured that Sophie was functioning at an age-appropriate level, but it also was indicated that Sophie would benefit from a program of individual tuition to improve her basic skills. Additionally, the parents were urged to encourage Sophie in more reading activity and to place limitations on the amount of television watching engaged in by their daughter.

As for the bedwetting, it was concluded that Sophie suffered from uncomplicated primary nocturnal enuresis. This condition became the focus of the intervention to be reported.

SELECTION OF TREATMENT

The treatment chosen to address Sophie's primary nocturnal enuresis was the standard conditioning procedure combined with the waking schedule taken from dry-bed training. This choice was based on the belief that Sophie's bedwetting represented a learning deficiency, and that the standard conditioning procedure has been amply demonstrated to be a highly effective treatment for this problem. There are few studies of the effectiveness of waking schedules in conjunction with the standard conditioning procedure, but those that have been performed offer support for this practice as a useful adjunct to the alarm (see Bollard & Nettelbeck, 1982). Sophie's previously unsuccessful trial with the bed buzzer was noted. However, it was considered that there were specific reasons for this failure—namely, technically inadequate equipment and a lack of appropriate supervision and follow-up. These shortcomings could be remedied by closer therapist involvement during treatment, by the use of more sophisticated equipment, and by the introduction of a systematic waking schedule.

COURSE OF TREATMENT

The first step in the treatment program was to emphasize to Sophie and her parents that bedwetting is a very common problem in childhood, that in the vast majority of cases it does not represent underlying emotional or physical pathology, and that with appropriate treatment the prospects of a complete recovery are high. After this reassurance, the following explanation of the problem was given. With the aid of a diagram, Sophie was asked to imagine her bladder filling up with urine during the daytime. It was explained that when her bladder collected a certain amount of urine, messages were sent to her brain to tell her that she needed to go to the toilet. These messages also enabled Sophie to tighten the muscle at the opening of her bladder so that she could hold urine until it was convenient to go to the toilet. She was asked to imagine what the feeling of a full bladder is like. It was then explained that her bladder worked the same way during sleep but that at the moment the feelings from her bladder were not strong enough to tell her brain to tighten the muscle at the opening (so she could hold urine throughout the night) or to awaken (so she could go to the toilet). The objective of the alarm procedure was to help her to learn how to take the "appropriate action" during sleep (that is, muscle contraction and/or awakening) when her bladder sent out its signals.

For a 2-week period prior to commencing treatment, Sophie was required to record her bedwetting frequency. This recording confirmed that Sophie was wetting the bed every night. The urine alarm equipment in this instance was manufactured by Ramsay Coote Instruments (Australia) Pty. Ltd. Technical details of this equipment are contained in Coote (1965). Arrangement of the equipment in the child's bed was explained, and then the alarm system was demonstrated by pouring a small amount of sterile saline onto the detector pad, thereby triggering the alarm. Sophie was encouraged to repeat this mock bedwetting procedure with one hand placed on the pad, thereby being assured that there was no subjectively experienced electric shock possible and nothing to fear.

The actual treatment procedure was then described in detail, and Sophie was required to role-play the various steps using a demonstration bed to ensure that the method was understood. The procedure involved placing the detector pad in her bed such that when the alarm was triggered by a wetting accident, Sophie would be awakened. The alarm unit was placed at a sufficient distance from the bed so that she could not switch it off while still in bed, but not so far away as to reduce the intensity of the signal. Once wakened in response to the alarm, Sophie was required to go quickly to the toilet in order to finish voiding. After returning to the bedside, she was required to remove the wet sheet, dry the detector pad thoroughly, and reset the alarm. Then she was to get back into bed and return to sleep. Sophie was encouraged to take responsibility for this procedure, but given her age, it was expected that the parents might need to give some assistance.

Next, the waking schedule was described. This was taken from the dry-bed training instructions. On the first night of training, Sophie was awakened every hour, using minimal prompting, and sent to the toilet to urinate. The practice of hourly awakenings throughout the night was given only during the initial training night. The following evening she was awakened only once, 3 hours after going to bed, and was sent off to the toilet. After each dry night, Sophie was awakened 30 mintues earlier than on the previous night. Waking was suspended when the schedule was down to within 1 hour of Sophie's going to bed. If she wet on 2 nights in 1 week, Sophie's training schedule required that she go back to being awakened 3 hours after bedtime. Thereafter, Sophie had to work her way through the schedule again—i.e., after each dry night to be awakened 30 minutes earlier than the previous night.

Sophie was encouraged to sleep in a summer nightie, without underpants, in order to minimize the delay between voiding and triggering the alarm. Written instructions for the above procedure and for recording were issued. Two records were kept. First, Sophie drew up a single calendar with the therapists, on which she recorded dry nights with the aid of reward stickers. Second, the parents kept a more comprehensive record, including details of Sophie's bedtime, time awakened by the alarm, time of self-awakening, size of the wet patch, dry nights, and any other information deemed to be relevant to the child's progress, such as illness or equipment malfunction.

In this particular case, the psychological preparation of Sophie and her parents, together with the motivation of all concerned to adhere to the parameters of the treatment program, resulted in the clinicians' having largely a monitoring and encouraging role in the subsequent programming. Sometimes, of course, issues of compliance failure either by the child and/or by the parents create special problems for the success of the treatment program, and in such instances these compliance matters may well become the focus of subsequent therapy. Nevertheless, in cases of uncomplicated enuresis, whether primary or secondary, in many instances the bulk of the work of the clinician is completed within a week or two of the implementation of the behavioral procedures applied herein. Sometimes, too, the issues involved in the emergence of secondary enuresis suggested during the assessment process create complications that require additional specialized handling and may involve some specific restructuring in the family dynamics. Such restructuring, if required, generally should be undertaken prior to the introduction of the conditioning paradigm together with the waking schedule recommended herein.

TERMINATION

Unlike the behavioral and other treatments of many conditions wherein a substantial period of therapy is required, as has been seen in the section headed "Follow-up and Evaluation," the treatment of Sophie had been completed largely within 2 weeks of implementing the procedures employed. Thus, while it was necessary for the clinicians to develop a substantial rapport with the patient and her family in order to ensure compliance in the present case, the process of termination largely involved a planned fading of the involvement of the clinicians in the life of the patient and her family. This fading occurred during the follow-up process.

FOLLOW-UP

Sophie was required to contact the therapists by telephone and report on her progress. A specific time for reporting was arranged. The parents were encouraged to make contact immediately if difficulties arose before the weekly designated contact time. A follow-up personal appointment was arranged for 4 weeks after treatment commenced. Treatment with the alarm was to continue until Sophie had achieved 14 consecutive dry nights. The parents negotiated with Sophie a separate reward (a new quilt for her bed) for achievement of this criterion.

Sophie's progress during treatment is summarized in Figure 1. She achieved a dry bed on the first night of training (largely because of the waking schedule). However, Sophie wet the bed on each of the 6 subsequent nights.

During the second week of treatment Sophie had 4 wet nights. Thereafter, she did not wet again until the criterion to stop using the alarm was reached. At this point the alarm was taken from the bed, though she continued to telephone each week, for a few weeks, with a progress report. Follow-up at 3, 6, and 12 months after reaching the initial dryness criterion established that Sophie had maintained her noctural continence with no relapses whatsoever.

Both parents and child were delighted with Sophie's achievement. While Sophie's bedwetting had not been a substantial problem prior to

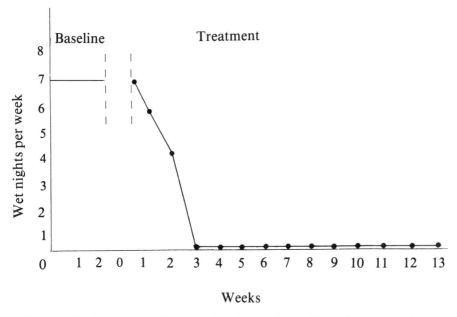

Figure 1.   Number of wet nights per week during baseline and throughout treatment.

treatment. Sophie's mother reported that Sophie appeared to gain further confidence and self-assurance following the enuresis program. Certainly, Sophie's social life became more active since she felt more able to sleep overnight at friends' houses and to have friends stay with her.

OVERALL EVALUATION

This case was chosen because it represents a typical example of primary nocturnal enuresis in terms of the history, presentation of the problem, and treatment response. Between us we have treated more than 1,000 bedwetters, and among these children there are some very commonly observed features. First, most of them present as normal, healthy, well-adjusted children. Even when there is evidence of emotional disorder, more often than not it seems secondary to the enuresis rather than a cause of the problem. Second, there is often a family history of enuresis involving a first-degree relative. Third, most parents report that their enuretic children are exceptionally deep sleepers. To date, the empirical data on the association between deep sleep and enuresis are equivocal. However, the frequent anecdotal reports of deep sleeping in enuretic children are constant reminders that an association of this kind may exist and be a fruitful area for further research. The standard conditioning procedure combined with a nighttime waking schedule in this instance was highly effective in arresting bedwetting.

REFERENCES

Azrin, N. H., Sneed, T. J., & Foxx, R. M. (1974). Dry-bed training: Rapid elimination of childhood enuresis. *Behaviour Research and Therapy, 12,* 147–156.

Bollard, J., & Nettelbeck, T. (1982). A component analysis of dry-bed training for treatment of bedwetting. *Behaviour Research and Therapy, 20,* 383–390.

Coote, M. A. (1965). Apparatus for conditioning treatment of enuresis. *Behaviour Research and Therapy, 2,* 233–238.

Cullen, K. J. (1966). Clinical observations concerning behavior disorders in children. *Medical Journal of Australia, 1,* 712–715.

Lovibond, S. H., & Coote, M. A. (1970). Enuresis. In C. G. Costello (Ed.), *Symptoms of psychopathology: A handbook.* New York: Wiley.

Mowrer, O. H., & Mowrer, W. M. (1938). Enuresis: A method for its study and treatment. *American Journal of Orthopsychiatry, 8,* 436–459.

CHAPTER 26

Encopresis

DANIEL M. DOLEYS

DESCRIPTION OF THE DISORDER

Encopresis is generally defined as the passage of fecal material into inappropriate or unacceptable places. As with many disorders, encopresis is primarily divided into those cases where definite organic pathology can be identified and those where it cannot. When no organic pathology can be identified, this is usually referred to as functional encopresis. According to DSM-III (APA, 1980), the essential feature is the "repeated voluntary or involuntary passage of feces of normal or near normal consistency into places not appropriate for that purpose in the individuals' own socio-culture setting, not due to any physical disorder." Functional encopresis can further be divided into primary and secondary. Primary functional encopresis describes a condition in a child who has never shown fecal continence. Secondary functional encopresis is applied to children who have demonstrated fecal continence of approximately 6 months or more. DSM-III uses a 1-year criterion.

Functional encopresis has also been referred to as fecal incontinence and, on occasion, as psychogenic megacolon. The term *psychogenic megacolon* is most applicable where soiling can be shown to be due, at least in part, to an enlarged colon.

There has been some disagreement as to the age when a child can be considered encopretic. It is sometimes difficult to differentiate between the child who is encopretic and the child who has never been totally

---

DANIEL M. DOLEYS • Behavioral Medicine Services, 3490 Independence Drive, Birmingham, Alabama 35209.

trained. Awareness of the child's general developmental rate and prior attempts at toilet training or of the presence of bladder control provides information in guiding the diagnosis. Most, however, agree that socialized children in this society should be bowel-trained by the age of 4.

In addition to the subclassification of encopresis as primary or secondary, it is also useful to divide these children into retentive and nonretentive type. The retentive type of encopretic has infrequent bowel movements and regularly uses purgatives. It is further necessary to differentiate those children who refrain from defecating because they are fearful of the toilet or pain from those who may demonstrate a "pot refusal" syndrome. The fearful group may respond to densensitization techniques, while those with pot refusal syndrome are often noncompliant children and may require a different therapeutic approach.

Overflow incontinence occurs when children have impactions and fecal material is forced around these impactions. This may present as diarrhea and in fact has been described as "paradoxical diarrhea," but the etiology involves the presence of impaction created by bowel retention or constipation. Treatment, therefore, must be focused upon maintaining a vacant colon, perhaps through the use of intermittent enemas.

The estimated incidence of functional encopresis varies from 1.5 to 7.5% of children. Bellman (1966) noted that 8.1% of 3-year-olds soiled their pants, 2.8% of 4-year-olds, and 2.2% of 5-year-olds. The incidence of functional encopresis seems to be substantially higher in males than in females and is more often found in children with developmental delays. In a very detailed study by Levine (1975) of 102 encopretics, 87 were found to be between the ages of 4 and 13, 85% were male, and 50% were incontinent during the day and night. The majority of the children described a sensory deficit in that they could not detect the urge to defecate and complained of abdominal pains, poor appetite, and lethargy. Fecal impactions were identified in 75%, and 40% were diagnosed as continuous encopretics. Familial, marital, and behavioral pathologies were uncommon.

An understanding of the physiology of fecal incontinence is necessary in the adequate treatment of these children. Briefly, the process is reflexive and is initiated by stimulation of receptors in the rectal mucosa (Anthony, 1963; Gaston, 1948). Defecation occurs in response to distention of the rectum, produced by mass peristalsis of fecal material about the colon. Filling and distention of the rectum results in (1) increased colonic peristalsis, (2) reflexive relaxation of internal anal sphincter, and (3) a desire to defecate. Voluntary contraction of thoracic and abdominal muscles and relaxation of the external anal sphincters bring about defecation. If defecation is voluntarily inhibited, rectal receptors adapt to the existing pressure and the urge to defecate diminishes. Subsequent urges may not occur until 24 hours later, when mass peristalsis begins again. During this retention interval, moisture from fecal mass can be absorbed, producing a hard stool and painful defecation.

From a learning theory perspective, the etiology of encopresis can be effectively described. The model emphasizes inadequate and/or inappropriate learning experiences. In the case of the primary encopretic, a learning model would evaluate the presence of preexisting skills, such as undressing, and the lack of sufficient reinforcement for proper toileting. It is usually assumed that cues emanating from rectal distention and internal anal sphincter relaxation have not become discriminative for temporary retention and bowel movements into the commode. Secondary encopresis, on the other hand, is often accounted for in terms of avoidance conditioning principals. It is often postulated that pain- or fear-arousing events have been associated with the onset of encopresis. Thus, retention becomes negatively reinforced by the delay of pain. This behavior often persists despite the fact that when a child does ultimately have a bowel movement, the pain is present to a higher degree than would have been the case without retention. Another possibility is the presence of inadvertent conditioning, which occurs when a child receives untimely reinforcement through parental attention and other reactions when soiling has occurred. In this way, the maladaptive behavior may actually be conditioned by the parental or significant others' attention devoted to the response.

A functional analysis can be used to isolate faulty environmental contingencies. Rearranging such contingencies is a major focus of therapy. However, understanding the physiology of the response is necessary to be assured that unreasonable expectations are not generated. Furthermore, nutritional evaluation to eliminate such factors as excessive caffeine, which can stimulate excessive bowel, is also quite important.

CASE IDENTIFICATION

The patient was a 9-year-old white male (M.C.). M.C. was the oldest of five children. His siblings were 8, 6, 4, and 3 years of age. The parents were middle to upper middle class. He was attending the fourth grade in a Christian elementary school that was considered to be rather difficult academically. He was known to be an A–B student. He was referred by a master's-level therapist who had done some evaluation of his encopresis and had also been working with M.C.'s parents on some family-related issues.

The patient had preschool experience from the age of 2. Reports of his teachers from the first, second, and third grades noted that he was performing well academically, but notes from the second grade showed that he was slow to obey and often refused to accept when and where he was wrong. During the third grade, his grades began to drop and it appeared as though he was becoming less compliant and attentive to his work. M.C. would reportedly not admit to any wrongdoing, even though his participation could be substantiated. He appeared to have fewer friends and on occasion engaged in baby talk. He participated in soccer in the first grade but otherwise was not involved in organized sports.

The child and parental referral source noted M.C.'s "weaknesses" to include wanting to control everything and requiring constant attention in order for him to follow through; low attention span and lackadaisical attitude toward his school work; marginal social skills regarding the acquisition and maintenance of friendships with his peers; desire to make all the rules; and tendency to be somewhat physically rough with his 6-year-old brother.

PRESENTING COMPLAINT

The presenting complaint was that of encopresis. The patient was noted to have bowel movements almost on a daily basis, but he would soil his underclothes up to four times a week. These accidents would sometimes involve a significant amount of fecal material and other times a stain.

HISTORY

The child had never been totally toilet-trained. At the age of 2, he was bladder-trained and only occasionally wet his pants. He then began to engage in some nocturnal enuresis about the age of 5 or 6, and it was felt that this was related to emotional upset and adjustment. Factors relevant in this situation involved the family's being transferred and the arrival of a new sibling. Between the age of 18 and 24 months, M.C. had a good deal of difficulty with milk allergies. He appeared to be plagued with an itchy rash, but this was ultimately resolved. There was no evidence of any delay in the usual developmental milestones. The patient had had somewhat of a history of impactions and was known on occasion to sit in the closet and to attempt to refrain from defecating.

His pattern of accidents tended to involve at least one to two during the course of the weekend and then perhaps one a day during the week-days. The longest period of time he had gone without accidents was 2 weeks. The amount of fecal material passed varied. It had a very strong odor to it. At various times, the parents had attempted talking with the patient, spanking him, using positive practice with a star chart, ignoring, and the use of milk of magnesia and fiber, along with periodic toileting. None of these systems produced significant results. M.C. reported that he could sometimes detect the need to defecate and at other times could not. When asked where he felt it, he appropriately identified the abdominal and rectal areas as focal points of attention. He claimed he could not feel the passage of feces into his clothes. When he was playing, he often did not respond to the urge to defecate. He denied any pain upon defecation. There was no evidence of any nocturnal accidents.

The patient's diet was fairly good and he was normal weight and had a normal amount of exercise and activity. Behaviorally, he would often challenge his parents, and discipline in the home involved yelling, spanking, and grounding. There was some suggestion of a rather immature style in that M.C. was very sensitive to comments made about him or discussions involving him.

M.C. had been examined by his own pediatrician. No abnormalities could be found. He was then seen by a pediatric gastroenterologist, who conducted anorectal manometry studies, the results of which were well within normal limits. He was again tried on dietary manipulations, involving the addition of milk of magnesia and scheduled toileting 15 minutes after each meal. This was ineffectual. M.C. had been seen briefly by a clinical psychologist with a specialty in pediatric psychology, who recommended some family counseling. The patient was then followed up by a master's-level counselor, who ultimately referred the patient to the author.

M.C. was intially seen for intake in April of 1986. The parents had been instructed to maintain a daily record sheet involving bowel movements and soiling episodes, which covered a 2-week period prior to the initial office visit. These records revealed that the patient had a total of 14 bowel movements during these 2 weeks, five episodes of pant soiling, and four episodes of staining. The baseline records were obtained by having one or both parents check M.C. every 2 hours when he was at home and available.

ASSESSMENT

The assessment of M.C. included an office visit with him and his parents. The baseline records were reviewed. He was asked very direct questions about his ability to detect the urge to defecate and his response to this detection. He was also interviewed as to his desire and motivation to resolve the problem. He was seen in conjunction with the parents, and then the parents were seen separately to observe the interaction. M.C. tended to be almost "hyperactive." He continually postured and moved about in his chair. He was mildly unruly and was often asked to quiet down or to sit quietly by his parents, especially his father. At times, he did seem almost antagonistic and challenging, especially to his father. During the interview with his parents, they described attempts to give M.C. enemas, as suggested by previous therapists. This was emotionally upsetting to the parents as well as to M.C., and it often resulted in a very physically uncomfortable situation. It was clear that their attempts at imposing treatment for the problem, although well intended, were often interrupted by other things in their life and that it had been especially difficult to follow through with the presence of four other younger children.

Following the interview, the author was fairly satisfied that M.C. had the potential to detect and respond to cues to defecate because there were numerous times when he did engage in self-initiated bowel movements. It was also apparent that the encopresis was primarily a response to inadequate motivation and perhaps was being maintained inadvertently by parental attention, even though much of this was "negative" attention involving scolding, ignoring, and restriction of privileges.

Medical assessment had clearly ruled out any organic pathology. Assessment of the diet did not reveal any significant difficulties, such as excessive caffeine or inadequate fiber. It was therefore decided to implement a previously researched and clinically effective program, which combined regular pant checks, supervised toileting, full-cleanliness training for accidents, and token reinforcement for appropriate toileting. Upon the introduction of the program, the parents and M.C. were shown a diagram and provided with an explanation as to the mechanism of defecation and various things, such as inadequate diet, that could contribute to problems. Written instructions regarding the treatment plan were given to the parents as well as to M.C., and these instructions were reviewed with everyone present so there could be no misunderstanding and all questions could be clarified.

SELECTION OF TREATMENT

The treatment plan for M.C. had several facets. The first involved periodic pant checks. Initially, he was to be checked every 2 hours by his parents. They were instructed to keep a diary and record the occurrence of soiling, staining, and clean pants. M.C. was toileted after each pant check for approximately 5 minutes. He was provided token reinforcement if he had a bowel movement into the commode. He was also provided reinforcement if he independently had a bowel movement. Rewards, however, were given only if the bowel movements were verified by parental check. The second was full-cleanliness training (FCT). Any episode of staining or soiling, no matter how small, was followed by FCT. This required M.C. to wash out his underwear and his trousers, and then to bathe himself. The whole process would encompass a 15- to 20-minute period of time. The instructions given to the parents and child were as follows:

> I know that this may seem like an awful lot of work. However, it is important each time a soil or stain is identified that we go through this procedure of cleaning. I'm sure that you think this is excessive punishment, M.C., for something that you cannot control. But at nine years of age we must realize that this problem is in large part yours and that it is your responsibility to clean up if there is an accident. You also need to keep in mind that if you don't have accidents and do have your bowel movements in the commode, then you won't have to do the cleaning. Mom and Dad, you must remember that this cleaning is to be done without a lot of emotional upset. I do not want you yelling or scolding M.C. If he has a stain or soils in his pants, simply point this out to him and tell him that he must go through the cleaning process as the doctor recommended. If M.C. resists or is noncompliant, you simply do what you can to encourage him to follow through with this and take him to the bathroom. If he falls on the floor, screams, and yells, do not get involved with a physical battle with him. Just indicate to him that privileges such as television will be removed until he does follow the cleaning. If, while he is doing the cleaning, he gets disruptive and yells, simply remind him that the rules are that he is to clean quietly before it can stop and that the longer he fusses and complains, the longer the cleaning will continue. If you have any difficulties with this at all, don't hesitate to give me a call. Now, Mom, Dad, M.C., do you have any questions at all?

At this point M.C. was asked to repeat back what would happen if he had a stain or soiled in his pants and then how he could avoid the cleaning episode. The parents were again instructed not to make this into some sort of "control battle" but to follow the directions that were laid out and to contact the therapist if there was a problem.

The third aspect of the treatment program involved the use of enemas. When there is some indication of retention that could lead to constipation, enemas become a necessary part of treatment to prevent the development of megacolon or impactions. The author's experience has suggested that parental application of enemas can often be abusive and complicate the treatment process. Indeed, M.C.'s parents noted that they were told to do this once in the past and it was very traumatic for them. M.C. would get resistant, and then one of the parents would have to hold him down while the other one gave the enema, and it resulted in a big emotional scene that did not help the encopresis problem at all. Rather, arrangements were made with the emergency room closest to the patient so that if he went 72 consecutive hours without a bowel movement, he would be taken to the emergency room and they would carry out the enema.

The fourth aspect of treatment was token reinforcement. Parents were instructed to make a chart containing 10 squares. Anytime M.C. had a bowel movement in the commode, whether it was prompted by the parents or carried out independently, he was to receive a star on his chart. This only occurred, however, if the bowel movement was confirmed. The chart was to be displayed in the bathroom. Upon leaving the therapy session, the parents were instructed to take M.C. to a local toy store, where he could select a reward to work for, the value of which could not exceed $5. This reward was to be kept in its package and attached somewhere in the bathroom, or to the chart, so that it could be seen by M.C. but where he could not have access to it. Immediately upon receiving his 10th star he was to be given the reward and a new chart created. M.C. was given his choice as to the type of backup reinforcer he wished to work for, be it an inexpensive toy, small amounts of money such as 10 or 25 cents for each star, or a visit to a fast food restaurant. No response cost was implemented at this point since the whole emphasis was to be on rewarding his success. In addition, the presence of FCT is a sufficient consequence for accidents.

Prior to leaving the office, the parents were provided with complete written instructions relating to the above, and data charts to keep. No matter how simplified the instructions are, it is always better to send something home with the patient and the parents so there can be no misunderstanding or confusion. They were informed that they would be called in a week or two, and a return visit was set up for approximately 2 weeks.

COURSE OF TREATMENT

During the first 4 weeks of treatment M.C. averaged five bowel movements a week into the commode, two bowel movements a week into his pants, and only one episode of staining his underpants. These data reflected improvement. However, he was having to be prompted and few of the episodes of bowel movements were self-initiated. Although occasionally upset about FCT, he was compliant with the task. The parents were encouraged to gradually reduce the frequency of their prompting to allow M.C. to become more independent in toileting behavior.

At the 6-week visit the number of stars required to obtain a backup reinforcer was increased from 10 to 15. Prompts were reduced to one to two per day. The 72-hour ER visit contingent upon the absence of a bowel movement was reinforced. M.C. expressed some frustration over having to do FCT even after a very small stain. Because the content of his verbalizations suggested the possibility of the development of a "control battle," he was reminded that the FCT was being carried out by his parents at the doctor's request and it was not their idea. He was also told, "You know, whether or not you do the full-cleanliness training is entirely up to you. When you get to the point where you are having bowel movements in the commode on a regular basis and you are no longer having accidents or stains in your pants, then you won't have to do the full-cleanliness training. So you should not be upset with your parents or even me, because everything that is happening to you is in your control." Reiterating that the child himself is in control of the contingencies helps to prevent potential difficult interactions between child and parents, and child and therapist. This helps to reinforce the notion that the child must accept the responsibility for his or her own actions, especially when it can be shown that the maladaptive behavior is controllable.

The next meeting was held approximately 5 weeks later. During the intervening weeks M.C. continued to have four to five bowel movements a week in the commode. There was one week when the family went camping and no data were collected, except that the parents reported that he had no accidents. The frequency of accidents at home was much more variable. There were 2 weeks when he had no accidents at all but the frequency would range from zero to six a week. In the weeks when he had no accidents at all, there were episodes of staining.

The next office visit noted that the parents were prompting him about twice per week. They had not assumed control of his underwear, as requested earlier in the program. They were therefore told to collect all of his underpants, to number them, and to provide them to M.C. only one pair at a time. Doing so would prevent any possibility of his hiding soiled underwear and avoiding the consequences. It also prevented situations where the parents would interrogate M.C. about his underwear and whether or not he had soiled. M.C. again seemed frustrated that he was having to do FCT even when there was a slight stain. Although he objected to this, he was compliant in carrying out the procedure at home.

Because M.C. had a tendency to "test limits," it was felt important to be very rigid about the contingencies. He was thus reminded that an agreement had been established that any indication of a bowel movement, no matter how slight, would have to be followed by FCT. He agreed that perhaps some of the stains might have been due to inadequate cleaning. He was reminded again that he was in control of this, and if he took time to clean himself appropriately there would then be no problem with having to do FCT. He understood the rationale but clearly wanted to manipulate his way out of the situation, as had been his pattern with the parents at other times.

The next visit some 6 weeks later showed that M.C. had had no episodes of soiling for 4 weeks. This was followed by four soiling episodes during a 1- to 2-week period. There had been increased prompting, which resulted in more frequent bowel movements in the commode. The contingency of going to the emergency room for an enema following 72 hours of no bowel movements was modified by the mother to 48 hours. M.C. noted that having to get 15 stars instead of 10 was a "drag." There had been evidence of independent toileting, and there was good compliance during the four cleaning episodes that were required. He was preparing to start at a new school in September. This particular visit also focused on some of M.C.'s feelings toward his younger brother, who is considered somewhat of an "all-American" boy. M.C. was questioned regarding any jealousy about his brother and any evidence of favoritism that he was aware of on the part of his parents. M.C. seemed to deny this as a significant problem, but the information presented by the mother suggested otherwise. M.C. was simply reinforced regarding his own capabilities and assets. No substantial changes were made in the program.

The next visit occurred in 6 weeks. Checking was reduced to one to two times per day. Parents found six pairs of underwear under M.C.'s bed. They acknowledged some responsibility for this because they were supposed to have secured all his underwear prior to the onset of the program. FCT training was executed by the parents for each pair of underwear found. Most of the underwear was found to be only slightly stained. M.C. continued to show evidence of independent toileting, and he had acquired 12 of 15 stars needed to receive his backup reinforcer. Some concern was generated because other children in the family asked for reinforcers. The following recommendations were made: (1) M.C. was to continue to work toward his rewards after 15 stars and then to increase the contingency to 20 stars, (2) the parents would monitor and control the underwear, (3) response-cost involving the loss of a star was to be implemented for accidents, and (4) separate reward systems would be set up for other children on the basis of appropriate behavior. It was pointed out, for example, that the children could be taken to a local restaurant as a treat for being compliant during the week. M.C. would be included in this if he had complied with his program. When it was noted that if he did not comply with the program or if he had a soiling episode he might be left at home while the rest of the family went for the treat, M.C. became somewhat upset, but it seemed to have the effect of heightening his motivation and desire to do well. The parents had neglected to keep systematic records for about 6 weeks. The necessity of maintenance of these records was emphasized, and they agreed to become more systematic.

The next visit was about 6 weeks later. M.C. had earned 20 stars for independent toileting and had received another reinforcer. There was no disruption during FCT. He had no episodes of bowel movements in his underwear; only stains were noted. In an attempt to further improve his motivation, the contingency was expanded so that if he was "perfect'— defined as being independent in his toileting and achieving an absence of any stains or bowel movements in his clothes—he would receive a large reinforcer, but if there were any episodes of encopresis, the next backup reinforcer would be somewhat diminished. Fading the star chart was discussed as being the next step in the program. M.C. was asked to call regarding his progress toward his next backup reinforcer.

About 3 weeks later M.C. successfully completed his contingency, achieved a "perfect," and received his large backup reinforcer. During the next 3 weeks there was a noticeable change in his behavior. Although he had only one episode of soiling, the frequency of bowel movements decreased to three per week. This was down from almost one per day. He had to lose a star, and the parents found themselves doing more prompting.

On his next visit it was determined that M.C. was perfectly capable of controlling his own bowel movements, and that the system was becoming somewhat cumbersome and perhaps in and of itself reinforcing M.C. in maintaining his soiling behavior. To remove the responsibility more from the parents and onto M.C. a behavioral contract was written. The contract stated: "I, M.C., agree to be admitted to the hospital if I have any problems with bowel movements, either not having enough per week, or by having accidents." The rationale for this contract was to further enhance the patient's motivation. It was clear that all that needed to be done had been done on an outpatient basis. If M.C. did not comply by remaining continent, it would mean one of two things: First, something had been missed regarding underlying organic pathology and reassessment would be required; second, there were some significant problems regarding motivation and compliance that would require evaluation on an inpatient basis. M.C. was quite taken aback by the idea of going into the hospital and vowed that he would give the program his best effort. He understood the rationale for making the recommendation and that at his age, especially after 8 months of treatment, there was no reason why he could not maintain total control of his own bowel activity. The parents were instructed to maintain control of his underwear by giving him one pair a day, thus enabling them to check for the presence of any soiling episodes. They were otherwise to impose no consequences or contingencies except for verbal feedback when M.C. appeared to be independently toileting himself. The exception to this was that he would be taken to the emergency room if he went 48 hours without a bowel movement.

TERMINATION AND FOLLOW-UP

Approximately 5 weeks after the behavioral contract was written, M.C. presented to the office. He continued to do very well in his program. He was occasionally prompted by his parents to have a bowel movement. No episodes of cleaning were required, and he was having bowel movements three or more times a week in the commode.

The follow-up schedule requires the patient to return for a brief office visit approximately every 3 months during the first year posttreatment. This would then be extended to every 6 months for the second year. Intermittent phone contacts would be made randomly. This schedule helps to give the patient and the parents the sense of continuity of care. Parents are encouraged to call if there are any problems.

OVERALL EVALUATION

In the case of M.C., the current treatment approach appears to have been effective. Except for a brief period of time when the parents did not collect data regarding soiling episodes, compliance with the program did not appear to be a problem. The parents were grateful for the frequency of contact and the intermittent phone calls, which allowed them to feel that the therapist was accessible.

M.C. seemed somewhat happier and certainly relieved not to be having to worry about cleaning his clothes. No specific assessment was made of the interaction pattern between M.C. and his parents, but casual observation suggested that it was more reinforcing than it had been in the past. It is interesting to note that M.C. never had to be taken to the emergency room for an enema. The possibility of this seemed to be powerful enough to encourage M.C. to do whatever was necessary to avoid retention.

M.C. was rather verbal and somewhat precocious. Like some children, he always had an explanation for everything that occurred and seemed to question each recommendation. It is very important that the therapist maintain control in this kind of a situation and not engage in a "verbal debate" with the patient. Specifying the contingencies in a clean precise manner with an expression of understanding and caring is important. "Verbal debates" are often reinforcing to this type of child and distract from the main emphasis of treatment.

REFERENCES

American Psychiatric Association. (1980). *Diagnostic and statistical manual of mental disorders* (3rd ed.). Washington DC: Author.

Anthony, C. P. (1963). *Textbook of anatomy and physiology* (6th ed.). St. Louis: Mosby.

Bellman, M. (1966). Studies on encopresis. *Acta Paediatrica Scandinavica, Supplement,* No. 70.

Gaston, E. A. (1948). The physiology of fecal incontinence. *Surgery, Gynecology and Obstetrics, 86,* 280–290.

Levine, M. D. (1975). Children with encopresis: A descriptive analysis. *Pediatrics, 56,* 412–416.

CHAPTER 27

Drug Abuse

GEARY S. ALFORD

DESCRIPTION OF THE DISORDER

Chemical substance use and misuse is a widespread and common practice among the adolescent population. According to surveys by the National Institute on Drug Abuse, some 70% of 1985 high school seniors admitted using alcohol at least once a month, 25% report such marijuana use, and 10 to 15% admit at least monthly use of stimulants (including cocaine). Percentages of at least monthly use are 2.5 for hallucinogens; 2.0 for sedative-anxiolytics, and 0.5 for narcotic analgesics. Approximately 5% of these students admitted *daily* use of alcohol and/or marijuana. All of these drugs, of course, exert potently disruptive effects on the central nervous system. Their abuse frequently results in maladaptive and dysfunctional cognitive and affectual as well as sensorimotor behavior, thereby impairing learning, memory, reasoning, emotional reactivity, and verbal, motor, and social skills. Some recent studies indicate that about 50% of young suicides involve chronic substance abusers (e.g., Fowler, Rich, & Young, 1986), while 80 to 90% of vehicular accidents among 16- to 20-year-old drivers is associated with drinking (Grundy, 1984). Such data support the conclusion that drug abuse has indeed reached epidemic proportions, resulting in a wide range of behavioral impairments and even catastrophic consequences for many adolescents.

In spite of its more operationalized format, the current *Diagnostic and Statistical Manual* (DSM-III; American Psychiatric Association,

GEARY S. ALFORD • Department of Psychiatry and Human Behavior, and Department of Pharmacology and Toxicology, University of Mississippi Medical Center, 2400 North State Street, Jackson, Mississippi 39216–4505.

1980) is far from satisfactory. For example, one DSM-III criterion for cannabis (marijuana) abuse, not to mention *dependence,* stipulates "use of cannabis nearly every day for at least one month." An adolescent who smoked marijuana heavily on weekends but only once in the middle of the week would not technically meet that test. However, since the metabolic half-life of delta-9 THC (the most potent psychoactive compound of the more than 450 chemical compounds in marijuana smoke) is some 60 to 70 hours, that student would, in fact, remain at least partially neurochemically intoxicated (although not necessarily subjectively perceived as "high") 100% of the time. The most fundamental and critical issue in chemical substance misuse is the extent to which chemical use of any amount on any schedule results in a pattern of significant adverse consequences in a person's life. Thus, the following definitions are suggested. *Misuse* is the self-administration of a psychoactive chemical compound of such a pharmacologic class and/or in such a manner in which a high probability of severe adverse consequences exists. *Dependence* is the continued use of such a compound and/or in such a manner in spite of severe adverse consequences that have occurred. Put another way, chemical dependency can be defined as *a relatively enduring pattern of use of some psychoactive substance, which use has contributed to or has directly resulted in severe, adverse, aversive consequences and which consequences have not led to reliable and enduring modification of usage pattern of that or similarly acting substances such that no further significant adverse consequences of use have occurred or have an objectively demonstrable high probability of resulting from such usage.* In contrast to DSM-III, this definition does not stipulate any specific quantity or frequency of use but focuses upon the pattern of use and the pattern of adverse consequences resulting from that use.

CASE IDENTIFICATION

The case chosen to illustrate assessment and treatment of adolescent drug dependency is that of a 16-year-old male, referred to in this chapter as "Tom." At the time of admission, Tom was 16 years old and lived at home with his mother, his father, and a younger brother, whose age was 12. A 19-year-old sister was away at college, but occasionally spent weekends at home. Both of Tom's parents were college graduates; his father owned a successful independent insurance agency where his mother worked part time, together providing the family with an above-average, though not lavish, income and standard of living. The parents appeared to be rather conventional and conservative in outlook, described themselves as light social drinkers, attended church "pretty regularly," and reported no history of alcoholism or drug abuse in their immediate forebears. Tom's medical history included the usual childhood diseases and a fractured right clavical from junior high football. This was his first hospitalization. His parents reported that up through the eighth grade Tom had been "not what you would call an ideal student, but most of his grades were above average." During his 10th-grade year, Tom's grades began to go down, and by the end of that year he had failed both Algebra II and English, which he then had to repeat in summer school. When the parents talked with a school counselor, they learned that Tom had several absences and occasions of leaving school early on the basis of forged notes from them. Further, the counselor reinforced the parents' own suspicions that several of Tom's friends were strongly suspected (by teachers and school counselors) as being involved in drug and alcohol abuse. Tom's behavior at home had gradually become more withdrawn and secretive, while his moods varied from pleasant and nonchalant to emotionally overreactive, angry, sullen, or depressed. Because of his declining school performance and "don't give a damn—general bad attitude," Tom's parents took him to a child psychiatrist, who reportedly diagnosed Tom as depressed and prescribed antidepressant medication and recommended weekly psychotherapy. Tom's parents were reluctant for Tom to take medication and subsequently took Tom to a psychologist, who worked out a therapeutic contract with Tom and his parents essentially involving a token economic program designed to increase Tom's study behavior. That lasted throughout the summer school session until he passed both algebra and English, receiving a D and a C, respectively. Both the psychiatrist and the psychologist had admitted to Tom's parents that he "probably" had used alcohol and marijuana "on occasion," but that he was not "dependent" or "what we would call an abuser" and that drugs were not the problem. The mood swings, along with the school problems, were attributed to "depression" by the psychiatrist and to "a developmental phase" by the psychologist.

Tom's grades for the first 6 weeks of his junior year were better but then declined, although he passed all his courses for the first semester. Shortly after the beginning of the second school semester, Tom was involved in a single-car automobile accident in which he was the driver. Police found beer cans, drug paraphernalia, and a small quantity of marijuana in the car. Although Tom, who subsequently had difficulty recalling the actual accident, adamantly claimed that the marijuana and paraphernalia belonged to his friends who had been with him in the car, his parents brought him in for a consultation and evaluation.

Tom and his parents were interviewed initially together, the parents recounting the history described above. Tom was then interviewed alone. Aside from minor disagreements about his parents' depiction of his moods, he acknowledged the essential accuracy of his parents' report. Tom also admitted that he drank, that he "got drunk sometimes," that he smoked marijuana "once in a while," and that he had "tried coke (cocaine) a couple of times." He stated that this was no more drinking or drug use than "any of the other guys."

ASSESSMENT

Initial assessment included a complete medical history and physical examination, chest X ray, SMA-18, and drug screen. Medical examination revealed a history of usual childhood illnesses, and an old healed fracture of the right clavical from a football injury. Review of systems was negative, except for some needle marks on his left arm. Drug screen revealed metabolites of amphetamine-type stimulant and of tetrahydrocannabinol (marijuana), but other laboratory studies were within normal limits or negative. On mental status examination, Tom appeared somewhat anxious and irritable, and tended to respond with vague answers when questioned about his chemical use history. When asked about the needle marks on his arm, Tom at first denied there were any needle marks but then admitted that he had used cocaine intravenously "a few times." He exhibited no primary symptoms or signs of major thought or major affective disorder, and mental status examination at time of admission was otherwise considered within normal limits. Although his drug history did not indicate that Tom had developed sufficient tolerance to a drug class that required systematic detoxification, the admitting physician placed Tom on a low dose of Tranxene—three doses the first day, two the second, and one the third, then discontinued.

With written consent and authorization of both Tom and his parents, all of Tom's school records were obtained for the 5 years immediately preceding admission (i.e., grades 7 through part of 11). Each parent was asked to give a careful and detailed history of Tom's behavior both through interviews and in written questionnaires. Tom's older sister was scheduled for similar interviews and questionnaires. Several days after completing the detoxification phase (in Tom's case, 3 days of "detoxification" on Tranxene), Tom was administered a Minnesota Multiphasic Personality Inventory (MMPI) and the Shipley Institute of Living Scale. In the Shipley, Tom scored in the above-average range on the vocabulary section but only in the average range on the abstract reasoning section.

Responses on the MMPI yielded an invalid profile, with an *F*-scale *T* score of 50 and a *K*-scale *T* score above 70.

As will be seen below, the bulk of information gathered about Tom indicated a relatively long history of chemical substance abuse and an associated pattern of significant adverse life experiences and events resulting from that chemical abuse. Both the chemical use pattern and the adverse consequences had intensified over time, particularly in the several months preceeding admission. Tom was diagnosed as chemically dependent.

SELECTION OF TREATMENT

I have elsewhere suggested (Alford & Fairbank, 1985) that problematic behaviors associated with various biobehavioral disorders can be usefully considered within four general categories of behavior:

Problems associated with behavioral skill repertoire include those behavioral problems that result from patients lacking specific *sets* of skills requisite to their natural environmental conditions (e.g., various types of educational, occupational, technical, or social skills deficits) and/or from patients having acquired and developed ineffectual, inappropriate, maladaptive behavioral skills (e.g., abusive child-rearing practices, offensive social behaviors).

Problems associated with conditioned emotional, autonomically mediated reactions include those behavioral events whose fundamental components entail essentially conditioned reflexive elements (e.g., simple, discrete phobic reactions; inadequate, inhibited, or deviant sexual arousal; excitatory arousal to drug paraphernalia). Specifically excluded from this category are affectual reactions that result directly from problems of other categories (e.g., frustration over unemployment due to occupational skills deficits), except, of course, where conditioned autonomically mediated elements can be demonstrated as a significant component of the overall behavioral problem (e.g., a client may have a conditioned anxiety response to the stimuli present in a job-interview setting *and* may also have anxiety secondary to lacking appropriate, effective job-interview social skills).

Problems associated with cognitive content and information processing, including secondary affectual behaviors, include maladaptive or aversive behaviors that result from inaccurate perception or interpretation of stimulus events; fallacious or illogical information processing; erroneous information or beliefs; and emotional reactions associated with those cognitive contents and processing (e.g., invalid, negativistic self-perceptions; lack of self-efficacy; nonpsychotic paranoid beliefs about other people).

Problems associated with identified or probable organic pathology include such problems as major thought and major affective psychoses, as well as physical addiction and drug-induced cognitive-affectual dysfunction.

Complex clinical problems may entail any combination or permutation of these categories. Thus, various behavioral systems and components of Tom's chemical dependency were examined within the context of these subcategories, each of which is addressed with different therapeutic strategies.

The treatment issue initially confronted in cases of substance abuse disorder is the question of physiological tolerance and need for detoxification (i.e., a Category IV biobehavioral problem). In Tom's case, his history did not indicate a need for a standard detoxification protocol. Nevertheless, the admitting physician did prescribe a brief course of a low dose of an anxiolytic, and Tom was monitored for any signs of abstinence syndrome. Such monitoring is customary since many patients, at the time of admission, tend to deny the actual nature and extent of their chemical use while some other patients tend to exaggerate their use. A second Category IV problem often present in chemical abusers is drug-induced acute organic brain dysfunction, which may vary from simple intoxication to schizophreniform psychosis. Chronic organic brain syndromes are relatively rare in adolescent abusers. Finally, with respect to behavioral problems associated with organic pathology, some adolescents do have a major thought disorder, schizophrenia, which will usually require pharmacotherapy during the course of treatment for their chemical dependency. It should be stressed, however, that many drug-abusing patients who exhibit signs and symptoms of major thought or major affective disorders, in fact, have drug-induced psychotic symptoms and do not have a chronic, endogenous psychotic disorder. It is, therefore, absolutely necessary for clinicians to evaluate such patients carefully in extended, drug-free conditions before assigning such a diagnosis. Fortunately, Tom's chemical abuse had not yet resulted in the active psychoses commonly associated with certain pharmacologic classes, especially stimulants, nor did he require a protracted, systematic detoxification in order to avoid a physiological abstinence syndrome.

During the week following detoxification, Tom, influenced by other patients on the adolescent unit as well as by his counselors, began to reveal more and more information about his drug history. He admitted that he started smoking marijuana and drinking alcohol "once in a while" during the spring of his 9th-grade year in school. The frequency and quantity of use increased substantially during the summer, subsided somewhat at the beginning of the school year, but then accelerated over the first semester of the 10th grade. By early in the spring semester, Tom was not only smoking marijuana regularly, "four to six joints on the weekend" and "once in a while during the week," but had begun using the stimulant "Ecstasy" or "X" (methylenedioxyamphetamine) at a frequency of "about one or two hits on weekends but not every weekend." This usage pattern reportedly persisted throughout the rest of that school year, across the summer months, and intermittently included alcohol intoxications and abuse of narcotic analgesics. During the fall of the 11th grade, Tom began "experimenting" with cocaine and subsequently turned to intravenous use of cocaine since neither "Ecstasy" nor "snorting" cocaine gave him the "rush" or "high" he desired.

This history, along with that provided by family reports and documented school records, formed the basis for initial evaluation and eventual intervention into many of Tom's Category III problem behaviors. First, Tom, like most adolescent patients, came into treatment with a kind of street-wise knowledge of pharmacology, most of which was incomplete, inaccurate, and even mythical. For example, while acknowledging that intravenous use of cocaine "might be a problem," Tom adamantly denied that marijuana smoking posed any more of a danger than "my old man's having a couple of cocktails." He thought "Ecstasy" was some sort of "pretty safe upper . . . it's not like speed, you know!" And "All my friends drink," he claimed." "I don't drink any more than anybody else."

Second, Tom tended to deny or minimize the relationships between his chemical use and many adverse life events. His decreasing school grades, he claimed, had more to do with his "being lazy," his loss of interest, and the "boring bullshit" being taught than with his drug usage. He admitted that he had experienced frequent feelings of depression, some profound and suicidal, but then argued that it was *because* of such feelings that he had increased his drug use. He viewed the conflicts with his family as normal and routine for any teenager. He denied any relationship between drug use and the automobile accident.

Third, at a more global level, Tom tended to talk and act as if external realities were true only to the extent that an individual personally believes them to be true. He did not, of course, explicitly endorse such a cosmology. However, such information processing was implicit in many of his statements. He would, for example, dismiss well-established scientific research findings with a cavalier "Well, that's what they think; everybody has a right to his own opinion," or "Maybe that's what marijuana docs to some people, but it doesn't affect my brain that way." Occasionally, he would come close to explicit acknowledgment of such thinking: "If somebody believes something, then, for them it's real." Similarly, Tom resented and tended to rebel against almost anything that he viewed as attempts to limit or constrain his personal freedoms: "Nothing and nobody is going to tell me what to do;" "I'm sick and tired of everybody else trying to run my life." In association with such attitudes, Tom reported and exhibited signs of much frustration, anger, and volatile temper.

The pattern of Tom's drug history, the development of dependence, and the multiple adverse, aversive consequences of that use are, in many ways, fairly typical (see Alford, 1981, in press). All drugs of abuse have properties of instating very pleasurable sensations and subjective states of well-being. Most are also capable of relieving aversive sensations or unpleasant moods and affectual states. Unfortunately, all such drugs when misused disrupt and impair normal neurological functioning, thereby resulting in abnormal and maladaptive sensory, cognitive, affectual, and overt behaviors. Dysfunctional behaviors further contribute to major problems in living. While most of the pleasurable, desirable (positively and negatively reinforcing) consequences occur immediately, are highly salient and detectable, and have a subjectively experienced high probability of occurring, most of the more aversive consequences tend to be delayed, tend to develop gradually, thus are often not initially easily detectable, and thus are frequently viewed by users as rather improbable. Therefore, by the time the more potent, salient, and highly aversive events do occur and chemical abusers enter treatment, there have usually been literally hundreds and sometimes thousands of pairings of chemical use stimuli (drug itself, paraphernalia, settings, cognitions, behavior of actual intake) with the pleasurable, reinforcing stimulus events. It should not be surprising, then, that chemical misuse has become a highly reinforced, well-established behavior pattern and one that entails components of classical conditioning as well.

Further, some drug-abusing adolescents have failed to develop the social skills appropriate to (therefore, necessary for) interaction with "normal," "straight" peers. Tom, for example, had begun dating in junior high school, but as his chemical use accelerated, he reportedly appeared to lose interest in dating, preferring to spend most of his free time with his male drug-using companions. During the course of his hospitalization, it became evident that Tom's behavior toward the age-equivalent female patients was unskillful and at times offensive. For example, he either avoided casual socializing with older female adolescents (preferring to interact with the 13- or 14-year-old girls) or he would, at times, engage in horseplay that the older girls found offensive (e.g., he once poured a cup of ice down inside a 17-year-old female patient's blouse). The 15- to

18-year-old female patients privately described Tom as "like a little kid," "immature," and "a nerd." Through the course of treatment, Tom eventually acknowledged that he was uncomfortable, unsure of himself, and "too nervous" around (age-equivalent) girls, although, he claimed, "I was never *this* uptight back when I was dating." He claimed a heterosexual arousal pattern and denied any homosexual feelings or experiences.

The high positive valence of drug using stimuli and the anxiety (aversive autonomic arousal) Tom reported and appeared to exhibit in heterosocial interactions were considered to be (but not exclusively) Category II-type problems. Some fraction of Tom's discomfort was considered to result from his Category I deficient and inappropriate social skills. Another Category I problem later discovered was grossly deficient study habits.

COURSE OF TREATMENT

The inpatient phases of Tom's treatment occurred in a 70-bed drug and alcohol unit located on the grounds of the 500-bed general hospital with which it was associated. The adolescent unit averaged 20 patients at a time whose ages ranged from 12 to 18. Many of the treatment activities, such as lectures, films, reading groups, and certain group therapy sessions, were conducted together with the adult patients. There were, however, special group therapy sessions and films—lectures followed by discussion groups specifically for adolescents. A typical day in this facility would include the following:

9:00 a.m.: Film or lecture presentation addressing some aspect of chemical abuse and dependency. These topics included elementary psychopharmacology (e.g., half-life and duration of action of tetrahydrocannabinol, drug effects on the brain and various behavioral systems, physical and medical pathology and diseases caused by drug toxicity), familial and social problems, legal and scholastic-occupational problems, and similar subjects.

10:30–12:00: Group therapy—with patients from the adult unit, 8 to 12 patients per group.

1:00–1:30: Reading group—small groups of patients discussing selected readings.

1:30–5:00: Free time—During free time patients may walk around on a special parklike portion of the hospital grounds, take scheduled trips to a local "Y" at which certain hours have been reserved for patients, and generally relax. However, it is during this "free-time" period that each patient meets for individual counseling, and patients are required to complete reading and written assignments at some time during the afternoon or evening free-time periods.

Individual Counseling: 30 minutes to 1 hour, 3 to 5 days a week. Occasional counseling sessions last 2 or more hours, such as during conferences with family members. These scheduled individual therapy sessions, of course, take precedence over any other free-time activity.

6:00–7:00: Film, lecture presentation, special group therapy/discussion, or Alcoholics Anonymous (AA) or Narcotics Anonymous (NA) speakers.

These daily activities are designed to address primarily Category III problems. For example, films and lecture presentations by staff psychologists, pharmacologists, and physicians not only educate patients in plain, straightforward language about chemical substances, their actions, and their effects, but they also disabuse patients of misinformation and erroneous beliefs. For example, it never occurs to most adolescents that such factors as chemical half-lives—hence, durations of action—play a major role in many drugs' adverse consequences. Tom's father's cocktail has a half-life of only a few minutes, with only a couple of hours' duration of action. Tom's marijuana (i.e., THC) has a 60- to 70-hour half-life, thus, several days' duration of action. It is impossible to smoke a couple of "joints" on Friday and Saturday and go to class Monday morning with no THC and metabolites on board. It is not true that "Ecstasy" is "not like 'speed,' you know." "Ecstasy" is methylenedioxyamphetamine. It *is* "speed"! Tom, like many patients, failed to understand fully that stimulant use produces depression and, more generally, that disruptive effects of most drugs of abuse are not confined to specific times of intoxication but occur during withdrawal phases and often well beyond. Most patients fail to appreciate the full range of adverse effects, that those effects are "natural law" properties of those compounds upon human brain and other tissues, and that they are thus not avoidable by individual personal attributes such as intelligence or willpower (i.e., that patients, as individuals, cannot abuse those compounds and somehow magically avoid the adverse, aversive effects of such abuse).

Information presented in film-lecture format is "personalized" for each patient within both group and individual counseling sessions. In group therapy, patients call attention, among other things, to how closely each other's personal histories correspond to the facts, figures, and realities presented. The individual counselor carefully and repeatedly reviewed with Tom all that had been learned of his drug history and its relationships to the variety of very aversive life events that resulted directly or indirectly from that use. Tom, as noted earlier, initially tended to deny such relationships, disassociating such things as declining school performance, family conflicts, and his automobile accident from his chemical abuse. He cited alleged statements by the psychologist and the psychiatrist he had briefly seen that it was the depression that caused him to abuse stimulants, not the stimulants that caused (or at least greatly exacerbated) the depression. He denied that he could not "control" his drug usage, pointing out that he sometimes went several days without using. His understandable ignorance of elementary pharmacokinetics contributed to his denial system, as did his own personal, subjective experience. He initially could not understand how smoking marijuana on weekends or in the evening could have exerted any influence "during the week" or "the next day when I wasn't high." He correctly noted that his drinking and marijuana smoking had begun long before there was any significant change in his grades. Through a cognitive-behavioral approach, counselors reviewed and rereviewed all of the scientific information, parental reports, school records and his own self-reports, concentrating on developing an accurate account of his drug-using history and its effects in his life. In addition, information provided in lectures, films, and reading material, or generated in group therapy was *personalized*. That is, the counselor repeatedly drew attention to how various facts from the patient's own life both exemplified and verified the scientific information and the life patterns reported by other patients and by outside NA speakers.

The following is a brief excerpt from a session with Tom that occurred approximately 2 weeks after admission. It exemplifies some of the stylistic and confrontational aspects of drug counseling.

THERAPIST: Let's talk some more about your drug history.

TOM: Shit, not again! How many times do we have to do that?

THERAPIST: We have gone over it several times, haven't we. But we keep getting more information and finding out new things. For example, you've now seen a couple of more films and heard Dr. Y's lectures on drug effects, and, last night, Bob C's story sounded a lot like your own. What do you think?

TOM: About that guy? I don't know whether to believe him or not. His story sounded kind of made up.

THERAPIST: How do you mean, "made up"?

TOM: Oh, all that shit about what a great athlete and good student and big success he was before he did drugs. How do we know he wasn't a dumb shit nerd before?

THERAPIST: Do you remember Bob saying he had once been a patient here about seven years ago?

TOM: Yeah, he said that.

THERAPIST: Well, I was on the staff here then, although I was not his counselor. I know he had gotten a football scholarship to college and I'm pretty sure that his grades had been at least average. What he tells in his "drug-alog" is pretty much what I remember about him.

TOM: O.K. but that doesn't mean what happened to him is what happened to me.

THERAPIST: Tom, do you still believe that you are somehow special or different, that drugs don't affect you the way they affect other people?

TOM: I never said I was special. I just said that everybody's not the same. Some people don't have much willpower.

THERAPIST: Yes, I remember your saying that you have a lot of willpower. Tom, do you think something like gravity affects people with a lot of willpower differently from the way it affects people with less willpower?

TOM: Of course not. But gravity is a physical force.

THERAPIST: So whether you have a lot or a little willpower or whether or not you even believe in the gravity makes no difference in gravity's effects on you.

TOM: No, but so what? I don't see what you are getting at.

THERAPIST: O.K., let me explain. Several films and Dr. Y's lectures have presented scientific evidence on the biochemistry and pharmacology of drugs. Now, chemistry and neurophysiology and psychopharmacology are not as neat, clean, and obvious as laws of gravity, but they too are what you called "physical." They also obey natural laws. If willpower can't stop gravity, how can willpower stop say, cyanide from killing you?

TOM: Who said anything about cyanide? I never used cyanide. Nobody uses cyanide.

THERAPIST: No you never used cyanide, but if you had, even just once to see what kind of high it might produce, you wouldn't be here now, regardless of all your willpower. You have used other drugs that have the chemical properties of disrupting normal brain functions and that can even kill you.

TOM: So, they change your brain.

THERAPIST: Tom, they not only change your brain, they change *your* brain in the *same* ways they change other people's brains. And, therefore, they produce the same kinds of effects on *your* thinking, *your* emotions, and *your* overt behavior that they produce in other people.

TOM: They do if you let them.

THERAPIST: What do you mean "if you let them"? Aren't you still trying to say that willpower, especially your willpower, can change natural laws, that you can will a drug not to react and not to affect your brain and thus your behavior the way that chemicals, obeying the laws of chemistry and biology, affect other people?

TOM: I never said that some of the effects weren't the same.

THERAPIST: Fair enough; let's look at some of those same effects. Dr. Y carefully described how drugs affect brain functions and the kinds of behavioral problems and problems in living that typically result. Bob's story fits that pattern pretty closely, wouldn't you agree?

TOM: Yeah, that's another reason why I wasn't sure whether to believe him or not. It's like, maybe Dr. Y told him what to say.

THERAPIST: Have you talked with some of the other patients here about their drug and life histories?

TOM: Sure.

THERAPIST: Don't most of their histories fit the pattern?

TOM: Some of them, I guess.

THERAPIST: Now, let's go over your own history again. (The therapist and Tom then review his own history and the particular problems Tom has experienced.)

THERAPIST: Dr. Y didn't tell *you* what to say, did he?

TOM: I've never talked with him.

THERAPIST: Yet doesn't your own history include many of the same kinds of things he described and that Bob and others have reported about their own lives?

Patients do not, of course, suddenly acknowledge, much less accept, all of the multiple and diverse relationships between and among substance abuse behaviors and internal and/or environmental adverse, aversive problems in living. Instead, it is usually a gradual process of examining and reexamining the facts and the evidence, a process during which the therapist also encourages patients to explore and talk about their feelings about those multiple, adverse experiences. The following are major aspects of film-lecture, reading assignments, and group and individual counseling:

1. Establishing a factual knowledge base about chemical substances and their multiple effects from brain to molar behaviors and to correct misinformation.

2. Fully identifying each patient's own drug use history and related problematic covert and overt behaviors.

3. Clarifying and making explicit as possible the relationships involving drug use, drug actions, and specific consequences in each patient's experiences and life; also, by encouraging emotive behavior associated with those life events, establishing and reinforcing cognitive-affectual mediation between drug abuse and negative, adverse, aversive consequences. Exposure to other patients whose personal histories usually share many elements further reinforces drug use–aversive consequence relationships. Older patients and outside speakers, whose personal histories closely parallel those of most younger patients up to a point, often report extremely painful, even catastrophic events that they subsequently personally experienced, but which most younger, adolescent patients have not yet suffered. Such exposure again exemplifies and supports what patients are learning about chemical abuse and its effects in their own lives, and also vividly exposes those patients to the kinds of further miseries that lie ahead if substance abuse continues. In addition to addressing Category III targets, it can be seen that these procedures also involve elements of Category II: Repeatedly emotion-laden review of personal drug abuse—adverse consequences histories can be viewed as involving covert conditioning, while exposure to other patients and to outside speakers from Narcotics Anonymous involves vicarious condi-

tioning (and, in the case of NA speakers, provides models for drug-free life-styles since those speakers also note their more adaptive, successful, and rewarding postdrug lives). Such therapeutic learning-conditioning procedures are intended to at least partially vitiate the long positive-reinforcement history of chemical abuse.

4. Identifying and modifying stylistic or "personality" factors that appear to play a role in maladaptive behaviors. In the brief vignette reproduced above, for example, the therapist addressed Tom's tendency to behave as if he believed that his own willpower could alter, if not obviate, natural biological laws, and Tom's related tendency to view himself as somehow different from the average human being such that what happens to normal, average people had little relevance to, or implication for, him. Both of these personality-type factors were related to an even more global cognitive behavior pattern. Tom argued quite logically and correctly that if people believe something to be true, they tend to behave as if it were true/real, i.e., in a fashion consistent with that belief (Tom's wording was "If somebody believes something, then for them its real"). The ambiguity in Tom's wording, however, suggests an incorrect, illogical component in his cosmology. He frequently spoke and acted in a manner that clearly implied that the actual external existence or validity of something was dependent upon his belief in it. Allied with this epistemological fallacy was his apparent assumption that external events could be directly affected by cognitive or emotive behavior. For example, Tom rather frequently made statements or comments such as the one cited in the dialogue above: When commenting on the behavioral pharmacologic properties of drugs and whether those drugs might affect his brain and behavior consistent with those properties, he had replied, "They do if you let them." Let me make clear that the issue here was not whether you take a drug or not, but, once it is ingested, whether one can volitionally *will* changes in the biochemical and physiological actions of those chemical compounds. Such notions are integrally involved in the belief that someone can habitually misuse chemical compounds but not suffer the aversive consequences because of his or her unusual willpower, intelligence, or other special personal characteristics. The fact that most of the highly aversive consequences indeed tend to be delayed, tend to develop relatively gradually, are often initially difficult to detect by the user, and even when detected tend to be misattributed to nondrug causes subjectively supports such notions. These and other Category III behavioral problems were addressed with Tom as briefly described above and as more thoroughly described in Alford and Fairbank (1985).

Tom progressed in becoming increasingly aware of his actual drug history and its central role in most of the adverse, maladaptive, and subjectively aversive events of his life since initiating drug abuse. He began to see that while he was of above-average intelligence and physically quite strong, he was fundamentally a rather ordinary, average mortal upon whom natural law (including chemical, biological, and psychological principles) acted just as it did upon other people. This received special reinforcement from an orthopedic surgeon who was in group therapy with Tom. This surgeon described how, being a physician and having had advanced training in pharmacology, he had somehow convinced himself that he could use medications (to treat his "stress' and "frequent headaches," which turned out to be alcohol hangovers) in ways ordinary people could not. He was in treatment for alcoholism and narcotic dependency. Tom went through a period of depression with feelings of guilt and remorse and with apprehension about his future, afraid that he had lost so much ground and was so far behind in school that he might be unable to catch up. Through adolescent group therapy and casual interaction on the unit, Tom became increasingly aware that most of the older adolescent females not only were not attracted to him but found him and his antics rather offensive. Tom was allowed to "grieve," and, of course, these negative affects were paired (cognitively affectually) with drug-abuse stimuli and behaviors. However, he was also encouraged about his "drug-free future" (aversion relief), along with guidance in developing practical plans. Continued exposure to NA speakers facilitated and reinforced these more optimistic views through hearing their various posttreatment, drug-free successes.

Approximately 6 weeks after Tom's hospital admission, he was transferred to a closely supervised halfway house operated by the hospital. In addition to continued daily group therepy and less frequent individual counseling sessions, several Category I and II problems were targeted. First, Tom reported that when seeing the small syringe a diabetic patient used to give herself insulin injections, he would feel a sudden excitement and transient urge to use "like just before I shot up coke." Second, he described a psychophysiological reaction (rapid heartbeat, dry mouth, muscle tension) when around female patients. In addition, Tom not only evidenced aversive-arousal-induced performance problems, he appeared to have repertorial social-skills deficits as well. Finally, through academic counseling in the special education program that halfway house adolescents attend, it was discovered that Tom had unusually poor study skills. Throughout the course of time in the halfway house, random drug screens are obtained on all patients.

A covert aversion procedure (e.g., Cautela, 1967) was designed to reduce the conditioned reflexive responses to sight of syringes. Put simply, images of syringes and other drug paraphernalia were repeatedly paired with aversive images drawn as much as possible from realistic events (e.g., scenes of overdose and death). During this treatment, Tom was also instructed to wear a rubber band on his wrist and to snap the rubber band whenever he saw or even thought about syringes or other paraphernalia (e.g., "roach clips"). Following 11 sessions of covert aversion, along with the rubber band tactic over a 3-week period, Tom reported few positive or negative feelings at seeing a syringe.

Because Tom's social behavior appeared to involve both a phobic component (Category II) and social-skill repertoire deficits and excesses (Category I), a brief course of systematic desensitization (Wolpe & Lazarus, 1966) was conducted. Tom was also enrolled in an adolescent skills training program with particular emphasis on heterosexual interaction and dating. This program was being conducted by a local medical school adolescent psychology division and entailed the usual behavioral social skills training methods (see Kelly, 1982).

Tom's study skills were addressed in straightforward fashion by applying simple human learning principles. For example, Tom was taught not only how to take effective notes from a teacher's lectures but also how to read and then reread while outlining or taking notes from reading material. The importance of not simply copying verbatim but of abstracting and translating material into his own language (i.e., idiosyncratic organizational and coding operations) was stressed, along with the most important human learning variable, *practice* (how to systematically review, rehearse, and associate-integrate new material into that previously learned).

TERMINATION AND FOLLOW-UP

After spending 3 months in the halfway house, Tom was discharged to return to live with his parents. He enrolled in summer school, taking two subjects, English and geometry, which he did not want to have to repeat the following school year. He earned a B in both courses and was given credit for a history course that he had completed in the special education program. However, to his disappointment, his regular high school required him to repeat the 11th grade, albeit with a lighter load since he received credit for 11th-grade English along with geometry and history. Tom reportedly attended NA meetings regularly, although not so frequently as had been recommended. He graduated from high school almost 2 years to the day after his discharge from the halfway house. Tom attended a local college for 2 years, then transferred to an out-of-state university, at which point follow-up contact ended. However, approximately 7 years after discharge, Tom's father renewed contact regarding some medical-psychological record he needed (he was giving Tom a paid-up life insurance policy as a wedding present). Tom, it turned out, had graduated from college and was working as a computer sales representative in another city. Tom was getting married, was quitting that job, which he did not like, and, having been accepted, was to begin law school the following fall. According to his father, Tom had shown no sign or evidence of subsequent drug use.

OVERALL EVALUATION

This case was chosen not only because it was, of course, a treatment success, but also because it exemplifies a multicomponent treatment package in which categories of problem behaviors are addressed with procedures most appropriate to the elements, processes, and behavioral systems involved in those diverse, but overlapping, categories of behavior. This patient's chemical dependency was not conceptualized either as a symptom of something else or as a natural consequence of environmental factors (i.e., as *influenced* but not *controlled* by environmental stimuli). Indeed, every effort was made to disabuse the patient of such notions. Instead, the patient was encouraged to view his drug-abuse history as having produced a biobehavioral disorder (by the way, considered no more or no less a "disease" than, say, anxiety, depressive, or eating "disorders"). While therapy focused on the cognitive, affectual, and overt behavioral components of chemical misuse and dependency, attention was also paid to additional behavioral problems the patient brought in, some, but not necessarily all, of which were significantly interactive with chemical abuse *per se*. Most chemically dependent adolescent patients bring into treatment similar arrays of behavioral problems and their chemical use–adverse life experience patterns share many elements with the present case.

REFERENCES

Alford, G. S. (1981). Hypnotics, sedatives, and minor tranquilizers. In S. J. Mulé (Ed.), *Behavior in excesses: An examination of the volitional disorders*. New York: Macmillan-Free Press.

Alford, G. S. (in press). Substance abuse disorders. In G. Hsu & M. Hersen (Eds.), *Recent developments in adolescent psychiatry*. New York: Wiley.

Alford, G. S., & Fairbank, J. A. (1985). Personality disorders. In M. Hersen (Ed.), *Practice of inpatient behavior therapy: A clinical guide* (173–199). Orlando: Grune and Stratton.

American Psychiatric Association. (1980). *Diagnostic and statistical manual of mental disorders* (3rd ed.). Washington, DC: Author.

Cautela, J. R. (1967). Covert sensitization. *Psychological Reports, 10,* 459–468.

Fowler, R. C., Rich, C. L., & Young, D. (1986). San Diego suicide study: Substance abuse in young cases. *Archives of General Psychiatry, 43,* 962–965.

Grundy, P. (1984). Deaths decline but drunk driving, other traffic safety hazards remain medical news. *Journal of the American Medical Association, 251,* 1645–1647.

Kelly, J. A. (1982). Social skills training: A practical guide for intervention. New York: Springer-Verlag.

Wolpe, J., & Lazarus, A. A. (1966). *Behavior therapy techniques: A guide to the treatment of neuroses.* New York: Pergamon Press.

CHAPTER 28

Somatoform Disorders

ANDRES J. PUMARIEGA and PAUL M. CINCIRIPINI

DESCRIPTION OF THE DISORDER

Somatoform disorders are a category of psychiatric diagnoses in which the symptomatology is suggestive of a physical disorder but supporting physical findings are not apparent. The symptoms seem involuntary, and positive evidence of contributing psychological factors are often present. In the *Diagnostic and Statistical Manual* (American Psychiatric Association, 1980), somatoform disorders refer to a family of diagnostic entities including somatization disorder (300.81), conversion disorder (300.11), psychogenic pain disorder (307.80), hypochondriasis (300.70), and atypical somatoform disorder (300.70).

Somatization disorder (300.81), also known as Briquet's syndrome, is chronic and polysymptomatic. It may involve multiple organ systems and span an individual's life history. Woodruff, Clayton, and Guze (1971) reported that the prevalence of somatoform disorders in the adult female population was 0.9 to 2%. Although the disorder is thought to begin in childhood and adolescence, prevalence statistics in this age group are lacking (Williams, 1985). The literature suggests that the incidence of single-symptom somatoform disorders in children and adolescents is probably quite high, possibly higher than in adults. Single-symptom somatoform disorders and psychogenic pain disorders, such as abdominal pain or headaches, have been extremely well documented in children (Driscoll, Glicklich, & Gallen, 1976; Oster, 1972; Bille, 1962).

ANDRES J. PUMARIEGA • Division of Child and Adolescent Psychiatry, University of Texas Medical Branch, Galveston, Texas 77550. PAUL M. CINCIRIPINI • Behavioral Medicine Laboratory, University of Texas Medical Branch, Galveston, Texas 77550.

One of the most frequently observed somatoform disorders in children and adolescents is the conversion reaction. This disorder involves a loss or alteration in physical functioning, characteristically involving sensory or voluntary motor function. Like other somatoform disorders, the disturbance is not under voluntary control. Moreover, conversion disorders feature a temporal relationship between symptom onset and some emotionally important event. The symptom often enables the individual to avoid circumstances surrounding that event. In addition, loss of physical function brings about additional reinforcement from the environment, which would not otherwise be forthcoming. Thus, both negative (removal of unpleasant consequences) and positive reinforcement paridigms may be involved in the maintenance of the conversion symptomaties. While a number of studies have shown a high prevalence of conversion disorders in children, effective treatment regimens have not been adequately developed (Proctor, 1958; Maloney, 1980; Rock, 1971). The most efficacious means of intervention involves the application of "contingency management" techniques. These techniques are particularly effective in eliminating environmental reinforcers that render the symptoms so resistant to other types of therapeutic intervention. The behavioral approach also allows the patient to learn more appropriate means to interact with the environment and to obtain normally available tangible and social rewards.

CASE IDENTIFICATION AND PRESENTING COMPLAINTS

Amy was a 9-year-old girl from a rural town in the southeastern United States. She had been previously treated at the Pediatric Neurology Clinic of a nearby university medical center for symptoms of akinetic seizure disorder. Amy's most recent clinic visit was precipitated by an increase in seizure frequency, from two or three times a month to five to seven times per week, during the month preceding her visit. Her seizure activity typically involved a sudden loss of consciousness and muscle tone with no tonic-clonic activity. The seizures were 1 to 2 minutes in duration. These symptoms were also accompanied by changes in her behavior, which included increased irritability and an exaggerated startle response to noise.

In the months preceding the visit, Amy's pattern of ambulation had also dramatically shifted from normal erect walking to crawling along the floor on all fours. Amy related her reasons for crawling to a fear that she would fall and sustain serious injury during normal walking. Her crawling behavior was observed both at home and at school, where she persisted in this form of ambulation in spite of teasing and ridicule by some of her peers. Amy attended a class with learning-disabled and handicapped youngsters, many of whom were unable to ambulate without assistance. Many times Amy was also transported around the school in a wheelchair in order to avoid a confrontation with her teachers about walking normally. Interestingly, both parents reported that Amy was able to run and even swim without difficulty when significant others were not in the vicinity. There was also a strong suspicion that many of her "seizures" involved a substantial behavioral component, since recent seizure episodes were not accompanied by expected neurological sequelae.

HISTORY

At age 5, Amy was evaluated for both seizurelike symptoms and a possible speech and communication disorder. At that time, her neurological examination was unremarkable. However, intellectual assessment suggested that Amy was mildly mentally retarded, achieving a Full Scale IQ of only 75. Both visual motor and auditory processing deficits were noted.

Amy's psychological and emotional development was punctuated by an important series of disruptions in her family environment. She was described by her natural mother as being more "clingy" than her other children. There was frequent marital conflict between Amy's natural parents, leading to a separation and eventual divorce when she was 2 years of age. Amy's natural father became her full-time custodian. He denied that Amy had any noticeable reaction to her mother's departure from the home. Amy's natural mother, however, reported that she was often whiny and demanding, sucked her thumb, and experienced frequent temper tantrums on subsequent visits with her following the divorce. When Amy was 4, her natural father remarried and his second wife developed a close relationship with her. The natural mother continued to exercise her visitation rights during this time. Amy's clinginess and regressive behaviors diminished over the next few years but resurfaced in the months preceding the most recent clinic visit. These changes coincided with increased marital conflict between the father and the stepmother, which eventually led to their separation 5 months prior to the consultation. In a manner similar to that described after the departure of the natural mother, Amy became clingy and anxious after visiting with her stepmother following the divorce. She refused to leave her stepmother's apartment, and at times she had to be physically carried away. Amy's father also described a return of the regressive behaviors at this time, such as whining, increased irrit-

ability, temper tantrums, and thumb sucking. The father seemed somewhat cognizant of the fact that the recent separation from the stepmother
might have been traumatic for Amy, in view of her close relationship with
her and her intermittent contact with the natural mother. However, he
minimized this effect and denied that Amy expressed much overt sadness
or distress concerning the divorce. The father also noted that Amy had
few friends her age, and usually sought out younger children as companions. In these relationships she was described as demanding and "bossy."
Frequent fighting and cursing were also reported between Amy and her
two older brothers and older sister.

ASSESSMENT

Prior to the behavioral intervention an extensive neurological assessment was undertaken. This included a complete neurological examination, a sleep and waking EEG, a computerized axial tomography scan
of the head, nerve conduction studies, and a urinary amino acid screen.
The results of these studies ruled out a degenerative neurological disease
or a metabolic disorder. Her electroecephalogram did not demonstrate
the characteristic pattern for akinetic seizures (spike and wave), although
this finding had been documented on previous EEGs obtained 2 years
earlier. Amy was maintained on Mysoline, 100 mg twice a day, for control
of the earlier documented seizure disorder.

On mental status examination, Amy appeared younger than her
chronological age and was somewhat unkempt in her appearance. She
was restless during the 40-minute interview and often fidgeted with her
hands and made alternate motions to stand and sit. She crawled from
room to room when the examiner left to interview the parents. Her affect
was inappropriate and was characterized by a superficially light and sometimes euphoric mood. However, there were occasions when she demonstrated some evidence of sadness, which was accompanied by increased motor movement. The content of her speech was appropriate but
her diction and pronunciation was immature. She had difficulty in forming
some words and phrases, and she often hesitated at the beginning of a
sentence. Periodic loose and disruptive associations were noted. However, she was able to retrace the association back to the previous topic,
with minimal prompting. She readily and without hesitation discussed her
fears about falling to the ground, fear of walking, and fear of noises.
However, she denied that her problems with ambulation presented any
serious limitations to her mobility. She also quickly described how she
was able to jump backwards off the edge of the swimming pool and "not

be afraid of the water.'' She then went on to describe how various members of the family were ''mean to her,'' especially her brother, who constantly ''picked'' on her. She related how she missed both her younger stepsister and her stepmother, but commented on the fact that this stepsister was also ''mean.'' When asked about her parents' marital separation, she said her father told her very little about it. She also indicated that it was unfair that her younger stepsister was able to live with her stepmother while she could not. She talked fondly about her classmates and teachers, but related that she had few friends outside of school. When asked about her family, she mentioned having ''two mothers,'' but was reluctant to talk further on the subject. She denied any evidence of hallucinations, unusual perceptual phenonema, symptoms of depression, or any feelings of overt sadness. At the close of the interview she agreed that talking with someone might help overcome her fears and her difficulty with walking. However, following this disclosure, her motor activity increased and she crawled abruptly out of the room.

The initial diagnosis for Amy was conversion disorder (300.11). Amy's inability to ambulate and the presence of seizure behavior in the absence of concurrent neurological changes were the most prominent features of this disorder. There was also a close temporal relationship between her father's separation from her natural mother and her stepmother and the initiation and exacerbation of these symptoms, respectively. Maternal figures were, at best, inconsistently available. The father was consistently available but appeared to lack any appreciation for the effect of maternal withdrawal on Amy's behavior. Amy's symptoms were reinforced by increased attention from her father and the natural mother, both of whom became increasingly more involved with the child when the symptoms occurred. Amy was exposed to handicapped peers, who may have served as models for the conversion symptoms; symptoms were readily followed by an increase in the level of attention and support from teachers and friends. The symptoms were also strengthened by the fact that few people challenged Amy in her refusal to walk normally.

Amy also expressed considerable anxiety about her relationship with her family, but little concern or distress was expressed about the symptoms themselves (e.g., her inability to ambulate and the frequency of her seizures). In fact, she appeared to be in an almost euphoric mood at times. A secondary diagnosis of separation anxiety disorder (309.21) was also made, given the role of the symptoms at maintaining maternal contact and reducing her opportunities to function independently outside the family.

Amy was admitted to the child psychiatry inpatient unit at the university medical center. Initial behavioral observations suggested that her incapacitation was significantly influenced by environmental factors. Prior to the onset of treatment, nursing observations were conducted on an occurrence/nonoccurrence basis for the target behaviors of crawling and correct (upright) ambulation. The first 10 minutes of successive 2-hour blocks were chosen for the daily observation intervals. The presence or absence of family, staff, or other children was recorded during each observation period. Observations were conducted unobtrusively by a third-party observer. A one-way mirror was used to observe Amy when she was alone or in the classroom or treatment settings. The preliminary observations suggested that Amy demonstrated erect posture and ambulation in approximately 25% of the intervals in which she was alone or in the presence of adults. The other 75% of the time Amy remained on all fours: crouching, crawling, or scooting. In observation intervals in which adults were present in her immediate surroundings, one or more of the target behaviors were observed in 95% of the intervals. During observations made in which family members were present, it was noted that they directly reinforced her inappropriate ambulation by either bringing objects to her at her request or readily carrying her from room to room. The differential reinforcement of this behavior was explicitly demonstrated by the family's lack of verbal and physical interaction with Amy in situations that *did not* involve some form of request for assistance. This behavior seemed consistent with the observation that both the family and Amy expressed some capitulation regarding her inability to ambulate. The father, in particular, continued to seek an organic cause for the disorder.

Within the first 2 days of admission, Amy also experienced two seizure episodes. These were sudden drop attacks, but without any noticeable loss of consciousness or postictal confusion. The staff on the unit managed the episodes matter-of-factly, not commenting on them and immediately redirecting Amy to the routine of the unit. No recurrence of the seizures was noted through the rest of the hospitalization.

SELECTION OF TREATMENT

A treatment strategy was designed to increase the frequency of standing, walking, and correct ambulation, while reducing the frequency of crawling and sitting. Social contact with peers and adults and tangible rewards were used to reinforce the occurrence of these target behaviors, through a contingency management program. Intervention consisted of daily 2-hour sessions with a physical therapist and a child psychiatrist or psychologist. The sessions focused on gradually increasing the frequency of locomotion in steps that followed a developmental continuum. Initially, the physical therapist began working with Amy to increase rapport and cooperativeness. Thus, when Amy followed simple directions, actively reached for objects, and stayed on task, she was given an opportunity to positively interact with the therapist and play a desired game or activity. Amy could also earn tokens for such desirable behaviors, which could be cashed in for a toy at the end of the week. During the course of therapy, Amy's opportunity to play games and earn tokens was made contingent upon her increasing the frequency of the following behaviors: standing up with supports, reaching for high objects, locomotion on two legs, using an erect posture while continually reclining on physical supports, upright locomotion with physical therapist or staff support, walking between two physical supports unassisted (for successive long distances), walking unsupported with staff or physical therapist nearby at arm's reach. These behaviors were viewed as part of a program to shape appropriate ambulation and were based on the naturally occurring sequence of motor development that precedes walking in normal children. As each new behavior was mastered, the next level in the sequence was then targeted.

A multiple-baseline design across behaviors was chosen to evaluate the effectiveness of the contingency management for walking and standing. During each 2-hour therapy session Amy was observed through a one-way mirror. The therapist worked with Amy on each of the behaviors described above, interacting and encouraging her throughout the session. At the end of each session, a 30-minute interval was chosen for evaluation. During that time Amy was asked to engage in standing or walking for as long as she could. Contingent praise was provided for correct responses, and the prompts to stand or walk were repeated every 5 minutes as needed. Crawling was always ignored. As Amy mastered standing, only prompts to walk were given. The distance walked within each session was also monitored, when Amy began to walk. Amy was also encouraged to locomote in a manner consistent with her therapy in situations outside the therapy setting. If she did so she was praised, but inappropriate behaviors were ignored.

COURSE OF TREATMENT

The results are summarized in Figures 1 and 2. Figure 1 depicts that period of time during the testing interval in which the target behaviors were observed. During the beginning of the shaping protocol, Amy was reluctant to comply with the expectations of the therapist. She was initially excited over the prospect of being able to earn a small toy and quickly chose a plastic pony as her reinforcer. However, when the ther-

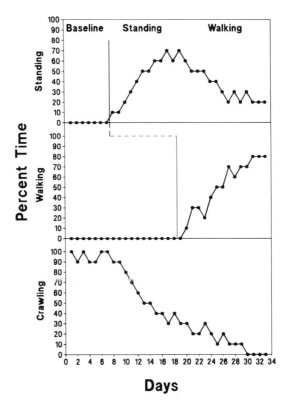

Figure 1.   The percent of time that each target behavior was observed is noted (see text for the details of the observation intervals). During baseline, no contingencies were in effect; from day 8 to day 18, standing was encouraged; and from day 19 until discharge, the patient was reinforced for walking. Crawling was always ignored.

apist explained that she would be required to stand, walk, and get things for herself in order to obtain the toy, she complained about "how difficult" this would be and that she "had no trouble" getting around now.

As shown in Figure 1, the target behaviors progressively increased as contingencies were introduced to enhance their occurrence. In a reciprocal fashion, crawling progressively decreased. Crawling had also disappeared outside the treatment setting.

When the contingencies were introduced to enhance standing with support and reaching objects by standing, Amy began complaining and whining. On day 9, she stated that "I never have to get up and reach for things that high up at home," and she accused the physical therapist of being "cruel" to her. He responded with encouragement and modeled how she could hold onto handles or edges on furniture to bring herself into an erect position and reach the desired objects. As she learned to do this more comfortably, her complaints were replaced by positive vocalization about her ability to perform the behavior. By day 12 standing erect was observed over 40% of the testing intervals, and by day 17 standing reached a 70% level of occurrence. Thus, on day 19 the contingencies were then shifted to walking with continual support. Amy again protested, this time expressing fears about "falling" and "hurting" her head. The physical therapist again responded with encouragement and modeled the target behavior. As shown in Figure 1, walking with support had reached a 40% level of occurrence by day 24. A concomitant decrease in standing and crawling was also noted during this period. The increase in walking was also accompanied a greater willingness to allow herself to be supported by the physical therapist as well as other staff. By day 33, Amy was able to walk with support in 80% of the observation intervals, crawling had dropped out completely, and standing remained between 20 and 30% which was appropriate for this time in therapy. As her walking increased, Amy also was able to participate freely in outside activities with the staff and other children, and she even allowed some of the other children to physically support her.

On day 34 contingencies were shifted to reinforce unsupported walking over a progressively increasing distance. Interestingly, Amy did not protest at this new demand, and even demonstrated genuine effort at achieving the new target behavior. As shown in Figure 2, Amy rapidly progressed from the initial distance of 1.5 feet on day 34 to the maximum required distance of 15.0 feet on day 43. She demonstrated unsteadiness only occasionally, and falls were infrequent. The physical therapist and staff dealt with falls in a nonreinforcing, matter-of-fact fashion. When walking appeared stable (day 43), the treatment team introduced Amy's father into some of the treatment sessions. This was done to train him and properly prepare Amy for home passes and discharge. The father required considerable direction and modeling on how to properly encourage Amy's ambulation without offering to physically assist her. As shown in Figure 2, Amy, sustained a number of falls and slightly decreased her unsupported distance to 13.5 feet by day 47, shortly after the father's introduction to the therapy setting. However, Amy was permitted short day passes off the unit with the father on days 48 and 52, and walking subsequently progressed back to a level of 15.0 feet. However, after the first overnight pass, Amy markedly regressed in her unsupported walking to a level of 6.5 feet on day 56. Multiple falls and a few crawling episodes were also reported at home. This turn of events prompted more intensive intervention for the father's behavior. The intervention focused on those

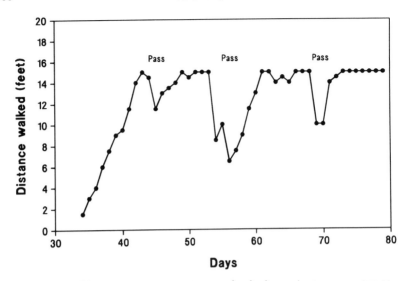

Figure 2.   The total distance walked per session is shown, beginning on day 32.

aspects of his interaction with Amy that reinforced inappropriate behavior (e.g., attention for falling, responding to requests for physical assistance). As shown in Figure 2, Amy's level of unsupported walking subsequently returned to a level of 15.0 feet by day 61. A second overnight pass on day 62 was not followed by an episode of falling. Weekend passes to the home were introduced on days 69 and 77, and again, no falling episodes were noted. Thus, by day 61 Amy was able to sustain walking for distances over 15 feet with only infrequent unsteadiness both in and outside the treatment setting.

Other therapeutic efforts were used in parallel to the contingency management program. Amy participated in individual therapy twice a week and learned how to express negative affect toward peers, siblings, and parents in a more direct and socially appropriate fashion. During these sessions, Amy was able to express her dislike of the special education classes and her anger toward her parents, particularly her natural mother, who related inconsistently to her. Family therapy was also pursued initially with Amy's father, but later Amy's natural mother and siblings were introduced. Both parents initially avoided verbal or affective interaction with Amy and chose instead to attend to her physical needs. In the session Amy's mother often paid attention to her physical appearance, fixing her hair or clothes, while the father attended more to the disuptive behavior of the older brothers. This pattern of intervention was discussed with the parents, and it was noted that they both reinforced inappropriate behavior and avoided discussion of any negative issues or emotions with Amy. The father began to recognize more clearly how his and his ex-wife's inconsistent interaction and lack of affective engagement with Amy contributed to her focus on somatic concerns. There was also some discussion of how the parents felt about their failed marriage and Amy's intellectual deficits, as well as discussion of how both could better coordinate their efforts as divorced parents. The stepmother was also invited to participate in the family sessions, but she refused, citing time conflicts and the demands of her natural child.

TERMINATION

After discharge from the child psychiatry unit, Amy continued to have two weekly sessions (2 hours each) with the physical therapist, and the family continued in once-a-week family therapy. In this outpatient phase, the contingencies were directed toward the reinforcement of more rapid ambulation, and even running during outdoor play. The sessions were scheduled in conjunction with Amy's recreational therapy sessions, where Amy was encouraged to engage in these activities.

FOLLOW-UP

Soon after her discharge, Amy experienced a recurrence of requests for supported ambulation (both at home and at school). Crawling, however, did not reappear. After subsequent consultation with the teachers and parents, Amy regained her predischarge level of unsupported walking by the end of her second week at home. She also showed more appropriate behavior with peers and relinquished inappropriate demands for physical assistance. After 6 weeks at home, the follow-up therapy sessions were reduced to once per week with the physical therapist and every other week with the family. By this point, Amy was taking more of a leadership role with her peers at school and in the recreation group. Her parents were also able to openly discuss her learning deficits and the need for special education. Four months after discharge, Amy's father indicated that he and his ex-wife felt far more comfortable dealing with Amy and questioned the need for further sessions. The treatment team agreed to discontinue therapy and to have follow-up visits with the family only as needed. Four follow-up visits were conducted subsequently at 3-month intervals, and no recurrence of Amy's symptoms was noted. In fact, Amy made considerable progress in her academic and social learning and continued to interact appropriately with family members. Upon mutual agreement, all follow-up sessions were discontinued 1½ years after the initial contact.

OVERALL EVALUATION

Behavioral intervention in Amy's case was particularly effective. The protracted nature of her symptomatology, its tendency to be reinforced by family members and others in her environment, and her cognitive limitations made her a difficult and challenging patient. A less focused and symptom-oriented form of therapy would probably have been of little value. A full analysis of reinforcement contingencies in the treatment of conversion or other somatic symptomatology appears essential to treatment.

Amother important aspect of Amy's case is the multidisciplinary nature of her treatment program. The involvement of other professionals who have expertise in motor development in children seems appropriate for this type of disorder. However, staff should have a full understanding of the behavioral treatment protocol in order to promote learning in a variety of settings. Other therapeutic techniques, such as assertion training, social skills training, and family therapy, may be used to enhance treatment effectiveness and the generalization of learning within the social milieu of the target behaviors.

REFERENCES

American Psychiatric Association. (1980). *Diagnostic and statistical manual of mental disorders* (3rd ed.). Washington, DC: Author.

Bille, B. (1962). Migraine in school children. *Acta Paediatrica Scandinavica, Supplement, 51* (136):1–151.

Driscoll, D., Glicklich, L., & Gallen, W. (1976). Chest pain in children: A prospective study. *Pediatrics, 57,* 648.

Maloney, M. J. (1980). Diagnosing hysterical conversion reactions in children. *Journal of Pediatrics, 97,* 1016–1020.

Oster, J. (1972). Recurrent abdominal pain, headache, and limb pain in children and adolescents. *Pediatrics, 50,* 429.

Proctor, J. (1958). Hysteria in childhood. *American Journal of Orthopsychiatry, 28,* 394–406.

Rock, N. L. (1971). Conversion reactions in childhood: A clinical study on childhood neurosis. *Journal of the American Academy of Child Psychiatry, 10,* 65–93.

Williams, D. T. (1985). Somatoform disorders. In D. Shaffer, A. A. Ehrhardt, L. L. Greenhill (Eds.), *The clinical guide to child psychiatry* (pp. 192–207). New York: Free Press.

Woodruff, R. A., Clayton, P. J., & Guze, S. B. (1971). Hysteria studies of diagnosis, outcome, and prevalence. *Journal of the American Medical Association, 215,* 425–428.

Index